Artificial Intelligence and Deep Learning in Pathology

Artificial Intelligence and Deep Learning in Pathology

Edited by

Stanley Cohen, M.D

Emeritus Chair of Pathology & Emeritus Founding Director
Center for Biophysical Pathology
Rutgers-New Jersey Medical School, Newark, NJ, United States

Adjunct Professor of Pathology
Perelman Medical School
University of Pennsylvania, Philadelphia, PA, United States

Adjunct Professor of Pathology
Kimmel School of Medicine
Jefferson University, Philadelphia, PA, United States

ELSEVIER

Elsevier
Radarweg 29, PO Box 211, 1000 AE Amsterdam, Netherlands
The Boulevard, Langford Lane, Kidlington, Oxford OX5 1GB, United Kingdom
50 Hampshire Street, 5th Floor, Cambridge, MA 02139, United States

Notices
Knowledge and best practice in this field are constantly changing. As new research and experience broaden our understanding, changes in research methods, professional practices, or medical treatment may become necessary.

Practitioners and researchers must always rely on their own experience and knowledge in evaluating and using any information, methods, compounds, or experiments described herein. In using such information or methods they should be mindful of their own safety and the safety of others, including parties for whom they have a professional responsibility.

To the fullest extent of the law, neither the Publisher nor the authors, contributors, or editors, assume any liability for any injury and/or damage to persons or property as a matter of products liability, negligence or otherwise, or from any use or operation of any methods, products, instructions, or ideas contained in the material herein.

Library of Congress Cataloging-in-Publication Data
A catalog record for this book is available from the Library of Congress

British Library Cataloguing-in-Publication Data
A catalogue record for this book is available from the British Library

ISBN: 978-0-323-67538-3

For information on all Elsevier publications visit our website at
https://www.elsevier.com/books-and-journals

Publisher: Dolores Meloni
Acquisitions Editor: Michael Houston
Editorial Project Manager: Sam W. Young
Project Manager: Niranjan Bhaskaran
Cover Designer: Alan Studholme

Typeset by TNQ Technologies

Working together
to grow libraries in
developing countries

www.elsevier.com • www.bookaid.org

This book is dedicated to the American Society for Investigative Pathology, and especially Mark Sobel and Martha Furie, for supporting my efforts to proselytize on behalf of artificial intelligence in pathology. It is also dedicated to the members of the Warren Alpert Center for Digital and Computational Pathology at Memorial Sloan-Kettering, under the leadership of David Klimstra and Meera Hameed, for nourishing my enthusiasm for this revolution in pathology. I am especially indebted to both Dean Christine Palus and the Departments of Computer Science and Mathematics at Villanova University for enabling me to get up to speed rapidly in this relatively new interest of mine while being so accommodating and friendly to a student older than his teachers. Most important, it is also dedicated to my wonderful wife and scientific colleague Marion, children (Laurie, Ron, and Ken), kids-in-law (Ron, Helen, and Kim respectively), and grandkids (Jessica, Rachel, Joanna, Julie, Emi, Risa, Brian, Seiji, and Ava). With natural intelligence like that, who needs artificial intelligence?

Contents

Contributors

Tanishq Abraham
Department of Biomedical Engineering, University of California, Davis, CA, United States

Ognjen Arandjelović, M.Eng. (Oxon), Ph.D. (Cantab)
School of Computer Science, University of St Andrews, St Andrews, United Kingdom

Peter D. Caie, BSc, MRes, PhD
School of Medicine, QUAD Pathology, University of St Andrews, St Andrews, United Kingdom

Stanley Cohen, MD
Emeritus Chair of Pathology & Emeritus Founding Director, Center for Biophysical Pathology, Rutgers-New Jersey Medical School, Newark, NJ, United States; Adjunct Professor of Pathology, Perelman Medical School, University of Pennsylvania, Philadelphia, PA, United States; Adjunct Professor of Pathology, Kimmel School of Medicine, Jefferson University, Philadelphia, PA, United States

Neofytos Dimitriou, B.Sc
School of Computer Science, University of St Andrews, St Andrews, United Kingdom

Michael Donovan
Department of Pathology, Icahn School of Medicine at Mount Sinai, New York, NY, United States

Gerardo Fernandez
Department of Pathology, Icahn School of Medicine at Mount Sinai, New York, NY, United States

Rajarsi Gupta, MD, PhD
Assistant Professor, Biomedical Informatics, Stony Brook Medicine, Stony Brook, NY, United States

Richard Levenson, MD
Professor and Vice Chair, Pathology and Laboratory Medicine, UC Davis Health, Sacramento, CA, United States

Bahram Marami
Department of Pathology, Icahn School of Medicine at Mount Sinai, New York, NY, United States

Benjamin R. Mitchell, BA, MSE, PhD
Assistant Professor, Department of Computing Sciences, Villanova University, Villanova, PA, United States

Daniel A. Orringer, MD
Associate Professor, Department of Surgery, NYU Langone Health, New York City, NY, United States

Anil V. Parwani, MD, PhD, MBA
Professor, Pathology and Biomedical Informatics, The Ohio State University, Columbus, OH, United States

Marcel Prastawa
Department of Pathology, Icahn School of Medicine at Mount Sinai, New York, NY, United States

Abishek Sainath Madduri
Department of Pathology, Icahn School of Medicine at Mount Sinai, New York, NY, United States

Joel Haskin Saltz, MD, PhD
Professor, Chair, Biomedical Informatics, Stony Brook University, Stony Brook, NY, United States

Richard Scott
Department of Pathology, Icahn School of Medicine at Mount Sinai, New York, NY, United States

Austin Todd
UT Health, San Antonio, TX, United States

John E. Tomaszewski, MD
SUNY Distinguished Professor and Chair, Pathology and Anatomical Sciences, University at Buffalo, State University of New York, Buffalo, NY, United States

Jack Zeineh
Department of Pathology, Icahn School of Medicine at Mount Sinai, New York, NY, United States

Preface

It is now well-recognized that artificial intelligence (AI) represents an inflection point for society at least as profound as was the Industrial Revolution. It plays increasing roles in industry, education, recreation, and transportation, as well as science and engineering. As one example of its ubiquity, a recent headline proclaimed that "Novak Djokovic used AI to Train for Wimbledon!"

In particular, AI has become important for both biomedical research and clinical practice. Part of the reason for this is the sheer amount of data currently obtainable by modern techniques. In the past, we would study one or a few enzymes or transduction pathways at a time. Now we can sequence the entire genome, develop gene expression arrays that allow us to dissect out critical networks and pathways, study the entire microbiome instead of a few bacterial species in isolation, and so on. We can also use AI to look for important patterns in the massive data that have already been collected, i.e., data mining both in defined datasets and in natural language sources. Also, we can take advantage of the power of AI in pattern recognition to analyze and classify pictorial data not only for classification tasks but also to extract information not obvious to an individual limited to direct observations through the microscope, a device that has never received FDA approval.

Radiologists have been among the first clinical specialists to embrace AI to assist in the processing and interpretation of X-ray images. Pathologists have lagged, in part because the visual content of the images that pathologists use is at least an order of magnitude greater than those of radiology. Another factor has been the delay of the major industrial players to enter this arena, as well as limited hospital resources based on perceived differences in hospital profitability between radiology and pathology practices. However, more and more pathology departments are embracing digital pathology via whole slide imaging (WSI), and WSI provides the infrastructure both for advanced imaging modalities and the archiving of annotated datasets needed for AI training and implementation. An ever-increasing number of articles utilizing AI are appearing in the literature, and a number of professional societies devoted to this field have emerged. Existing societies and journals in pathology have begun to create subsections specifically devoted to AI.

Unfortunately, existing texts on machine learning, deep learning, and AI (terms that are distinct, but loosely overlap) tend to be either very general and superficial overviews for the layman or highly technical tomes assuming a background in linear algebra, multivariate calculus, and programming languages. They do not therefore serve as a useful introduction for most pathologists, as well as physicians in other disciplines. The purpose of this monograph is to provide a detailed understanding of both the concepts and methods of AI, as well as its use in pathology. In broad general terms, the book covers machine learning and introduction to data processing, the integration of AI and pathology, and detailed examples of state-of-the-art AI applications in pathology. It focuses heavily on diagnostic anatomic pathology, and thanks to advances in neural network architecture we now have the tools for extraction of high-level information from images.

We begin with an opening chapter on the evolution of machine learning, including both a historical perspective and some thoughts as to its future. The next four chapters provide the underlying framework of machine learning with special attention to deep learning and AI, building from the simple to the complex. Although quite detailed and intensive, these require no knowledge of computer programming or of mathematical formalism. Wherever possible, concepts are illustrated by examples from pathology. The next two chapters deal with the integration of AI with digital pathology and its application not only for classification, prediction, and inference but also for the manipulation of the images themselves for extraction of meaningful information not readily accessible to the unaided eye. Following this is a chapter on precision medicine in digital pathology that demonstrates the power of traditional machine learning paradigms as well as deep learning, The reader will find a certain amount of overlap in these chapters for the following reasons; each author needs to review some basic aspects of AI as they specifically relate to his or her assigned topic, each presents their own perspective on the underpinnings of the work they describe, and each topic considered can best be understood in the light of parallel work in other areas. The next two chapters deal with two important topics relating to cancer in which the authors utilize AI to great effect and discuss their findings in the context of studies in other laboratories. Taken together, these latter chapters provide complementary views of the current state of the art based upon different perspectives and priorities.

The book concludes with an overview that puts all this in perspective and makes the argument that AI does not replace us, but rather serves as a digital assistant. While it is still too early to determine the final direction in which pathology will evolve, it is not too early to recognize that it will grow well beyond its current capabilities and will do so with the aid of AI. However, until "general AI" is attained that can fully simulate conscious thought (which may never happen), biological brains will remain indispensable. Thus, for the foreseeable future, human pathologists will not be obsolete. Instead, the partnership between artificial and natural intelligence will continue to expand to form a true partnership. The machine will generate knowledge, and the human will provide the wisdom to properly apply that knowledge. The machine will provide the knowledge that a tomato is a fruit. The human will provide the wisdom that it does not belong in a fruit salad. Together they will determine that ketchup is not a smoothie.

Stanley Cohen, MD
Emeritus Chair of Pathology & Emeritus Founding Director
Center for Biophysical Pathology
Rutgers-New Jersey Medical School, Newark, NJ, United States

Adjunct Professor of Pathology
Perelman Medical School
University of Pennsylvania, Philadelphia, PA, United States

Adjunct Professor of Pathology
Kimmel School of Medicine
Jefferson University, Philadelphia, PA, United States

The evolution of machine learning: past, present, and future

Stanley Cohen, MD [1,2,3]

[1]*Emeritus Chair of Pathology & Emeritus Founding Director, Center for Biophysical Pathology, Rutgers-New Jersey Medical School, Newark, NJ, United States;* [2]*Adjunct Professor of Pathology, Perelman Medical School, University of Pennsylvania, Philadelphia, PA, United States;* [3]*Adjunct Professor of Pathology, Kimmel School of Medicine, Jefferson University, Philadelphia, PA, United States*

Introduction

The first computers were designed solely to perform complex calculations rapidly. Although conceived in the 1800s, and theoretical underpinnings developed in the early 1900s, it was not until ENIAC was built that the first practical computer can be said to have come into existence. The acronym ENIAC stands for Electronic Numerical Integrator and Calculator. It occupied a 20 × 40 foot room, and contained over 18,000 vacuum tubes. From that time until the mid-20th century, the programs that ran on the descendants of ENIAC were rule based, in that the machine was given a set of instructions to manipulate data based upon mathematical, logical, and/or probabilistic formulas. The difference between an electronic calculator and a computer is that the computer encodes not only numeric data but also the rules for the manipulation of these data (encoded as number sequences).

There are three basic parts to a computer: core memory, where programs and data are stored, a central processing unit that executes the instructions and returns the output of that computation to memory for further use, and devices for input and output of data. High-level programming languages take as input program statements and translate them into the (numeric) information that a computer can understand. Additionally, there are three basic concepts that are intrinsic to every programming language: assignment, conditionals, and loops. In a computer, x = 5 is not a statement about equality. Instead, it means that the value 5 is assigned to x. In this context, X = X + 2 though mathematically impossible makes perfect sense. We add 2 to whatever is in X (in this case, 5) and the new value (7) now replaces that old value (5) in X. It helps to think of the = sign as meaning that the quantity on the left is replaced by the quantity on the right. A conditional is easier to understand. We ask the computer to make a test that has two possible results. If one result holds, then the computer will do something. If not, it will do something else. This is typically an IF-THEN statement. IF you are wearing a green suit with yellow polka dots,

Artificial Intelligence and Deep Learning in Pathology. https://doi.org/10.1016/B978-0-323-67538-3.00001-4

PRINT "You have terrible taste!" IF NOT print "There is still hope for your sartorial sensibilities." Finally, a LOOP enables the computer to perform a single instruction or set of instructions a given number of times. From these simple building blocks, we can create instructions to do extremely complex computational tasks on any input.

The traditional approach to computing involves encoding a model of the problem based on a mathematical structure, logical inference, and/or known relationships within the data structure. In a sense, the computer is testing your hypothesis with a limited set of data but is not using that data to inform or modify the algorithm itself. Correct results provide a test of that computer model, and it can then be used to work on larger sets of more complex data. This rules-based approach is analogous to hypothesis testing in science. In contrast, machine learning is analogous to hypothesis-generating science. In essence, the machine is given a large amount of data and then models its internal state so that it becomes increasingly accurate in its predictions about the data. The computer is creating its own set of rules from data, rather than being given ad hoc rules by the programmer. In brief, machine learning uses standard computer architecture to construct a set of instructions that, instead of doing direct computation on some inputted data according to a set of rules, uses a large number of known examples to deduce the desired output when an unknown input is presented. That kind of high-level set of instructions is used to create the various kinds of machine learning algorithms that are in general use today. Most machine learning programs are written in PYTHON programming language, which is both powerful and one of the easiest computer languages to learn. A good introduction and tutorial that utilizes biological examples is Ref. [1].

Rules-based versus machine learning: a deeper look

Consider the problem of distinguishing squares and rectangles and circles from each other. One way to approach this problem using a rules-based program would be to calculate relationships between area and circumference for each shape by using geometric-based formulas, and then comparing the measurements of a novel unknown sample to those values for the best fit, which will define its shape. One could also simply count edges, defining a circle as having zero edges, and use that information to correctly classify the unknown.

The only hitch here would be the necessity to know pi for the case of the circle. But that is also easy to obtain. Archimedes did this somewhere about 250 BCE by using geometric formula to calculate the areas of two regular polygons; one polygon inscribed inside the circle and the other the polygon with which the circle was circumscribed (Fig. 1.1).

Since the actual area of the circle lies between the areas of the inscribed and circumscribed polygons, the calculable areas of these polygons set upper and layer bounds for the area of the circle. Without a computer, Archimedes showed that pi is between 3.1408 and 3.1428. Using computers, we can now do this calculation for polygons with very large numbers of sides and reach an approximate value of pi

FIGURE 1.1

Circle bounded by inscribed and circumscribed polygons. The area of the circle lies between the areas of these bounds. As the number of polygon sides increases, the approximation becomes better and better.

Wikipedia commons; Public domain.

to how many decimal places we require. For a more "modern" approach, we can use a computer to sum a very large number of terms of an infinite series that converges to pi. There are many such series, the first of which having been described in the 14th century.

These rules-based programs are also capable of simulations; as an example, pi can be computed by simulation. For example, if we have a circle quadrant of radius = 1 embedded in a square target board with sides = 1 units, and throw darts at the board so that they randomly land somewhere within the board, the probability of a hit within the circle segment is the ratio of the area of that segment to the area of the whole square, which by simple geometry is pi/4. We can simulate this experiment by computer, by having it pick pairs of random numbers (each between zero and one) and using these as X-Y coordinates to compute the location of a simulated hit. The computer can keep track of both the ratio of the number of hits landing within the circle quadrant and the total number of hits anywhere on the board, and this ratio is then equal to pi/4. This is illustrated in Fig. 1.2.

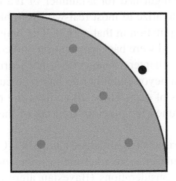

FIGURE 1.2

Simulation of random dart toss. Here the number of tosses within the segment of the circle is 5 and the total number of tosses is 6.

From Wikipedia commons; public domain.

In the example shown in Fig. 1.2, the value of pi is approximately 3.3, based on only 6 tosses. With only a few more tosses we can beat Archimedes, and with a very large number of tosses we can come close to the best value of pi obtained by other means. Because this involves random processes, it is known as Monte Carlo simulation.

Machine learning is quite different. Consider a program that is created to distinguish between squares and circles. For machine learning, all we have to do is present a large number of known squares and circles, each labeled with its correct identity. From this labeled data the computer creates its own set of rules, which are not given to it by the programmer. The machine uses its accumulated experience to ultimately correctly classify an unknown image. There is no need for the programmer to explicitly define the parameters that make the shape into a circle or square. There are many different kinds of machine learning strategies that can do this.

In the most sophisticated forms of machine learning such as neural networks (deep learning), the internal representations by which the computer arrives at a classification are not directly observable or understandable by the programmer. As the program gets more and more labeled samples, it gets better and better at distinguishing the "roundness," or "squareness" of new data that it has never seen before. It is using prior experience to improve its discriminative ability, and the data itself need not be tightly constrained. In this example, the program can arrive at a decision that is independent of the size, color, and even regularity of the shape. We call this artificial intelligence (AI), since it seems more analogous to the way human beings behave than traditional computing.

Varieties of machine learning

The age of machine learning essentially began with the work of pioneers such as Marvin Minsky and Frank Rosenblatt who described the earliest neural networks. However, this approach languished for a number of reasons including the lack of algorithms that could generalize to most real-world problems, the primitive nature of input storage, and computation in that period. The major conceptual innovations that moved the field forward were backpropagation and convolution, which we will discuss in detail in a later chapter. Meanwhile, other learning algorithms that were being developed also went beyond simply rule-based calculation and involved inferences from large amounts of data. These all address the problem of classifying an unknown instance based upon the previous training of the algorithm with a known dataset.

Most, but not all, algorithms fall into three categories. Classification can be based on clustering of data points in an abstract multidimensional space (support vector machines), probabilistic considerations (Bayesian algorithms), or stratification of the data through a sequential search in decision trees and random forests. Some methods utilizing these techniques are shown in Fig. 1.3.

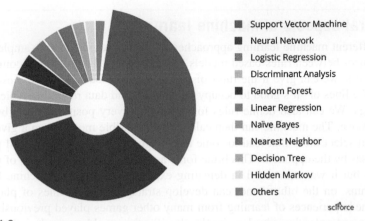

Legend:
- ■ Support Vector Machine
- ■ Neural Network
- ■ Logistic Regression
- ■ Discriminant Analysis
- ■ Random Forest
- ■ Linear Regression
- ■ Naïve Bayes
- ■ Nearest Neighbor
- ■ Decision Tree
- ■ Hidden Markov
- ■ Others

sciforce

FIGURE 1.3

Varieties of machine learning.

Reprinted from https://medium.com/sciforce/top-ai-algorithms-for-healthcare-aa5007ffa330, with permission of Dr. Max Ved, Co-founder, SciForce.

All of those latter approaches, in addition to neural networks, are collectively known as "machine learning." In recent years, however, neural networks have come to dominate the field because of their near-universal applicability and their ability create high-level abstractions from the input data. Neural network-based programs are often defined as "deep learning." Contrary to common belief, this is not because of the complexity of the learning that takes place in such a network, but simply due to the multilayer construction of a neural network as will be discussed below. For simplicity, in this book we will refer to the other kinds of machine learning as "shallow learning."

The evolution of the neural network class of machine learning algorithms has been broadly but crudely based upon the workings of biological neural networks in the brain. The neural network does not "think"; rather it utilizes information to improve its performance. This is learning, rather than thinking. The basics of all of these will be covered in this chapter. The term "Artificial Intelligence" is often used to describe the ability of a computer to perform what appears to be human-level cognition, but this is an anthropomorphism of the machine, since, as stated above, machines do not think. In the sense that they learn by creating generalizations from inputted training data, and also because certain computer programs can be trained by a process similar to that of operant conditioning of an animal, it is easy to think of them as intelligent. However, as we shall see, machine learning at its most basic level is simply about looking for similarities and patterns in things. Our programs can create high levels of abstraction from building blocks such as these in order to make predictions, and identify patterns. But "asking if a machine can think is like asking whether a submarine can swim" [2]. Nevertheless, we will use the term artificial intelligence throughout the book (and in the title as well) as it is now firmly ingrained in the field.

General aspects of machine learning

The different machine learning approaches for chess provide good examples of the differences between rules-based models and AI models. To program a computer to play chess, we can give it the rules of the game, some basic strategic information along the lines of "it's good to occupy the center," and data regarding typical chess openings. We can also define rules for evaluating every position on the board for every move. The machine can then calculate all possible moves from a given position and select those that lead to some advantage. It can also calculate all possible responses by the opponent. This brute force approach evaluated billions of possible moves, but it was successful in defeating expert chess players. Machine learning algorithms, on the other hand, can develop strategically best lines of play based upon the experiences of learning from many other games played previously, much as prior examples improved a simple classification problem as described in the previous section. Early machine learning models took only 72 h of play to match the best rules-based chess programs in the world. Networks such as these learn to make judgment without implicit input as to the rules to be invoked in making those judgments.

What most machine learning programs have in common is the need for large amounts of known examples as the data with which to train them. In an abstract sense, the program uses data to create an internal model or representation that encapsulates the properties of those data. When it receives an unknown sample, it determines whether it fits that model to "train" them. A neural network is one of the best approaches toward generating such internal models, but in a certain sense, every machine learning algorithm does this. For example, a program might be designed to distinguish between cats and dogs. The training set consists of many examples of dogs and cats. Essentially, the program starts by making guesses, and the guesses are refined through multiple known examples. At some point, the program can classify an unknown example correctly as a dog or a cat. It has generated an internal model of "cat-ness" and "dog-ness." The dataset composed of known examples is known as the "training set." Before using this model on unlabeled, unknown examples, one must test the program to see how well it works. For this, one also needs a set of known examples that are NOT used for training, but rather to test whether the machine has learned to identify examples that it has never seen before. The algorithm is analyzed for its ability to characterize this "test set."

Although many papers quantitate the results of this test in terms of accuracy, this is an incomplete measure, and in cases where there is an imbalance between the two classes that are to be distinguished, it is completely useless. As an example, overall cancer incidence for the period 2011−15 was less than 500 cases per 100,000 men and women. I can create a simple algorithm for predicting whether a random individual has cancer or not, by simply having the algorithm report that everyone is negative. This model will be wrong less than only 500 times, and so its accuracy is approximately 99.5%! Yet this model is clearly useless, as it will not identify any patient with cancer.

As this example shows, we must not only take into account the accuracy of the model but also the nature of its errors. There are several ways of doing this. The simplest is as follows. There are four possible results for an output from the model: true positives (TP), false positives (FP), true negatives (TN), and false negatives (FN). There are simple formulas to determine the positive predictive value and the sensitivity of the algorithm. These are known as "precision" (Pr) and "recall" (Re), respectively. In some publications, an F1 value is given, which is the harmonic mean of Pr and Re.

Deep learning and neural networks

For many kinds of machine learning, the programmer determines the relevant features and their quantification. Features may include such things as weight, size, color, temperature, or any parameter that can be described in quantitative, semiquantitative, or relative terms. The process of creating feature vectors is often known as feature engineering. There are some things that have too many features to do this directly. For example, a picture may have several megabytes of data at the pixel level. Prior to machine learning, image analysis was based upon specific rules and measurements to define features, and a rules-based program detected patterns based on edges, textures, shapes, and intensity to identify objects of such as nuclei, cytoplasm, mitoses, necrosis and so on, but interpretation of these was up to the human pathologist. Before neural networks, machine learning also needed humans to define features, a task often referred to "feature engineering." These more powerful networks could make specific classification and predictions from the image as a whole. Neural networks consisting of layers of simulated neurons took this a step further; a large part of the strength of these algorithms is that the network can abstract out high-level features from the inputted data all by itself. Those are based on combinations of initial data inputs and are often referred to as representations of the data. These representations are of significantly lower dimensionality than the original feature vectors of the input. The representations are formed in the network layers that are between input and output which are referred to as hidden layers. Training refines these representations, and the program uses them to derive its own internal rules for decision-making based on them. Thus, the neural network learns rules by creating hidden variables from data.

Within the inner layers of the neural network, the process of abstraction leading to a representation is based on an iterative model often initiated by random variables, and so is partially unexplainable to the human observer (which is why the term "hidden" is used for these inner layers). This lack of explainability is uncomfortable for some researchers in the field. However, if you were to ask an experienced pathologist how he or she arrived a diagnosis based upon examination of a biopsy slide, they would find it difficult to explain the cognitive processes that went into that judgment, although if pressed, they could define a set of features consistent with that diagnosis. Thus, both neural networks and humans base their decisions on processes not readily explainable.

The simplest neural net has at least one hidden layer. Most neural nets have several layers of simulated neurons, and the "neurons" of each layer are connected to all of the neurons in the next layer. These are often preceded by a convolutional set of layers, based loosely on the architecture of the visual cortex of the brain. These transform the input data to a form that can be handled by the following fully connected layer. There are many different kinds of modern sophisticated machine learning algorithms based on this kind of neural network, and they will be featured predominantly throughout this monograph. Not all machine learning programs are based on these deep learning concepts. There are some that rely on different interconnections among the simulated neurons within them, for example, so-called restricted Boltzmann networks. Others, such as spiking neural networks, utilize an architecture that is more like biological brains work. While these represent examples of the current state of the art in AI, the basic fully connected and convolutional framework are simpler to train and more computationally efficient, and thus remain the networks of choice as of 2019.

It should also be noted that it is possible to do unsupervised or weakly supervised learning where there is little to no a priori information about the class labels and large datasets are required for these approaches as well. In subsequent chapters we will describe these concepts in detail as we describe the inner workings of the various kinds of machine learning, and following these we will describe how AI fits into the framework of whole slide imaging (WSI) in pathology. With this as baseline, we will explore in detail examples of current state-of-the art applications of AI in pathology. This is especially timely in that AI is now an intrinsic part of our lives. The modern safety features in cars, decisions on whether or not we are good credit risks, targeted advertising, and facial recognition are some obvious examples. When we talk to Siri or Alexa we are interacting with an AI program. If you have an iWatch or similar device, you can be monitored for arrhythmias, accidental falls, etc. AI's successes have included natural language processing and image analysis, among other breakthroughs.

AI plays an increasingly important role in medicine, from research to clinical applications. A typical workflow for using machine learning for integrating clinical data for patient care is illustrated in Fig. 1.4.

IBM's Watson is a good example of the use of this paradigm. Unstructured data from natural language is processed and outputted in a form that can be combined with the more structured clinical information such as laboratory tests and physical diagnosis. In the paradigm shown here, images are not themselves interpreted via machine learning; rather they are the annotation of those entities (diagnostic impression, notable features, etc.) that are used. As neural networks have become more sophisticated, they can take on the task of interpreting the images and, under pathologist and radiologist supervision, further streamline the diagnostic pathway. In Fig. 1.4, AI is the term used to define the whole process by which the machine has used its training to make what appears to be a humanlike judgment call.

FIGURE 1.4

The incorporation of artificial intelligence into clinical decision-making. Both precise quantifiable data and unstructured narrative information can be captured within this framework.

Reprinted from https://medium.com/sciforce/top-ai-algorithms-for-healthcare-aa5007ffa330, with permission of Dr. Max Ved, Co-founder, SciForce.

The role of AI in pathology

It has been estimated that approximately 70% of a clinical chart is composed of laboratory data, and the pathologist is therefore an important interpreter of those data in the context of the remaining 30%. Even in the age of molecular analysis, the cognitive skills involved in the interpretation of image-based data by the pathologist remain of major importance in those clinical situations where diagnosis occurs at the tissue level. This has become increasingly difficult because of the complexities of diagnostic grading for prognosis, the need to integrate visual correlates of molecular data such as histochemical markers based on genes, gene expression, and immunologic profiles, and the wealth of archival material for comparative review. For these and many other reasons, research and implementation of AI in anatomic pathology, along with continuing implementation in clinical pathology, is proceeding at an exponential rate.

In many ways, the experiences of radiologists are helping to guide us in the evolution of pathology, since radiologists continue to adopt AI at a rapid pace. Pathologists have been late in coming to the table. For radiologists AI is mainly about analyzing images, and their images are relatively easy to digitize. In pathology, acquisition and annotation of datasets for computer input was not possible until WSI at appropriate scale of resolution and speed of acquisition became available. Some of the drivers of WSI are efficiency, data portability, integration with other diagnostic modalities, and so on, but two main consequences of the move from glass microscopy to WSI are the ability to incorporate AI and the incorporation of computer-intensive imaging modalities. Although AI plays important roles in clinical pathology, in the interpretation of genomic and proteomic arrays, etc., where inference and prediction models are important, the focus of this book will be on the use of AI in anatomic pathology, with specific attention to the extraction of maximal information from images regarding diagnosis, grading, prediction, and so on.

Limitations of AI

While recognizing the great success of AI, it is important to note three important limitations. First, for the most part, current algorithms are one-trick ponies that can perform a specific task that they have been trained for, with limited capability of applying that training to new problems. It is possible to do so-called transfer learning on a computer, but it is still far removed from the kind of general intelligence that humans possess. Second, training an algorithm requires huge datasets often numbering in the thousands of examples. In contrast, humans can learn from very small amounts of data. It does not take a toddler 1000 examples to learn the difference between an apple and a banana. Third, computation by machine is very inefficient, in terms of energy needs as compared with the human brain, even though the brain is much more complex than the largest supercomputer ever developed. A typical human brain has about 100 billion neurons and 100 trillion interconnections, which is much bigger than the entire set of neural networks running at any time across the globe. This has a secondary consequence. It has been estimated that training large AI models produces carbon emissions nearly five times greater than the lifecycle carbon emissions of an automobile.

There are several new approaches that have the ability to address these issues. The first is neuromorphic computing, which attempts to create a brainlike physical substrate in which the AI can be implemented, instead of running solely as a software model. Artificial neurons, based upon use of a phase-change material, have been created. A phase-change material is one that can exist in two different phases (for example, crystalline or amorphous) and easily switch between the two when triggered by laser or electricity. At some point the material changes from a nonconductive to a conductive state and fires.

After a brief refractory period, it is ready to begin this process again. In other words, this phase-change neuron behaves just like a biological neuron. Artificial synapses have also been created. These constructs appear to be much more energy efficient than current fully software implementations such as both conventional neural networks and spiking net algorithms that more directly simulate neuronal behavior.

Much further in the future is the promise of quantum computing that will be orders of magnitude faster than the most powerful computers presently available. These are based on three-state "qubits" (0, 1, and an indeterminate superposition of these) rather than binary bits, and these states can hold multiple values simultaneously. A quantum computer can also process these multiple values simultaneously. In theory, this allows us to address problems that are currently intractable and could lead to major advances in AI. Although current quantum computers have only a small number of interacting qubits, it is conceivable that a quantum computer of the future could approach the complexity of the human brain, with far less numbers of interacting qubits (unless, of course, the brain itself functions in part as a quantum computer, as some have speculated). This is not as far-fetched as it seems, as photosynthetic processes have been shown to exhibit quantum properties at physiological temperatures [3,4], thus demonstrating the feasibility of maintaining quantum coherence at room temperatures, based on technologies that have had millions of years to evolve.

Even with current technology, however, both the potential and current applications of AI have demonstrated that it will play as powerful a role in pathology and medicine in general, as it has already done in many other fields and disciplines. For both a good overview and historical perspective of AI, see Ref. [5].

General aspects of AI

For any use of AI in solving real-world problems, a number of practical issues must be addressed. For example,

a. For the choice of a given AI algorithm, what are the classes of learning problems that are difficult or easy, as compared with other potential strategies for their solution?

b. How does one estimate the number of training examples necessary or sufficient for learning?

c. What trade-offs between precision and sensitivity is one willing to make?

d. How does computational complexity of the proposed model compare with that of competing models?

For questions such as these there is no current analytical approach to the best answer. Thus, the choice of algorithm and its optimization remains an empirical trial and error approach. Nevertheless, there are many aspects of medicine that have proven amenable to AI approaches. Some are "record-centric" in that they mine electronic health records, journal and textbook materials, patient clinical support systems, and so on, for epidemiologic patterns, risk factors, and diagnostic predictions. These all involve natural language processing. Others involve signal classification, such as interpretation of EKG and EEG recordings. A major area of application involves medical image analysis. Just as they have for the digitization of images, our colleagues in radiology have taken the lead in this field, with impressive results. Pathology has embraced this approach with the advent of whole slide imaging, which in addition to its many other benefits, provides the framework in which to embed machine learning from biopsy specimens.

Because of the increasing importance and ubiquity of WSI, in the chapters to follow, there will be a focus on image interpretation, with some additional attention to the use of AI in exploring other large correlated data arrays such as those from genomic and proteomic studies. Interestingly, although genotype determines phenotype, using AI we can sometimes work backward from image phenotype to genotype underpinning based on subtle morphologic distinctions not readily apparent to the naked eye. Natural language understanding, which is another major area of current AI research, is a vast field that requires its own monograph and is largely outside the scope of the present volume though important for analyzing clinical charts, electronic health records, and epidemiologic information, as well as article and reference retrieval. By removing the mysticism surrounding AI, it becomes clear that it is a silicon-based assistant for the clinical and the research laboratories rather than an artificial brain that will replace the pathologist.

References

[1] Jones MO. Python for biologists. CreateSpace Press; 2013.
[2] Dijkstra, E.W. The threats to computing science (EWD-898) (PDF). E.W. Dijkstra Archive. Center for American History, University of Texas at Austin. [transcription].
[3] Fassioli F, Olaya-Castro A. Distribution of entanglement in light-harvesting complexes and their quantum efficiency (2010). New Journal of Physics 2010;12(8). http://iopscience.iop.org/1367-2630/12/8/085006.
[4] O'Reilly EJ, Olay-Castro A. Non-classicality of the molecular vibrations assisting exciton energy transfer at room temperature. Nature Communications 2014;5:3012.
[5] Sejnowski TJ. The deep learning revolution: artificial intelligence meets human intelligence. MIT Press; 2018.

The basics of machine learning: strategies and techniques

Stanley Cohen, MD [1,2,3]

[1]*Emeritus Chair of Pathology & Emeritus Founding Director, Center for Biophysical Pathology, Rutgers-New Jersey Medical School, Newark, NJ, United States;* [2]*Adjunct Professor of Pathology, Perelman Medical School, University of Pennsylvania, Philadelphia, PA, United States;* [3]*Adjunct Professor of Pathology, Kimmel School of Medicine, Jefferson University, Philadelphia, PA, United States*

Introduction

To begin, it is important to note that the term "artificial intelligence" is somewhat nebulous. It is usually used to describe computer systems that normally require human intelligence such as visual perception, speech recognition, translation, decision-making, and prediction. As we will see, pretty much all of machine learning fits under this broad umbrella. This chapter is a guide to the basics of some of the major learning strategies. To avoid repetition, I will use only hypothetical clinical examples that I am certain will not be covered elsewhere.

Machine learning refers to a class of computer algorithms that construct models for classification and prediction from existing known data, as compared to models based upon a set of explicit instructions. In this sense, the computer is learning from experience, and using this experience to improve its performance.

The main idea of machine learning is that of concept learning. To learn a concept is to come up with a way of describing a general rule from a set of concrete examples. In abstract terms, if we think of samples being defined in terms of their attributes, then a machine language algorithm is a function that maps those attributes into a specific output. For most of the examples in this chapter, the output will involve classification, as this is one of the major building blocks for all the things that machine learning can accomplish.

In most cases, large datasets are required for optimal learning. The basic strategies for machine learning in general are (1) supervised learning, (2) unsupervised learning, and (3) reinforcement learning. In supervised learning, the training set consists of data that have been labeled and annotated by a human observer. Unsupervised learning does not use labeled data, and is based upon clustering algorithms of various sorts. In both of these, improvement comes via sequential attempts to minimize the difference between the actual example (ground truth) and the predicted

Artificial Intelligence and Deep Learning in Pathology. https://doi.org/10.1016/B978-0-323-67538-3.00002-6

value. In reinforcement learning, the algorithm learns to react to its environment and finds optimal strategies via a reward function.

Although we tend to think of deep learning and neural networks as the newest forms of machine learning, this is not the case. The primitive ancestors of modern neural network architectures began with the work of Rosenblatt [1] in 1957. These neural networks were loosely based upon the model of neuronal function described by McCulloch and Pitt [2] about a decade earlier (see Ref. [3] for a review of the history of deep learning). Basically, it involves a sequence of simulated neurons arranged in layers, with the outputs of one layer becoming the input of the next. Each layer thus receives increasingly complex input from the layer beneath it, and it is this complexity that allows the algorithm to map an unknown input to an outputted solution. Note that the term "deep learning" does not refer to the sophistication of the program or to its capacity to mimic thought in any meaningful way. Rather, it simply refers to the fact that it is built of many layers of nonlinear processing units and their linear interconnections. At its most fundamental level, deep learning is all about linear algebra with a little bit of multivariate calculus and probability thrown in.

Meanwhile a number of other models of machine learning were being developed, which are collectively referred to, by many though not all, as shallow learning. Just as is the case of deep learning, in all of these models, the program is presented with a large dataset of known examples and their defining features. In the simplest case, there are two classes of objects in the training set, and the program has to construct a model from these data that will allow it to predict the class of an unknown example. If the two classes are bedbugs and caterpillars, the useful features might be length and width. To distinguish between different faces, a large number of different morphometric features might have to be determined. The development of these architectures progressed in parallel with that of neural networks. A major advantage of neural networks is that they can derive their own features directly from data (feature learning) while shallow learning required the programmer to explicitly create the feature set (feature engineering). Another advantage of deep learning is that it can be used for reinforcement learning in which the algorithm learns to react to an environment by maximizing a reward function.

In spite of this obvious advantage, the field of deep learning languished for many years, partially because the early models did not live up to the hype (they were billed as thinking machines) but mostly because the computational power and storage capacities available were insufficient until relatively recently. Deep learning tends to be more computationally "needy" than shallow learning.

In all forms of machine learning, the computer is presented with a training set of known examples. Once the program has been trained, it is presented with a validation set. This is another set of known examples. However, this is withheld until training is complete. At that point, the program is tested with the examples in the validation set, to determine how well it can identify these samples that it has never seen. It is important to note that accuracy alone is not a valid measure of performance. As an example, if I know that the incidence of a disease is 1%, I can design a simple program with an accuracy of 99%. Simply call every example healthy. Obviously, this is not very useful. Since accuracy does not give a complete picture, two other measures are usually used; precision and recall. For a typical classification problem, "precision" is defined as the number of true positives divided by the sum of true and false positives. It is also known as the positive predictive value (PPV) and is essentially a measure of a classifier's exactness. In other words, what proportion of positive identifications was actually correct? "Recall" is the number of true positives divided by the sum of true positives and false negatives. This is also known as sensitivity. There are a number of other ways of determining how good a given machine learning model is, including (1) the F1 score, which is twice the product of precision and recall divided by the sum of precision and recall, and (2) AUC (area under the curve) which estimates that a classifier will rank a randomly chosen positive instance higher than a randomly chosen negative instance. Finally, a confusion matrix allows visualization of the performance of an algorithm. Each row of the matrix represents the instances in a predicted class, while each column represents the instances of an actual class. These concepts are important in allowing one to evaluate results in the published literature and to compare the efficacy of different models of machine learning applied to the same dataset.

With a bit of simplification, we can say that the basic aim of a machine learning strategy is to discover differences and/or similarities as well as patterns among sets of things. This can lead to high-level behaviors that mimic biological intelligence such as finding associations and correlations among patterns, interpreting and acting upon sensory information, processing language, and so on. While, in general, the datasets for machine learning must be large, it is impossible to overstate the importance of the quality of that data. For example, a study of patients with sepsis at a Chicago hospital (cited in 4) concluded that patients with low pH levels in their blood were less likely to return to the hospital soon after being discharged! This is counter to the known fact that metabolic acidosis in sepsis is associated with increased risk. It turned out that the data included patients who died during their hospital stay and who were obviously not candidates for readmission. The patients least likely to be readmitted were the ones who had already been discharged to the funeral home. When the deceased were excluded, it turned out that patients with low pH were in significantly greater danger than those with pH closer to normal, as expected. This was a classic example of data bias.

Shallow learning

Shallow learning algorithms can be broadly classified as geometric models, probabilistic models, and stratification models. Since much of machine learning is based on linear algebra, it makes sense that the data itself are best represented as a matrix (Fig. 2.1). This is also a data representation for deep learning.

Sample	Feature 1	Feature 2	Feature 3	Feature 4	CLASS
1	a1	b1	c1	d1	Class 1
2	a2	b2	c2	d2	Class 1
3	a3	b3	c3	d3	Class 2
4	a4	b4	c4	d4	Class 1
5	a5	b5	c5	d5	Class 2
6	a6	b6	c6	d6	Class 2
7	a7	b7	c7	d7	Class 1
8	a8	b8	c8	d8	Class 1
9	a9	b9	c9	d9	Class 1

FIGURE 2.1

A dataset in matrix form. Each feature set is written as a letter with a number that shows which sample it belongs to. Note that these need not be unique; for example, a1, a3, a7 can be identical. In fact, there *must* be shared feature values for learning to occur. In this dataset, four attributes define each sample. When samples in a training set are presented to a machine learning program, they are generally arranged in random order.

In this example, there are nine samples, representing two distinct classes. Each sample is defined in terms of its feature set (in this example, 4). In machine learning jargon, samples (or examples) are also known as "instances," and features are also known as "attributes." The set of features for a given sample is called its "feature vector." In this context, a vector is defined as an ordered collection of n elements, rather than as a directed line segment. The features (a1, a2, etc.) can be anything that can be amenable for computer manipulation. If one feature is color, we would have to define that feature by assigning each color to a different number (red would be coded as 1, blue as 2, and so on). We can refer to the dimensionality N of the feature vector (here 4) or, in some cases, the dimensionality of the entire dataset. In order for this to be a usable training set, no sample can have a completely unique feature set, since if that were the case, the computer would have no basis for generalization to new unknown samples; all it could do would be to memorize the list.

Geometric (distance-based) models

These fall into the category of clustering algorithms. They will be discussed in detail as to illuminate many of the concepts involved in more complicated forms of machine learning.

The best way to begin to talk about clustering is with an example. Bloodletting was a widely accepted therapeutic practice for a variety of diseases beginning about 3000 years ago and still is practiced for conditions such as polycythemia vera and hemochromatosis [5]. Back in the good old days of medicine this was accomplished by the use of bloodsucking leeches. There are both bloodsucking leeches and nonbloodsucking leeches (I assume the latter are vegetarians). You are given the unenviable task of distinguishing between these two different species when presented with an unknown sample. Luckily, the leeches can be identified morphologically as well as functionally, and the two classes are of different sizes. You accept the challenge, with the proviso that you also will be given a list consisting of a number of different samples of each, with their respective weights and lengths as known examples. This will be the training set. We will ignore the validation step in this example.

You are then presented with the unknown leech. Unfortunately, you do not remember how to calculate standard deviations, so high school statistics is out. A good approach might be to plot the lengths and weights of your known samples (instances) as seen in Fig. 2.2, where reds and blues correspond to the two different classes. The colored shapes on the graph are the examples, and their coordinates represent their attributes. In this example, it is possible to draw a straight boundary line exactly separating the classes. All that is now necessary is to weigh and measure the unknown leech and see on which side of the line it falls, which tells you which of the two leech classes it belongs to. This is a geometric model since the distance between two points tells you how similar they are. It has learned from data how to predict the class of an unknown sample from its attributes. While this may seem needlessly complicated for a situation with samples such as this that have only a few attributes and fit into only two classes, consider the more general case where there may be multiple distinct classes, and the number of attributes may run into the hundreds or thousands.

Unfortunately, life is not as simple as has just been described. There are obviously many possible lines that can separate the two classes, even in this simple example. How do we treat novel samples that are on or close to the line? In fact, how do we know where to draw the line? What happens if we cannot find a simple line i.e., there might be a nonlinear boundary? Finally, is it possible to extract information from the data if we do not have a priori knowledge of the classes of our samples (so-called unsupervised learning)?

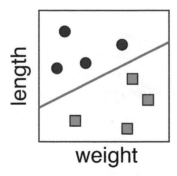

FIGURE 2.2

Plot of length and weight of the two different leech species.

To treat novel samples on or close to the line, we look for a point in the training space closest to the novel point and assume that they are in the same class. However, the points may be exactly halfway between two points in two different classes, the test point itself might be inaccurate, and the data might be "noisy." The solution is the **K-nearest neighbor algorithm (KNN)**, which, though simple, is a strong machine learning strategy. Just use several (K) nearest neighbors instead of one and go with the majority, or use an average or weighted average.

It has already been noted that this may, at first glance, seem no better than a rules-based algorithm involving statistical analysis. However, consider the situation where the number of attributes (feature vector) has hundreds or thousands of attributes rather than just two.

Even with more complex but still linearly separable plots, there are often many different ways to draw the boundary line, as illustrated in Fig. 2.3A. In fact, there are an infinite number of linear separators in this example. The best line is the one that provides the greatest separation of the two classes. For this purpose, we obviously need to consider only the closest points to the line, which are known as support vectors. Using these, the algorithm creates a line that is farthest away from all the points in both the clusters (Fig. 2.3B). The algorithm that does this is known as a **support vector machine (SVM)**.

An SVM can do much more than finding optimal linear boundaries. It can even transform nonlinear data to a linear form by transforming the data in a new coordinate system in a higher dimensional space by means of a kernel function, which itself involves only linear operations. This is known as the "kernel trick."

Fig. 2.4 shows, in the right, an example of two classes without a linear boundary that can separate them. In this example, there are two classes, each with two defining attributes. Clearly there is no linear boundary that can separate them. In this case, a circle (nonlinear boundary) will do the job. However, if you imagine pulling one class up into the third dimension, as shown on the left of Fig. 2.4, then it is easy

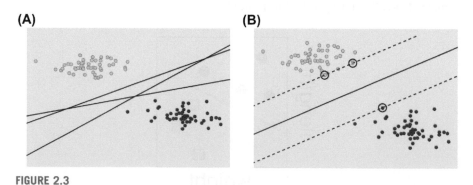

FIGURE 2.3

A): Possible linear separators for the clusters shown. (B): Support vectors are used to construct the line that best separates them.

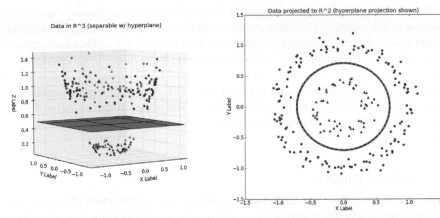

FIGURE 2.4

Creating a linear separator for the data by adding a dimension to it. The separating plane shown in the 3D space on the left is analogous to a line drawn in 2D space. In general, for any N-dimensional space, a linear construct such as this is defined as a hyperplane.

Reprinted with permission from Eric Kim (www.eric-kim.net).

to see that a flat plane can divide them. In general, an SVM can raise the dimensionality of the data space until an (N-1) hyperplane can separate the classes. In this example, the two-dimensional plot is transformed into a three-dimensional space such that an $N = 2$ hyperplane can provide a boundary.

The K-Means Algorithm (KM)

This is also a classic clustering algorithm, but it is discussed in a separate section because it important not to confuse it with KNN, and so they are presented separately for pedagogical rather than conceptual reasons. This is another important distinction, in that unlike the K nearest neighbor algorithm, it involves unsupervised learning. As such, it has important applications not only on its own but also in conjunction with some deep learning methods.

The K means algorithm attempts to find clustering in unlabeled data. One starts by making a guess as to how many clusters there are (this will be refined later). A centroid is the arithmetic mean position of all the points in a cluster. Next make a random guess as to where the central points of each cluster are so as to create k pseudo-centers. These should be reasonably distant from each other, but need have no relationship to the actual clusters and can be chosen randomly (unless there is some prior knowledge about the data structure). Next assign each point of the dataset to its nearest pseudo-center. We now form clusters with each cluster comprising all of the data points associated with its pseudo-center. Next update the location of each cluster's pseudo-center so that it is now indeed in the center of all its members. Do this recursively until there are no more changes to cluster membership.

We can determine the best choice for K by plotting within-cluster scatter as a function of the number of clusters. As an extreme example, if K equals the number of data points, there is obviously no variance within each cluster, as they each consist of one element. The smaller the number of clusters, the greater the variance within the clusters. When variance is plotted as a function of K, the equation is reminiscent of exponential decay, and it is easy to pick a value of K such that larger values do not appreciably change the overall variance. This is analogous to the so-called "scree plots" used in principal component analysis (PCA), described in a separate section below.

Probabilistic models

In the previous section, the basic building blocks of clustering and distance were used to learn relationships among data and to use those relationships to predict class labels. We can also approach this problem by asking the following question; given the feature set for an unknown example, what is the probability that it belongs to a given class? More precisely, if we let X represent the variables we know about, namely our instance's feature values, and Y the target variables, namely the instance's class, then we want to use machine learning to model the relationship between X and Y.

Since X is known for a given instance, but Y is not (other than in the training set), we are interested in the conditional probabilities; what is the probability of Y given X. This is another way of saying that given a sample's feature set (X), predict the class it belongs to (Y). In mathematical notation, this is written as $P(Y|X)$ which is read as "the probability of Y given X. As a concrete example, X could indicate the phrase" my fellow Americans" and Y could indicate whether the speaker is a member of the class politician (thus using the words "class" and "politician" in the same sentence, possibly for the first time).

The classification problem is thus simply to find $P(Y|X)$. The probabilities of several kinds of occurrence can be calculated directly from the training set. In the data matrix in Fig. 2.1, for any given feature X, we can simply count the number of times its value appears divided by the total number of variables, giving $P(X)$. For any given value of Y, we can count similarly count the ratio of the number of times that class appears relative to the overall number of classes. In this manner, we can calculate values for the sets X,Y to get $P(Y)$ and $P(X)$.

There is one more thing we can do, and that is to calculate $P(X|Y)$, the probability of the feature, given the class, which is simply based on looking only at that class and determining how many times the feature value X appears in samples of that class in the training set. We now know $P(X|Y)$. Given this information, we can calculate the probability of the class given our knowledge of its feature set, $P(Y|X)$ by means of the easily proven Bayes theorem (the only equation used in this chapter):

$P(Y|X) = (P(X|Y)*P(Y))/P(X)$ which, if a Venn diagram is drawn, becomes intuitively obvious.

In practice this formula is too simple, since in order to make predictive assignments from attributes to class, each sample must have more than one attribute, and in real-world problems, many more than one. The procedure for dealing with multiple attributes is more complicated [6]. In any case, the Bayes theorem is a formulation of one of the basic rules for conditional probabilities. However, the problem with computing probabilities in this way is that some of the features in a feature set may be dependent on each other (for embryos, mass and cell number are dependent variables), which makes the calculations difficult. In practice, this complication is ignored, and the features are treated as if they were independent. This algorithm is known as **Naïve Bayes** where naïve means that we are foolish enough to assume independence. Surprisingly Naïve Bayes works remarkably well in spite of this limitation, and so it has become an important machine learning model. There are much more complex models that deal with dependency relationships; these are known as Bayesian optimal classifiers. There is also a middle ground that is based on the idea that some things are conditionally dependent but some things are not.

These approaches fall into the framework of probabilistic graphical models that are known as Bayesian Belief Networks or Directed Graphical Networks. These are networks that represent a set of variables and their conditional dependencies via the use of a directed graph. A simple network of this kind is shown in Fig. 2.5. Rain influences whether the sprinkler is turned on, and both rain and the sprinkler influence whether we get wet. Bayesian Belief Networks are beyond the scope of this chapter, but additional information may be found in Ref. [7]. All these algorithms learn from probability distributions within their sample space, rather than spatial metrics, as was the case for SVMs and other geometrical models.

FIGURE 2.5

Relationships among three objects. Whether it is raining or not determines whether the sprinkler gets turned on, but not vice versa, so this is a directed graph. Similarly, either rain or the sprinkler will get something wet, but the state of wetness does not cause either rain or the sprinkler to happen, so these arrows are also directional.

All machine learning algorithms have problems of some sort. For example, KNN does not handle large sets of multivariate data very well. Naïve Bayes works on discrete attributes, but only if there are enough examples to get good estimates for all the probabilities that have to be estimated from the training dataset.

Decision Trees and Random Forests

The Decision Tree algorithm is a simple classic supervised learning model that works surprisingly well. The classifiers discussed above all expect attribute values to be presented at the same time. To make a diagnosis, we usually begin with symptoms, then obtain historical information and look for signs based on physical examination. Based upon this sequence of events, laboratory tests and radiologic examinations are ordered. Within the laboratory there may be reflexive testing; an initial test result may influence the choice of the next set of tests to be performed. Thus, information may be accumulated sequentially. A decision tree will be given its data all at once, but utilizes it in a sequential manner such as that described above. The game of "twenty questions" is a good example of a binary decision tree.

A decision tree uses a treelike graph that represents a flow-chart-like structure in which the starting point is the "root." Each internal node of the tree represents a test on an attribute or subset of attributes. Each branch from the node represents the outcome of the test, and the final node is a "leaf" that represents a class label. One can construct a simple decision tree by hand. However, it is easy to design an algorithm that learns the tree from data. As is the case for other kinds of machine learning, in the decision tree approach supervised learning takes labeled examples and builds a classifier by computing the sequence of branch choices. Decision trees, as the name implies, can be used for decision-making as well as classification. In that case, each of the classes represents different decision choices; for example, should I complete this chapter or watch the political debate? An example of a decision tree is shown in Fig. 2.6, which predicts an output based on a set of binary decisions. The tree proceeds from left to right.

There are lots of different ways that a decision tree can be constructed from the dataset, based upon which attributes to choose for each node, and what conditions are to be used for splitting at that node. The problem is to look at the available attributes and pick whichever are best to make a decision fork at each branch of the tree. The algorithm chooses "best" as that choice that maximizes the information gain for that step. It does so by the use of equations from information theory that are based on the concept of entropy and attempts to minimize entropy. Unlike the situation in physics, entropy in information theory is a measure of how random a set of things are. A set of things that are all the same has low entropy, and a set of things that are completely random has high entropy. Trying to minimize entropy is a good way of generating decision trees. However, measures other than entropy can also be used; in practice they tend to perform similarly. The process is terminated when there are no attributes left to test on, or when the remaining examples are of a single class. When it gets to that node the program returns a class label.

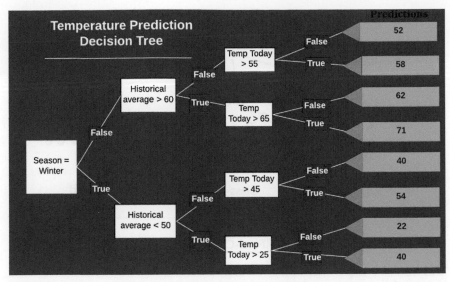

FIGURE 2.6

A decision tree for predicting tomorrow's maximum temperature. Seattle, 12/27/2017. From Koehrsen, Random forest simplified. In this tree, there is a binary decision made at each branch, so each parent node gives rise to two children nodes.

https://medium.com/@williamkoehrsen/random-forest-simple-explanation-377895a60d2d.

One can construct decision trees for a given dataset in a variety of ways (a) using different subsets of the data for different trees, (b) using different decision criteria, (c) limiting the depth of each tree, and so on. For (a) a technique called bagging is commonly used. In bagging, multiple new training subsets are taken by sampling from the main dataset with replacement after each sample is generated. Each subset is used in a different tree. A **Random Forest** consists of a set of several of such decision trees, with majority voting or some other consensus criterion determining final output values (Fig. 2.7).

The curse of dimensionality and principal component analysis

Intuitively, adding more features to the data would seem to improve our ability to classify it, but in many applications, this can make things worse [8]. As the dimensionality of the feature set increases, the space in which the samples reside increases with the power of the dimension, and so the sample density at any given point falls below that which is needed for an accurate prediction. The obvious solution is to get more data, but this may not always be possible in practice. There are techniques for dimensional reduction that minimize the loss of information that comes from this

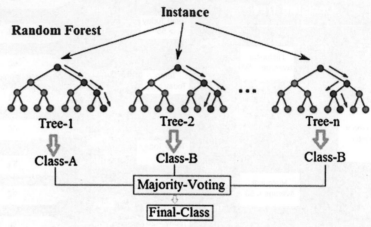

FIGURE 2.7

A random forest composed of three decision trees. Koehrsen, Random forest simplified.
https://medium.com/@williamkoehrsen/random-forest-simple-explanation-377895a60d2d.

reduction. The classic example, from statistical models, is known as PCA, which was first described in the 1930s, way before the onset of machine learning. PCA operates by finding the direction of maximum variance in the data. This is the dimension along which the data are most spread out and is the first principal component. The next one is the line perpendicular to this component that has the next best spread of the data, and so on. This process is repeated until there are as many principal components as the original data have dimensions. In essence, it is simply a linear transformation of the data from one n-dimensional space to another n-dimensional space that retains the information in the original set. In order to reduce the dimensionality of this transformed set, we must discard some of these components. Since the n components have already been ordered according to importance, if we want to project down the k dimensions ($k < n$) we just keep the first k components and discard the rest. We can plot the loss of information by a graph showing variance as a function of component number (in mathematical terms, the curve shows the eigenvalues of the covariance matrix on the y-axis and the component number of the x-axis). This construct is known as a scree plot.

Deep learning and the artificial neural network

Shallow learning works well in those situations where one can explicitly define the feature vectors of the problem. Problems involving image interpretation and classification as well as those requiring natural language processing are examples where these models perform poorly because of the complexity of the data. The human brain is very good at this because it makes use of a series of processing levels or "layers", each one doing a more complex analysis than the previous one. Deep learning computational approaches patterned on the brain deal with this issue very well. Although not the only form of deep learning, neural network—based models are the ones most currently employed at present.

As we shall see, ANNs develop increasingly complex internal representations of the data, and in the process automatically extract the relevant salient feature vectors of the dataset. In this chapter we will cover the basics of fully connected and convolutional networks. More advanced architectures will be covered in the next chapter. The aim is to present the inner workings of ANNs in detail (the second-floor view), rather than merely providing the descriptive 30,000 feet overview that appears in most of the medical literature, while avoiding the underlying mathematics and programming details that become apparent at ground level. There is only one equation in the entire exposition, and it is easily derived. It should be noted that there are many other deep learning algorithms that are not based on connected layers in linear sequences such as those described here (for example, Boltzmann machines). As these have only rarely been employed in pathology applications, they will not be covered here.

In the examples provided, the emphasis will be placed on image interpretation, but the principles can also be applied to genomics and expression arrays, as well as natural language processing. Natural language processing and semantic understanding are not covered; at the current state-of-the-art programs such as IBM's Watson and similar efforts have proven disappointing in the clinical setting. The focus will be entirely on supervised models. Just as there are shallow network models for unsupervised learning, there are a number of unsupervised deep learning strategies, and some of these will be covered in later chapters.

Neuroscience 101

As indicated above, models for deep learning are (very) loosely based upon the neural network architecture of the mammalian brain and how the neurons within the networks comprising the brain process signals both inside the neuron and from one neuron to another. The first mammalian neural nets came into being about 200 million years ago. Through a process of "continuous performance improvement," we now have the cellular structure shown in Fig. 2.8.

The neuron receives signals at its dendritic end, usually from multiple other neurons. Those signals are integrated within the cell, and if they rise past a threshold value, they are passed through the axon as an action potential. Signals are propagated via electrical pulses or spikes generated via the modulation of ion channels at the cell membrane and are transduced across the synapses that separate the neurons via electrochemical reactions involving a variety of chemical mediators. Each action potential is a simple on-off burst of electrical energy. The only exception is

FIGURE 2.8

Schematic of a typical neuron. The cell can receive signals from many other neurons via its dendrites. If the sum of these exceeds a threshold value, the neuron passes the integrated signal on to other neurons. The human brain has approximately 100 billion neurons. LadyofHats, Creative Commons.

for sensory neurons that terminate in a transducer. For example, in the Pacinian corpuscle, the action potential varies with stimulus intensity.

Since each dendritic input interacts with the others via multiple interacting electrochemical events, there may be a nonlinear sum of inputs, especially since the spatial separation of the inputs affects their interaction. For this reason, the neuronal threshold for firing can be an all-or-none event (in mathematical jargon, this is a Heaviside ramp function) while the total process is nonlinear. Moreover, information can move backwards in a neuron through current flow. In other words, the neuron has an internal feedback system. A single backpropagating action potential can activate slow dendritic voltage-gated ionic currents, which in turn flow back toward the spike initiation zone in the axon, resulting in additional action potentials. Effectively this gives us a two-layered neural network that resides in a single neuron. There are experiments that show that directional selectivity and coincidence detection may be implemented even at this basic computational level.

The pulses of electrical activity that mediate interneuron signaling can be modulated on the basis of pulse frequency, pulse width, or pulse arrival time in relation to other incoming signals. A neuron can receive either excitatory or inhibitory signals.

Additional modulation of signals comes at the synapses between two brain cells. A synapse between two neurons is strengthened when the neurons on either side of the synapse (input and output) have highly correlated outputs. This is known as Hebbian learning. In essence this means that if one neuron repeatedly excites another, then the connection between them is facilitated. Hebbian learning allows modification of the flow of information within the network. In the brain, the synaptic connections are constantly being remodeled, based upon the integrated set of signals they are responding to at any given moment. Remodeling is not well understood, but appears to be based on the accumulation and depletion of chemical gradients. Some synapses can be completely eliminated via interaction with astrocytes or glia, presumably via cytokines.

This picture is further complicated in that the neuron, taken as a whole, can show bistable behavior. Bistability is a property of a dynamical system that exhibits more than one stable point. A model proposed by Lowenstein and Sompolinsky [9] involves bistability with respect to the dendritic concentration of Ca++. If it is forced to be in the up state at one end of the dendrite, and in the down state at the other, then a standing wave of Ca++ concentration is created, instead of a gradient. As long as no further input occurs, the wave front will maintain its position. This model is very important. Although the process of activating and firing a neuron occurs at very short time scales, working memory requires longer time scales, and this model is one simple way of integrating transient effects into a persistent trace, which is essentially a definition of working memory.

Since each neuron receives inputs from many other neurons, and transmits its output to many other neurons, the neurons essentially work as aggregators; the total amount of output is controlled by the total input from all its dendritic connections. Since the axon can also connect to multiple neurons, this allows a complex, multi-layer structure to develop. The human brain has approximately 100 billion neurons. Even though arranged as subsystems, there are huge numbers of possible interconnections.

The rise of the machines

After approximately 1.9 million years and 3 months (author's note: It was 1.9 million when this chapter was begun, 3 months ago) of brain evolution, human scientists began to model the brain. Rosenblatt's single layer perceptron [1] was based upon the first mathematical model of a neuron by McCullough and Pitts [2], the MCP neuron. This was inspired by the Hebbian concept of synaptic plasticity based on the adaptation of brain neurons during the learning process. Applying different relative weights to the inputs affects the output, Rosenblatt developed a supervised learning algorithm for this modified MCP neuron that enabled it to figure out the correct weights by learning from data all by itself. Such an artificial neuron, which is a mathematical abstraction rather than a physical construct, is diagrammed in Fig. 2.9 and compared to a simple representation of a biological neuron.

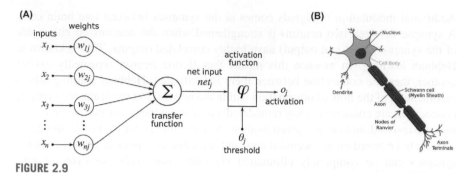

FIGURE 2.9

An artificial neuron (which is an abstraction in a computer program, rather than a physical entity) is diagrammed in 9A. Each of the inputs x are modified by a weights w and then summed just as the synaptic inputs would be in a real neuron. This sum Σ is passed to an activation function, φ and if it exceeds the value of the function's threshold θ it is passed on as an output o. In this schematic, (Σ and φ) together are the analogs to a biological neuron. Chrislb, Creative Commons. For comparison, a biological neuron is shown in 9B.

(NickGorton-commonswiki).

    This artificial neuron, which is the basic building block of most of the artificial networks of deep learning, is a great oversimplification in the following ways. Since the mathematical analysis of pulse-based coding is difficult, the model neuron receives as input a single steady value at each dendrite that is connected to an upstream neuron (there are spiking artificial neural networks (ANNs), but they are not in widespread use). The signal variability during learning is represented by a set of weights associated with the signals, and these weights change as the neural network learns. Another important difference between a biological and a modern ANN is that in the former, the threshold is based upon a simple off-on ramp, whereas in the latter, a smooth curve such as a sigmoid or similar kind of function is used.

    Initially, sigmoid functions were used as the transfer function. The curve for a typical sigmoid function is shown in Fig. 2.10. The sigmoid's value ranges from zero to one. The sigmoid is a continuous, nonlinear differentiable function. Note that, unlike the Heaviside, the activation threshold can be any value we choose in its range. Current ANNs often use other functions, such as the hypertangent function or the rectified linear function (ReLU) as well. As we shall see, in a neural network weights are adjusted by a process that involves finding the minimum of a loss function through the use of calculus, and so the threshold must be a continuous function. Additionally, the function must allow the network to deal with nonlinear relationships. One of the criticisms of the earlier neural networks shortly after they were published was related to their inability to deal with nonlinear relationships. Although there was a great deal of hype surrounding the Rosenblatt perception, in 1969, Minsky [10] published a book that not only showed how limited Rosenblatt's perception (and indeed, any single layer perceptron) actually is but also led to an intellectual climate change among the "artificial intelligentsia," namely the

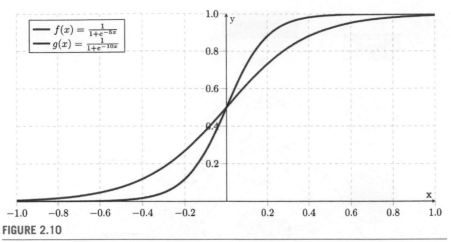

FIGURE 2.10

Plot of a sigmoid function. The slope of the curve can be adjusted by the choice of the multiplier for x in the equation. The curve's bounds on the x-axis are from 0 to 1, thus making it a reasonable substitute for a ramp activation.

M. Thoma, Wikimedia Commons.

so-called AI-winter in the 1980s. However, major contributions by many investigators brought back ANNs into the forefront of AI research, based on the multilayer concept, nonlinear activations, backpropagation, and convolution. The beauty of a modern ANN and its many advanced variants that will be covered in the next chapter is that it can represent the output of any continuous bounded function, and thus can mimic the output of any algorithmic structure that uses mathematics for its underlying implementation (i.e., most, if not all of them). Thus, in addition to its own unique abilities, an ANN can do anything a shallow learning network can do, but for data that are not too complex, shallow learning can be more computationally efficient. However, these modern artificial networks, in evolving beyond these humble beginnings, have become truly sophisticated models employing concepts from linear algebra, multivariate calculus, mathematical statistics, game theory, reinforcement learning, and evolutionary theory. In order to emphasize how much further we have to go to achieve true general intelligence in an artificial substrate, it is humbling to note that the human brain contains many billion neurons and rather than being merely passive devices, each function as an independent small computer in the way that it processes data. If we think of the brain as a set of giant interacting networks, the number of possible connections is literally astronomically large.

The basic ANN

A typical neural net is composed of several layers of nodes, as shown in Fig. 2.11.

Each neuron in the net has the properties described for perceptrons. However, in addition to the input and output layers, there are a variable number of "hidden" layers that connect the input to the output layers. They are called hidden layers

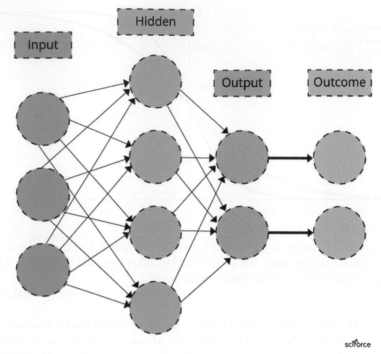

FIGURE 2.11

The multilayer construction of a neural network. Each colored circle represents a neuron (which passes the aggregated signal through an activation function) and the lines are the inputs and output connecting them. In this example, only a single hidden layer is shown. In practice, multiple hidden layers are used.

From SciForce: white paper on Top Algorithms for Health", by permission of M. Ved, "Top Algorithms for Healthcare" SciForce-Medium.

for the following reason: since we know the inputs and receive output data, both these layers are known to us. In contrast, the layers in between are not readily accessible to the observer. Since the computer has no cognition, each run of the algorithm is, in essence, a double-blind experiment. This has raised philosophical issues about the explainability of deep learning models.

The basic features of an ANN are as follows:

- Each input neuron gets only one input, directly from outside; those of the hidden layers get many.
- Neurons in a layer do not connect to each other.
- Each neuron in one layer connects to all the neurons in the next layer.
- The ANN is a synchronous model; all nodes in a given layer receive their inputs and calculate their activities at the same time. This means that all the calculations in the n layer must be calculated before we can start the calculations for the (n+1) layer.

Thus, the output of one layer becomes the inputs of the next. Because of the summing process, each layer receives increasingly complex inputs. At any given layer, the network creates an internal representation of the data that incorporates relationships among the feature vectors of each sample. Basically, a neural network utilizes multiple levels of representation to model both simple and complex relationships among data. They are powerful classifiers and can extract relations, predict outcomes, and make inferences from data, all without the need to manually define the feature vectors for that set. For example, instead of inputting the eye-snout ratios and other defining characteristics of dogs versus cats to classify an unknown image as to it dog-ness or cat-ness, one can simply present multiple known examples of each to the program.

The weights in an ANN

As was the case for the Rosenblatt perception, every input within an ANN is associated with a weight that represents the relative importance of that input with respect to its contribution to the sum of signals received by the neuron. For a node receiving input from two nodes of the previous layer, the total input is the sum of the output of the first node times its weight plus the output of the second node times its weight. This is the product of two vectors. In general, one can set up the computation of each layer of nodes as a single matrix-vector product. Basically, there is a matrix of weights multiplied by the input vector, which produces the aggregated output when acted upon by the activation function. When these calculations are generalized to multilayer networks with many nodes, they are seen to be the result of simple multiplicative steps in linear algebra. In some ANNs a bias term is also added; this is a scalar that is added to the input to ensure that a few nodes per layer are activated regardless of signal strength. It is because the weighted inputs summed is a linear function that a nonlinear activation function must act upon them so that the ANN is not restricted to linear problems. Both weights and biases are modified throughout the training of an ANN.

Learning from examples; Backprop and stochastic gradient descent.

The traditional learning method for feed-forward networks such as the ANN is to take a fixed network architecture and then use the examples to find appropriate values for the weights that lead to correct performance. The fact that each node in a layer has an incoming connection from every node in the previous layer does not interfere with this adjustment, since any unnecessary connection can be set to zero during this process.

The network learns the proper weights from the training set using a gradient-descent algorithm based upon The Error Back-Propagation algorithm (Backprop). The basics of backpropagation were derived in the context of control theory by multiple researchers in the 1960s. Subsequently, in the 1980s, a number of investigators proposed that it could be used for neural networks. Thus, it is difficult to assign priority to this fundamental technique that is the basis for neural network training (see Ref. [3] for historical details).

The way Backprop works is as follows: We initially pick a training instance and set the activity of the input nodes to the values from that instance. Activities are then propagated through the ANN in its initial state (the initial weights, within certain constraints, are arbitrary, and often are randomly chosen). The output is then examined. At this point, the output values are compared to the correct answer, which we know, since the example is from the labeled training set. The labels are known as "ground truth" and the object is to generate a result that matches this ground truth. If this turns out to be the case, then a miracle occurred. If not, the difference between ground truth and the prediction is quantified by a so-called "loss" or "cost" function. This is often, but not always, a mean square error function. The task is now to minimize the cost function by adjusting the weights in an iterative manner. This is not a straightforward process, since each weight contributes to more than one output, and so we cannot simply apply corrections evenly among all the weights. In practice, we work backwards from the output layer through the hidden layers rather than starting at the beginning of the net. This is known as gradient descent.

Fig. 2.12 shows a simple diagram of an error curve, where J(w) is the loss function and w is a weight. The gradient, or slope, shows the direction of change in the weight needed to reach either a minimum or a maximum. That is the point at which the gradient (slope) is zero. At each step of the gradient descent method, the iterative steps are proportional to the negative of the gradient of the function at the current point. The gradient is calculated from the partial derivatives of the loss function with respect to the weights (multivariate calculus to the rescue).

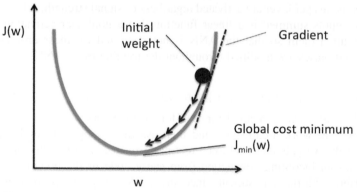

FIGURE 2.12

The gradient is given by the slope of the curve directly above the point we are interested in. Lines that go up as we move right have a positive slope, and otherwise they are negative. The weight is adjusted in a stepwise manner as shown.

Mixtend, Creative Commons. license.

The actual situation is not that simple. As the dimensionally of the space increases, the loss function curve can get complex. In Fig. 2.13 it can be seen that there is no single minimum; instead there are local minima that can be reached by different starting trajectories. There is no computationally efficient way of calculating the true global minimum. However, in practice, local minima are good enough for excellent algorithmic performance. One can always take different starting points for the weights and compare outputs as a way of sampling the local minima.

This process is refined over the set of training examples. Backpropagation is one of the reasons that training sets for deep learning must be large. Interestingly, if the network has too many layers, training can suffer. As we proceed further and further backwards down the net the weighting corrections get smaller and smaller and they will become closer and closer to zero. This is known as the vanishing gradient problem. It can be overcome in a specialized ANN known as a residual neural network, which will be covered in the next chapter.

Finally, it is important to note that this algorithm assumes that tweaking all the weights independently and simultaneously actually leads to a reduction in this error. This is not intuitive, since changing one weight could cause ripple effects throughout

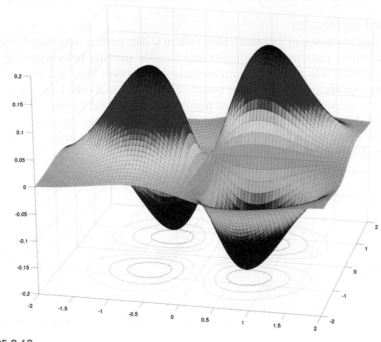

FIGURE 2.13

A complex 3D curve showing multiple local minima and saddle points. The situation is even more complex in multidimensional space.

Wikimedia Commons.

the rest of the network. It turns out, however, that if we make the changes to the weights small enough the assumption generally holds true, and the weights do, in fact, reach good error reduction.

Convolutional Neural Networks

Overview

Convolutional Neural Networks (CNNs) are sufficiently complex so that a brief overview will be helpful prior to a more complete discussion. In brief, images are too large to be analyzed at the input pixel level. Arguable, the first CNN was "Alexnet" in 2012 by A Krizhevsky et al. [11]. The CNN extracts image features to create increasingly complex representation. It uses feature extraction filters on the original image, and uses some of the hidden layers to move up from low level feature maps to high level ones. CNNs have two kinds of layers, convolutional and pooling (subsampling). Convolutional filters are small matrices that are "slid" over the image. The matrix is combined with the underlying image piece and the maximum value from each convolution is obtained. In the CNN, the convolutional layers are not fully connected, but their output is usually passed to one or more fully connected layers that perform the final classification. An overview of the process is seen in Fig. 2.14.

Detailed explanation

CNNs take advantage of the hierarchical pattern in data such as images and assemble more complex patterns using smaller and simpler patterns before moving these representations into traditional fully connected networks. They are loosely based upon the organization of the visual cortex of the brain. Individual cortical neurons respond to stimuli only in a restricted region of the visual field known as the receptive field. The receptive fields of different neurons partially overlap such that they cover the entire visual field. The CNN mimics this, in that its layers are not fully connected. This is shown in Fig. 2.15.

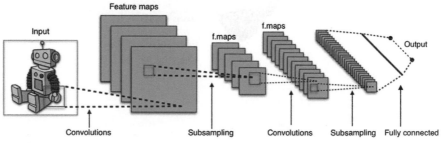

FIGURE 2.14

Schematic of a typical convolutional network diagramming convolutions and subsampling. The image representation at the final layer is passed to fully connected layers and a classification prediction is made.

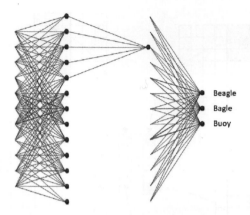

FIGURE 2.15

This figure illustrates the beginning and end of a CNN. Not all the neurons of one hidden layer will connect to each neuron in the next layer. However, in all cases there are neurons that share connections from the previous layer so as to create overlapping fields (not shown). The output of neuronal fields is down-sampled to further reduce the dimensionality of the sample space.

Wikimedia Commons.

As noted above, in the CNN a convolutional matrix (also called filter or kernel) is "slid" across the image and applied at each position. The resulting value then becomes the value for that pixel in the result. This is shown in Figs. 2.16 and 2.17.

The convolution is then followed by a pooling layer that down-samples the feature maps by summarizing the presence of features in patches of the feature map. Max pooling simply involves using the largest value rather than averaging them. This makes the resulting representations more robust with respect to changes in the position of the feature in the image (local translation invariance). CNN trained on similar data produce similar internal representations, and so they are useful for transfer learning, which will be discussed in subsequent chapters.

As seen above, the filters themselves are just matrices of numbers. By proper choice of values, they can detect specific features in the images such as horizontal and vertical lines, edges, shapes and so on. These numbers can be modified by back-propagation. The filters in Photoshop are convolution filters, and can be used to experiment with these concepts. Under "other" in the Filter tab there is an entry labeled Custom. Fig. 2.18 is a screenshot showing a convolution filter applied to a portrait of my face.

Overfitting and underfitting

In all of the examples of machine learning discussed above, their central purpose is to generalize. Generalization is the model's ability to give correct outputs to set of inputs that it has never seen before. Underfitting simply means that the algorithm has

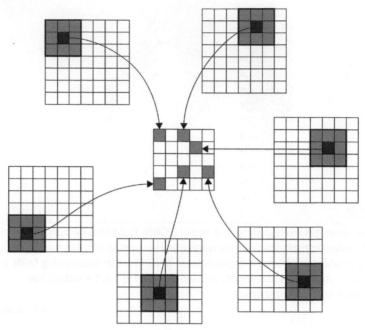

FIGURE 2.16

To convolve an image with a filter, the filter is moved across the image and applied at each position. In practice, blank rows and columns are added at each end so that there is no loss of coverage when the filter reaches the farthest position in the row or column. If padding (blank grids around the perimeter) was added to the grid being scanned by the 9×9 convolution filter, there would have been no dimensional reduction at this step.

-1	1	-1		1	1	0			-1	1	0	
-1	1	-1	×	0	0	0	=		0	0	0	⇨ −3 + 1 = -2
-1	1	-1		1	0	1			-1	0	-1	

-1	1	-1		0	1	0			0	1	0	
-1	1	-1	×	0	1	0	=		0	1	0	⇨ 3
-1	1	-1		0	1	0			0	1	0	

FIGURE 2.17

Applying the filter to an image. The filter is on the left. The section of the image currently overlaid by the filter is in the middle. The result of multiplying each pixel by its corresponding filter value is shown on the right. Adding up the nine values gives the final sum on the right.

FIGURE 2.18

Closeup of part of my face. (A) mild convolution (most detail remains). (B) after more convolution. In (B), the filter was chosen so as to detect line boundaries. In (A), the filter was chosen so as to simply make me look better. Your results may vary.

not learned well enough from the data. The concept of overfitting is a bit more complicated because it means that the algorithm learns too well! A model so powerful that it "memorizes" the data (overfitting) would cause each sample to define a separate class, while a model that is too weak cannot find any reliable class distinctions (underfitting). For a given model, finding the balance between overfitting and underfitting is more art than science.

Instead of these extremes, consider an actual scenario, as shown in Fig. 2.19, which depicts the results of a clustering model. In case A, there is a smooth boundary line, with only one error. This model has high accuracy. Moreover, we can easily place a novel unknown point on either side, accepting the fact that we will occasionally make a mistake. The model generalizes well. In contrast, in case B we have a boundary line that has separated both classes perfectly. In this case, when the model sees a novel point, it will simply bend the boundary again so as to accommodate it, rather than generalize it for prediction. Perfection is the enemy of the truth. The subject of overfitting is a complex one and the details are beyond the scope of this chapter. For a complete discussion of overfitting and mechanisms for dealing with it, see Ref. [12].

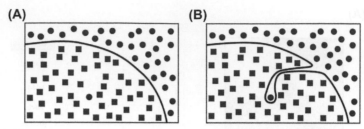

FIGURE 2.19

(A): there is a smooth boundary line that does a good job of separating the two classes, with only one error. This is a good fit from which we can generalize well. (B): the boundary curve distorts itself to accommodate a single aberrant point (overfitting).

Things to come

While the many models for deep learning are impressive in their sophistication and power, we are only at the beginning of the age of artificial intelligence. Our human brains still have a number of obvious advantages over ANNs as presently implemented. For example, we can learn complex patterns from a very small training set of examples, and we are much better than machines at avoiding both overfitting and the increase of errors with multiple processing layers due to vanishing gradients during backpropagation. In fact, backpropagation itself seems biologically unlikely, based in part on measures of latency during biologic learning, and because very few neurons have taken courses in multivariate calculus. For these reasons, there has been an increasing interest in models for deep learning that more closely mimic our current understanding of biological neural function. This includes both the development of spiking neural networks, and attempts to replace backpropagation in more traditional models, the latter via synthetic gradients, random feedback, or direct feedback alignment. With respect to spiking networks, the notion of a set of weighted inputs across layers is replaced by an integrate-and-fire model that integrates incoming pulses based upon pulse coding. Such models lend themselves well to synaptic plasticity, by which is meant that there is a correlation between pre- and postsynaptic neurons based upon long-term depression and potentiation effects. They have intrinsic temporal information processing activity, and are amenable to implementation of unsupervised learning strategies. Current spiking models are relatively simplistic and are not yet competitive with traditional ANNs for practical applications, but there is a great deal of ongoing research on optimizing them.

Of great potential significance is the creation of artificial neurons and synapses that will allow for the construction of spiking networks in hardware as well as software. For example, Tuma et al. [13] have described an artificial stochastic phase-change neuron in which membrane potential is represented by a reversible amorphous-to-crystal phase transition. More recently, Schneider et al. [14] have described an artificial synapse in which the strength of an electrical current flowing across it can be precisely controlled analogous to the way ions flow between neurons. This "synapse" is based on nanotextured magnetic Josephson junctions. Advances in the design of spiking network architecture implemented in hardware such as this may lead to a true artificial brain, assuming that we can also model the hierarchical architecture, modular structure, and cascading networks of the real thing, as will be done in 2338 for Chief Operations Officer Data in Star Trek TNG using an alloy of platinum and iridium. (Wikipedia)

At the current state of the art, ANN and CNN are one-trick ponies that are trained to do specific tasks, and they find it difficult to generalize this learning to novel tasks. They can only do this in a limited manner. If one trains a CNN to recognize prostatic cancer and another to recognize breast cancer, they will only work on prostate and breast cancer, respectively. Using so-called transfer learning it is possible to use the weights of the early layers of the trained prostate CNN to replace the initial random weightings in the training of the breast CNN. A human, however, can generalize across problems to a much greater degree. We use the term "artificial general intelligence" (AGI) to mean the representation of generalized human cognitive abilities in software (or ultimately in hardware) so that, faced with an unfamiliar task, the AI system could find a solution. What is currently known as AI is more correctly called weak AI. Most of the artificial intelligentsia feel that AGI will come about within this century. We will recognize the arrival of AGI in academic circles when it asks for (and is granted) tenure.

References

[1] Rosenblatt F. The Perception-a perceiving and recognizing automaton. Cornell Aeronautical Laboratory; 1957. Report 85-460-1.

[2] McCulloch WS, Pitts W. A logical calculus of the ideas immanent in nervous activity. Bulletin of Mathematical Biophysics 1943;5:115−33.

[3] Sejnowski TJ. The deep learning revolution. Cambridge, MA: MIT Press; 2018.

[4] Smith G, Cordes J. The 9 pitfalls of data science. Oxford University Press; 2019.

[5] Greenstone G. The history of bloodletting. BC Medical Journal 2010:12−4.

[6] A. Wasilewska. Bayesian classification. https://www3.cs.stonybrook.edu/∼cse634/19Bayes2.pdf.

[7] Koller D, Friedman N. Probabilistic graphical models. Cambridge, MA: MIT Press; 2009. See also, https://ai.stanford.edu/∼koller/Papers/Koller+al:SRL07.pdf.

[8] B Carter, Typical sets and the curse of dimensionality Stan blog 2017 https://mc-stan.org/users/documentation/case-studies/curse-dims.html Refs. [For PCA, overfitting and underfitting].

[9] Loewenstein Y, Sompolinsky H. Temporal integration by calcium dynamics in a model neuron. Nature Neuroscience 2003;6:961−7.

[10] Minsky M, Papert SA. Perceptions: an introduction to computational geometry. Cambridge, MA: MIT Press; 1969.

[11] Krizhevsky A, Sutskever I, Hinton GE. Imagen et classification with deep convolutional neural networks. In: Advances in neural information processing systems; 2012. p. 1106–14. https://arxiv.org/pdf/1803.01164.pdf.

[12] Glassner A. Chapter 9: overfitting and underfitting. In: Deep Learning: from basics to practice; 2018. p. 334–49. Kindle ASIN: B079XSQNRX.

[13] Tuma T, et al. Stochastic phase-change neurons. Nature Nanotechnology 2016;11: 693–9.

[14] Schneider ML, et al. Ultra-low power artificial synapses using nano-textured magnetic Josephson junctions. Science Advances 2018;4(1):e1701329. https://doi.org/10.1126/sciadv.1701329.

Overview of advanced neural network architectures

3

Benjamin R. Mitchell, BA, MSE, PhD

*Assistant Professor, Department of Computing Sciences, Villanova University, Villanova, PA,
United States*

Introduction

The field of deep learning has expanded rapidly over the past few years, and modern practitioners now use a wide range of methods and techniques to achieve state-of-the-art performance. Many of the best performing systems now use architectures that are significantly more complex than the fully connected feed-forward networks used in the past. These techniques draw inspiration from a range of different fields, including statistical methods, time series analysis, game theory, information theory, operant conditioning, genetic evolution, and modern neuroscience (though for the last few it is worth a reminder that "inspired by" is not the same as "accurately modeling").

This chapter will cover some of the most popular variations, including residual connections (ResNet), unsupervised pretraining (Autoencoders), transfer learning, generative models (GANs), recurrent networks (LSTMs), reinforcement learning, ensemble methods, and evolutionary algorithms. When reading this chapter, keep in mind that the methods presented are largely ways of modifying or expanding on the basic techniques presented in the previous chapter. This is done to address problems where those basic techniques are insufficient. The techniques described here can be used to address problems such as computational efficiency, classifier accuracy, and lack of large amounts of labeled training data.

Network depth and residual connections

The "depth" of a deep neural network can be highly variable depending on the task. In the earliest days of artificial neural networks, most networks were "shallow," meaning they did not have hidden layers. This was not because the early network designers did not want to have deeper networks; rather, it was because early researchers had no reliable method for training these deeper networks. As time progressed, developments in the field have allowed for the successful training of deeper and deeper networks. Today, some networks may have hundreds of hidden layers.

Artificial Intelligence and Deep Learning in Pathology. https://doi.org/10.1016/B978-0-323-67538-3.00003-8

The primary advantage of adding more hidden layers is that it allows the network to encode more complex functions. Since each layer takes the output of the previous layer as its input, each layer can be thought of as computing some sort of abstract "features" of the previous layer. Thus, each additional layer can compute a more abstract and complex function of the original data. A deeper network has more computational power than a shallower one, at least in theory.

In practice, this theoretical power may not always be easy to realize. There are several practical problems that can arise from adding extra hidden layers. The first, and simplest, is the fact that adding more hidden layers means adding more connections. Those extra connections give the network more representational power, but they also represent extra parameters which we must propagate information through and learn good values for. In other words, more connections means the network will operate more slowly and may take more epochs to train.

Even if we are willing to pay the computational cost of adding more connections, there is another phenomenon which can arise with too many hidden layers: the *vanishing gradient* problem. Since the standard method for learning weights in a neural network is using error backpropagation via the chain rule, the more hidden layers there are the more times we must "chain" the derivatives together. This can lead to the gradient becoming flattened and "diffused" as we get farther and farther away from the output units. This problem is particularly severe when using sigmoid activation functions, since the sigmoid function will always have a derivative between 0 and 1, and multiplying small numbers yields even smaller numbers. This is the primary reason that most modern neural networks use a rectified linear (ReLU) activation function [1]; the ReLU activation is less prone to gradient diffusion, allowing deeper networks to be used successfully.

However, even with the use of ReLU units, there are practical limits to how deep a simple feed-forward network can be successfully trained. In order to push depth beyond that limit, more advanced network architectures are required. One method which has become very popular in recent years is the use of *residual* connections [2]. This involves creating connections which "skip" one or more layers (also sometimes called "skip connections") (Fig. 3.2). In typical modern practice, these residual connections do not have tunable weights, but rather are a way to simply copy the activation from a lower level.

The key mathematical insight behind making these connections "skip" a layer is that it makes it much easier for that layer to "learn" to replicate the input of the previous layer; with the addition of the residual connections, simply outputting 0 will result in the output value being equal to the node the residual connection originates from. In effect, any nonzero output of the node is now added to the value from the earlier layer, rather than replacing it (as would be typical in a standard feed-forward network).

The term "residual" means the leftover or remaining error. In the case of residual connections, the idea is that each additional layer of the network now only has to try to fit the residual error, which simplifies the learning process. The result is that networks that make use of residual connections can be made much deeper than are possible otherwise, without falling prey to gradient diffusion or other optimization difficulties. The term ResNet may be used to refer to the original network

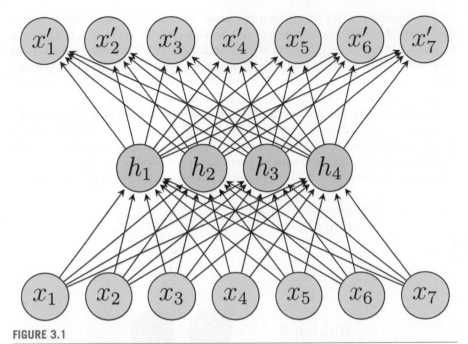

FIGURE 3.1

An autoencoder network is trained to reproduce its inputs with as little reconstruction error as possible. Since the hidden layer has fewer units than the input and output layers, this means the network learns to produce a reduced dimensionality encoding in the hidden layer. This is an "unsupervised" training process, since it requires no additional human annotation to the raw data.

proposed using this type of connection [2], but the term is also sometimes used to refer to any network making use of residual connections.

Autoencoders and unsupervised pretraining

One of the known drawbacks of deep neural networks is that they require very large amounts of data to train. This is a natural consequence of the power of the model; the more connections a network has, the more "power" it has to encode complex functions. However, it has long been known that the more parameters we need to estimate, the more data necessary to estimate good values for them. Since deep neural networks can have millions of free parameters, it is unsurprising that very large datasets may be needed to train them. As a few examples, the MNIST data set is a classic benchmarking set that is been around for over 20 years [3,4]. These days, it is considered a "toy" problem due to its comparatively small scale and the ease of achieving high performance. However, even this "small" data set has 60,000 images for training. The ImageNet data set, which is a more modern benchmarking set, consists of over 15 million high-resolution images [5]. In practice, many authors use only a subset of this full set, but even the subsets tend to have over a million training images.

This requirement for very large training sets would already be enough to potentially limit the problems that deep neural networks can be applied to, but the true scenario is even worse. Not only do we need very large amounts of data, most deep networks are trained using backpropagation, which is a supervised learning method. This means that we need a human-annotation giving the correct label (i.e., desired output) for each and every one of our millions of training examples.

For some tasks, this process can be crowdsourced; for instance, the ImageNet data set was created using Amazon's Mechanical Turk to pay large numbers of unskilled annotators to label images which had been scraped from the web [5]. Unfortunately, for many problems of interest, it is not possible to rely on unskilled annotators. In fields like medical imaging, it is common that humans require a

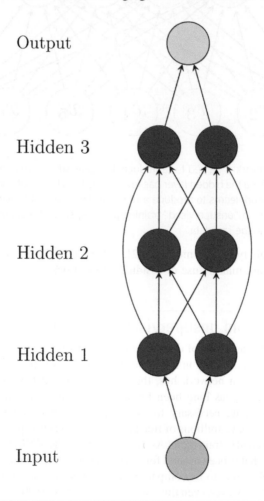

FIGURE 3.2

Many modern deep networks make use of skip connections, which allow for easier optimization in very deep networks. Here, the units in the first layer have direct connections to corresponding units in the third hidden layer, in addition to their "normal" connections to units in the second hidden layer.

significant amount of training to be able to correctly and reliably annotate images. Thus, even if a large set of images can be collected, it may not be practical to annotate them all. In this scenario, in which a large amount of data is available but only a small portion can be annotated, pure supervised learning is unlikely to succeed. Fortunately, we do have other options.

One method for handling this scenario is called *unsupervised pretraining*. The idea behind unsupervised pretraining is that, prior to applying a supervised learning technique, we will first apply an unsupervised learning technique in an attempt to make the final supervised optimization problem easier.

A classic example of this is to first train one or more layers of a neural network as an *autoencoder* [6]. The autoencoder is trained simply to reconstruct its input; that is, the desired output is merely a copy of the input (Fig. 3.1). If the network has enough hidden nodes, this task becomes trivial, but if the network is restricted in capacity then it is forced to learn some low-dimensional encoding. This can be thought of as analogous to a lossy compression scheme; the "compressed" data are encoded by the activations of the hidden nodes.

A single autoencoder layer is trained using backpropagation, which is a supervised learning technique; however, the "correct output" values are just a copy of the input values, meaning no human annotation or labeling is required. Thus, the method as a whole is considered an unsupervised technique. If an even more abstract and compressed representation is desired, we can use the output of one autoencoder layer as the input for another. The result is called a *stacked autoencoder*.

A similar style of network can be generated using a restricted Boltzmann machine (RBM) instead of a feed-forward network; the result of stacking RBMs is sometimes called a *deep belief network*. The training method for RBMs is quite different (see Ref. [7] for details), but for the purposes of unsupervised pretraining, the end result is functionally similar.

Once the unsupervised model has been trained, it is then used as the basis for a supervised model, typically by simply adding one or two extra fully connected layers to the top. At that point, the entire network is trained using a standard supervised approach. The intuition behind the use of unsupervised pretraining is that the "unsupervised" step is essentially finding a feature-based representation of the data suitable for reconstructing the original inputs. So long as a similar set of features is useful for classification, pretraining the network in an unsupervised setting can allow the supervised learning stage to achieve good convergence even in cases where the amount of labeled data would otherwise be too small to allow it.

It should be noted that unsupervised pretraining is not a magic bullet; in particular, it can reduce the amount of labeled data required to a point, but there will still be a point at which there is simply too little labeled data to learn a model which generalizes well. Additionally, it is nearly always the case that unsupervised pretraining will be outperformed by fully supervised training using the same amount of data (i.e., if you have labels for all your data, you are better off simply doing supervised training from the beginning).

That said, this is still a potentially useful method, particularly in cases where acquiring large amounts of labeled data is considerably more expensive than acquiring large amounts of unlabeled data. Additionally, there are a number of more recent variations on the autoencoder idea which may have advantages on certain tasks. Variational autoencoders [8] and sparsity [9] are some examples.

Transfer learning

Another potential way around the problem of not having enough data to train a deep neural network is the process of *transfer learning* [10]. Similar to unsupervised pretraining, transfer learning is a method to "start" learning on your data set using a network with weights that have already been pretrained. The difference is that in transfer learning, the "pretraining" is achieved by simply doing regular, supervised learning on a different-but-related problem. Here, the key insight is that if two problems involve similar data, then the low-level features needed to solve one problem are likely to be useful for the other as well.

To perform transfer learning, the first step is to train a deep neural network on some data set which is large, and as similar as possible to the task you ultimately want to do. In particular, the similarity of the data is the most important. What this means in practice is that if you want to train a digit classification network, MNIST is a reasonable data set to start out with. However, if you want to classify natural images of the world, a network trained on MNIST is likely to transfer poorly. Instead, a network trained on the ImageNet data set would likely give a much better result, since that data set is already composed of natural images of the world.

One potential issue here is that training a large, complex network on a large, complex data set requires a large amount of computational hardware (and/or a lot of training time). Fortunately, in many instances, it is possible to use a pretrained network created by someone else. Several prominent "pretrained" networks are available to download for a variety of deep learning toolkits; check the information for the deep learning library you are using to find out what is available.

The actual transfer learning process involves taking a pretrained network, removing the fully connected "topper" on the network that does the classification, and replacing it with a new fully connected "topper" (with randomly initialized weights). At this point, the network is trained as usual using your data set. Again, the primary advantage is that the training can succeed with a much smaller labeled training set than would be required to train the same network "from scratch" (i.e., starting with randomly initialized weights).

It is also possible to selectively update only part of the network. This is primarily useful if you are using a large pretrained network and have limited computational power available, as it will speed up training, but can result in lowered accuracy if done too aggressively. Here, the idea is that when performing the training for your data set, the uppermost layers of the pretrained network are the ones most likely to be significantly changed by the secondary training process. Therefore, it is possible to "freeze" the weights of the lower layers of the pretrained network, and only update the weights for the top few layers. Since many architectures have a lot more connections at lower levels than they do at higher levels, this can often result in a significant speedup of training.

Generative models and generative adversarial networks

The type of network we have dealt with so far is aimed at the task of classification. While classification networks are by far the most popular type, they are not the only type used. There are several other types of problems that can be tackled using machine learning, and one of them is the problem of generative modeling. A *generative model* is one which can be used to "generate" new examples. The basic task is to take in a set of examples and then construct new examples that are unique, but are similar to the examples the system was trained on. In statistical terms, the goal is to model the distribution that the training samples were drawn from and then generate new samples drawn from the same distribution.

There are several cases in which it might we worthwhile to train such a generative model. Firstly, we might directly want the outputs, that is, the generation of plausible synthetic examples may be useful in its own right. Second, we may view the generative model as another way of finding potentially useful features, which we could then exploit as a method of unsupervised pretraining. Third, we may be interested in a conditional generative model, which is a fancy way of saying that we are interested in transforming inputs, rather than creating them from whole cloth. For instance, taking an image and generating a version in the style of some famous artist. All three of these things are possible using generative models.

In the context of deep neural networks, the most popular generative model is called a *generative adversarial network* (GAN) [11]. GANs work by creating two networks and training them in competition with one another. The first network is called the *generator*, and it is responsible for generating plausible synthetic examples. The second network is called the *discriminator*, and it is responsible for distinguishing between "real" examples (taken from the training set) and "fake" examples (created by the generator). These two networks are effectively playing a zero-sum game, in which each player's success must come at the expense of the other. The only way for the generator to win is to come up with examples that the discriminator cannot tell apart from real examples; the only way for the discriminator to win is to figure out how to recognize the generator's artificial examples.

Training proceeds by first initializing each network randomly, and then alternately updating first one, then the other. Updating the discriminator network is simple, since it is a basic application of backpropagation; since we know which examples are real and which are fake, we have "ground truth" labels. Updating the generator, however, would seem to be more difficult; how do we define an error function for the generator?

The answer is at the heart of what makes GANs such a clever idea: since the output of the generator is used as the input to the discriminator, we can view the combined generator-plus-discriminator as being just one big network. If we take this view, we can then propagate error from the discriminator back all the way down to the bottom of the generator. Of course, when we are training the generator, we want to *minimize* the performance of the discriminator, so we cannot update the weights for the discriminator when we are training the generator. By alternating which network gets updated (always freezing the weights of the other), the overall performance of both players will slowly improve. Every time the generator finds some loophole in the discriminator, the discriminator is forced to fix the loophole. Every time the discriminator discovers flaws in the generated content, the generator must make its output more realistic to fix the flaws.

Thus, over many iterations, the generator slowly converges toward producing synthetic examples that are indistinguishable from the real examples. Of course, in practice there are several complicating factors that mean the system may not always converge as well as we would like, especially if the distribution we are trying to simulate is highly complex. Nevertheless, GANs are useful in many domains where generating synthetic examples is desirable.

Recurrent neural networks

While convolutional networks perform very well on image and imagelike data, convolution is not always the best choice for all types of problems. One popular alternative for sequential data is a *recurrent* network. The basic idea behind a recurrent network is that for sequential or time-series problems, the "current" input may not be sufficient to successfully solve the problem. In other words, the problem requires some access to past information to solve correctly.

It is possible to address this by simply feeding the network multiple time points concatenated together as a single 'input," but this approach has some limitations. In particular, the size of the temporal window is fixed; for example, if we use a window of size 4 (i.e., feed the network the last 4 timesteps as its input), then we cannot capture temporal dependencies longer than 4 timesteps. Additionally, for every extra timestep of history we add, the complexity of the network (i.e., number of nodes and weights) increases dramatically, which often makes the use of long temporal windows impractical.

It is possible to do convolution in the time domain (see, e.g., Ref. [12]), but if longer temporal histories are required, the classic approach is to use a recurrent network. The term "recurrent" here refers to the fact that the hidden nodes have some access to their own previous states; that is, the value of a hidden node at time t is dependent on its inputs at time t as well as its own state at time $t - 1$ (and possibly the states of other hidden nodes at time $t - 1$).

In the earliest recurrent networks, this was a direct dependence, meaning that the previous states were treated just like any other input to a node; however, this proved to be somewhat inflexible. More recent work typically uses a type of node called a *long-short term memory* (LSTM) [13]. In modern parlance, there are some who use the terms "LSTM" and "recurrent network" interchangeably, though this can sometimes lead to confusion. It is also worth noting that there are a number of minor variations on LSTMs which may be encountered, but at a high level they have fairly similar properties (see Ref. [14]). The GRU [15] is probably the most well known of these.

These modern recurrent networks make use of "gates" to allow a context-dependent decision about when to make use of the prior value of a hidden node, and when to ignore it. This allows, for example, a sequence delimiter (such as a punctuation mark in text data) to be handled intelligently by the network. In general, LSTMs are significantly more flexible and powerful than their older counterparts, and in the context of modern work it would be highly unusual to use units without some sort of gate in any type of recurrent network.

As with any other architectural building block, LSTM units are typically arranged in layers, and in modern practice these layers are often stacked to create deep recurrent networks.

The operation of LSTMs is not quite as well suited to massively parallel GPU implementations as their convolutional counterparts, so training LSTMs is typically slower than training convolutional neural networks (CNNs). However, for some types of tasks, they are still the right choice. For example, most modern machine translation systems make use of LSTMs (see Ref. [16] for a popular example from Google).

Reinforcement learning

Most neural network models are trained in a "supervised" fashion, meaning that the system is given a labeled training set consisting of hand-labeled input-output pairs. However, for some types of task this is not practical. In particular, for sequential decision problems, it is often the case that we can only accurately assess the performance of the system at certain points. A common example is trying to train a network to play a game like chess or Go; until the game is over, we do not know whether the strategy being employed is a good one or not. This means we cannot train the network to decide what moves to make in the middle of the game using standard supervised learning.

The idea of *reinforcement learning* was developed for situations like this. Inspired by operant conditioning, reinforcement learning works by providing a "reward" signal that tells the system when it is doing well and when it is doing poorly. Over time, the system experiments and through trial and error discovers a policy that will maximizes its expected reward.

The classic formulations of this algorithm are based on the formalism of a Markov decision process (MDP). An MDP encodes a problem as a discrete set of possible states and actions, along with a transition model that specifies a probability distribution over possible "next" states, given a current state and choice of action. Given a "reward" function that specifies what reward the agent receives for being in any given state, it is possible to use an iterative approximation algorithm to determine the optimal action to take in any state, where "optimal" is defined as the action that leads to the highest expected future reward. It is also common to add a "discount" factor, which allows us to downweight future expected gain based on how distant it is; by tuning this parameter, we can make the agent optimize for more short-term or more long-term reward.

Unfortunately, this method is limited by the fact that the transition model needs to be fully specified as an input; in real-world problems, this is often not the case. If we need to discover the transition probabilities, the problem becomes more difficult. It can still be solved, using algorithms like adaptive dynamic programming and Q-learning, but these algorithms tend to converge very slowly. Furthermore, there is an additional difficulty that arises, which is that the agent's own decisions control which state-action sequences it gets observations from. As a result, there is a need to ensure sufficient "exploration" of the state-action space that takes place to avoid converging to poor local optima. Simply taking random actions will result in a high degree of exploration, but in most real-world problems, some areas of the state-action space are more productive than others, so it is inefficient to spend a lot of time exploring choices that we already know lead to bad outcomes. This is known as the "exploration/exploitation dilemma," and it is yet another reason that convergence is so slow; if we are too aggressive, we can get premature convergence to a bad solution.

These classic reinforcement learning algorithms are limited in that they tend to work best on small, discrete state spaces, and do not scale well to complex, high-dimensional problems. One of the fundamental issues is that reinforcement learning treats each state in the state-space as atomic, meaning that information about each state must be learned separately, even if the states appear to be "similar" to a human. The combinatorics means that for large state-action spaces, the number of training runs needed to get good estimates can become intractable.

The solution to this is to use a technique known as *function approximation*, which means that instead of directly learning the expected utility of taking a given action in a given state for each state, we use some sort of regression techniques to learn an approximation. The primary advantage of function approximation is that, in addition to making the combinatorics less bad, it can also allow a means to treat states as nonatomic, meaning we can learn based on similarity between states (i.e., if we have encountered a similar state in the past, we may assume that this state will have a similar expected reward).

It is particularly convenient to use a neural network as the function approximator for reinforcement learning because neural networks can be trained in an online fashion (i.e., one training example at a time), allowing them to be updated after each action. In recent years, deep neural networks have become increasingly popular for this, allowing for better scaling to large and complex problems. Many recent successful solutions to games have made use of reinforcement learning for training, including results on Atari games [17] and Go [18].

The primary downside of reinforcement learning is its lack of computational efficiency; training via reinforcement learning is very slow compared with fully supervised learning. For problems where fully supervised learning is an option, it is typically preferred. However, reinforcement learning opens up the possibility of solving an entire class of problems that would otherwise be intractable, making it a very valuable technique for that class of problems.

Additionally, there are cases in which the two methods can be combined. This typically occurs when we have some training labels for our data, but they do not fully capture the behavior we want. For example, many machine translation systems are trained to optimize BLEU score [19], even though it is acknowledged to be an imperfect model for human evaluation of translation quality. Training a machine translation system fully using reinforcement learning and human evaluation would require so much time as to be entirely infeasible. However, it is possible to first train the system in a supervised fashion using BLEU scores, and then refine the system using reinforcement learning. Since it is only a refinement, much less training data are required, making this more practical. However, it is worth note that there is no guarantee this will actually improve the performance of the final system; some experiments done using Google Translate showed that the benefits of this approach were not as great as had been hoped [16].

Ensembles

A classic machine learning method for boosting the performance of classifiers is to combine several of them together into an *ensemble* classifier. The inspiration is the same as that behind crowdsourcing; in both cases, each individual member may be wrong, but so long as enough of them are right, the "group" gets the correct answer. This relies on the assumption that the members of the ensemble are sufficiently diverse, since if they all make the *same* mistakes, there is no benefit. However, there is enough randomness in the standard neural network training algorithms to allow for a reasonable degree of independence, which can be increased if necessary through methods like boosting or bagging.

Even without these methods, ensembles of deep neural networks tend to outperform their members. Thus, a reliable way of increasing the performance of a deep neural network is to simply train four or five different copies of the network and then allow them to "vote" for the correct answer. There are limits to how much performance can be gained this way, but it is a fairly simple means of eking out a few more percentage points of accuracy.

This is an example of the simplest way to build an ensemble, simply training multiple copies of the *base* classifier and then combining their output. The simplest way of combining classifier output is to allow each classifier to make its own prediction and then choose the plurality prediction as the "final" output. This simple *voting* scheme is easy to implement and easy to understand, but it does not always produce the best possible results. In particular, it gives equal weight to all members of the ensemble, which may not be a good idea. If we have reason to believe that a particular member of the ensemble is likely to be unusually trustworthy (or untrustworthy) for a given example, it would make sense to do *weighted voting*. Here, each classifier still gets to vote, but not all votes count equally. Instead of each classifier contributing $+1$ to the vote tally for their respective choice, they will contribute an amount proportional to some confidence measure. At the end, the answer with the largest total score is then the one chosen as the ensemble's joint answer. The choice of confidence measure will be problem dependent, but for artificial neural networks one common choice is to train the networks to produce pseudo-likelihood scores for the various classes as their outputs. The score associated with the "winning" class can then be used as a confidence measure; if the network predicts a class with a value of 0.99, we give it more weight than if the highest output value is only 0.6.

The performance of an ensemble depends on the members making *different* mistakes; therefore, ensemble performance can often be boosted by forcing the member classifiers to be more different from each other, even if that comes at the cost of a small accuracy penalty to each individual member. The simplest example of this is a method called *bagging*, which works by ensuring each member is trained using a slightly different training set. Rather than training each classifier with all of the available training data, each classifier is trained using some fraction of the examples, chosen at random. This ensures different classifiers will have different strengths and weaknesses, and helps ensure the ensemble as a whole does not overfit the training data. The smaller the fraction of the training data given to each classifier, the more diverse they will be, but the lower their performance will tend to be as well. At some point, the individual performance degradation overcomes the benefit from increased diversity. Unfortunately, exactly where the sweet spot is located is problem dependent.

One alternative to bagging is a method called *boosting*. Boosting makes the observation that the goal is to ensure that every example is classified correctly by a sufficient number of members, and tries to build an ensemble to ensure this is the case. In boosting, the first member classifier is trained normally, but after that each classifier is trained as follows. First, test the performance of the existing ensemble on the training data; for each example, count how many classifiers get it right, and how many get it wrong. Then, weight the examples based on how often they were predicted correctly by the existing ensemble. The more times an example was guessed incorrectly, the more importance weight is put on that example. Then, a new classifier is trained factoring in the example weights; this means that the new classifier will be pushed to do well on the examples that other classifiers are getting wrong and will have less incentive to perform well on examples that other classifiers are getting right.

Boosting often performs very well in practice, but it does have a few downsides. In particular, bagging is an algorithm that makes use of data parallelism, meaning all the member classifiers can be trained simultaneously if enough parallel compute power is available. Boosting, on the other hand, is an iterative method; each new classifier needs to know the performance of the previous ones, so they must be trained one at a time. Additionally, boosting works best for classifiers that can easily make use of the importance weights on the examples, which not all possible base classifiers can do.

The only real downside of ensembles is their computational cost; each member of the ensemble must be trained from scratch, since otherwise they will not be sufficiently independent. As a result, producing an ensemble with five members will require five times the total amount of computational resources to train. Since deep neural networks are already expensive to train, this can make the technique impractical. If training a network takes 10 days, most researchers are unwilling to wait another 40 days to build an ensemble. However, the members of the ensemble can be trained in parallel, so if enough computational hardware is available the extra copies can all be trained simultaneously.

Since the gain from forming an ensemble is reasonably consistent, it is common practice for researchers to simply compare single classifiers with each other; whichever wins is likely to win as an ensemble as well, and this saves compute time. When creating production systems, however, it is typically a good idea to make use of ensembles, since the training time is a one-time cost and will improve the performance of the system.

Finally, it is worth mentioning that many types of ensembles have developed their own names over the years. For instance, a "random forest" is typically a bagging ensemble of decision trees. AdaBoost (Adaptive Boosting) and XGBoost (eXtreme Gradient Boosting) are two common implementations of boosting, also typically using decision trees as their base classifiers.

Genetic algorithms

Genetic algorithms (GAs) are a part of the field of evolutionary computation (EC), a field which draws inspiration from the biological process of Darwinian evolution. In addition to inspiration, practitioners in this field often use the terminology of biological evolution to describe their algorithms; it is important to understand that these terms are used metaphorically, not literally. Thus, when a term like "genotype" is used, it should be understood as meaning something like "the part of our algorithm analogous to a genotype." As with all computations inspired by biology, the computational models are a massive oversimplification of the actual biological process.

That said, the goal of evolutionary computation is to make use of inspiration from nature to solve difficult computational problems. Genetic algorithms in particular are a method for performing a type of search. For the purposes of training artificial neural networks, GAs are typically used to find good values for the connection weights; in effect, GAs are an alternative to the error backpropagation method. The primary advantage that a GA has over backprop is that the backprop method is a local gradient descent method, making it vulnerable to local minima and bad initializations. GAs operate as a distributed search and as such are much more robust against these issues. The primary drawback is computational; GAs are computationally expensive and do not scale as well as backprop to very large numbers of weights. As a result, they are more likely to be applied to smaller networks. Additionally, GAs have a large number of user-tunable hyperparameters, several of which are qualitative, to which they are highly sensitive. As such, the successful deployment of a GA may be more challenging than the use of backprop. However, for some problems the gains from the distributed search process allow GAs to reach levels of classification performance not possible using backprop.

A GA begins with an initial "population" of "individuals," each of which represents a candidate solution to the problem. Each individual is generated at random, and the population size is a user-tunable parameter. In the case of a neural network, each "individual" will be a complete network. The individual is encoded with a "genome," which is simply a numeric representation of the individual. In some applications, there may be complex encoding functions needed to transform between "genotype" and "phenotype," while in other applications the two forms might be identical. The key factor is that the genotype encoding must support the functioning of the rest of the genetic algorithm; a poorly chosen encoding can handicap the entire process.

Each individual is evaluated using a "fitness function," which is another term for the thing we are trying to optimize. In the case of a neural net, this is typically just the inverse of the loss function used for backprop (we invert the value because a GA maximizes, where backprop minimizes). In other applications, more complex or interesting notions of "fitness" may be used, including relative measures such as tournament-based selection.

The overall operation of the GA proceeds in rounds, or "generations." In each round, all the individuals are evaluated using the fitness function, and then some of them are selected to "reproduce." The most common selection criterion is fitness proportionate, which simply means the likelihood of selection is proportional to the fraction of the total population's net fitness accounted for by the given individual. Again, the GA literature contains many alternatives, and the choice of a selection strategy is up to the user.

Selected individuals are then used to produce "offspring," or new individuals, using the genetic operators of "mutation" and "crossover." The exact implementation of these operators is defined with respect to the chosen genotype encoding and must be selected on a per-problem basis, but the underlying idea is always the same. Mutation makes a small, random change to the encoding; for a neural network, this might mean adjusting some randomly selected weights with small random perturbations. Crossover operates on two selected individuals and creates one offspring genome by combining the two parent genomes. For a convolutional neural network, this might involve something like taking half the filter kernels at random from one parent and the other half from the other parent. It is important that whatever operators are used must be well suited to the problem; they need to have some reasonable likelihood of producing a child that is better than the parent(s), or the GA will not converge. For this reason, in some applications, only one or the other is applied. If no useful definition for crossover is available, it is better to simply rely on mutation.

Once a number of offspring have been produced, some number of individuals in the "parent" generation are selected for replacement, and removed from the population. Again, the choice of how many are replaced at each generation and how they are selected is a user-choosable parameter, but typically the population size is kept fixed, meaning that for each individual that is removed, a new offspring is added. It is possible to replace the entire population at each generation, known as "full replacement," but partial replacement can yield better results for some types of problems, as it makes for a slower and more conservative search process.

This process of fitness-based selection, reproduction, and replacement is then repeated for many iterations, until the GA converges on a solution. Depending on the problem, this may require dozens, hundreds, or even thousands of generations. Typically, the highest-fitness individual discovered by the end of the process is taken as the final "output" of the algorithm.

References

[1] Nair V, Hinton Geoffrey E. Rectified linear units improve restricted Boltzmann machines. In: Proceedings of international conference on machine learning (ICML); 2010.

[2] He K, Zhang X, Ren S, Sun J. Deep residual learning for image recognition computing research repository. CoRR; 2015.

[3] LeCun Y, Bottou L'eon, Bengio Y, Haffner P. Gradient-based learning applied to document recognition. Proceedings of the IEEE 1998;86:2278−324.

[4] Yan LC, Cortes C, Burges C. The MNIST database of handwritten digits. 1999. http://yann.lecun.com/exdb/mnist/.

[5] Krizhevsky A, Sutskever I, Hinton GE. ImageNet classification with deep convolutional neural networks 2012;25:1097−105.

[6] Hinton GE, Salakhutdinov R. Reducing the dimensionality of data with neural networks. Science 2006;313:504−7.

[7] Hinton GE. Training products of experts by minimizing contrastive divergence. Neural Computation 2002;14:1771−800.

[8] Kingma DP, Welling M. Auto-encoding variational bayes. In: The international conference on learning representations (ICLR); 2014.

[9] Ranzato M, Boureau Y, Yan LC. Sparse feature learning for deep belief networks. In: Proceedings of neural information processing systems (NIPS); 2007.

[10] Bengio Y. Deep learning of representations for unsupervised and transfer learn- ing. In: Guyon I, Dror G, Lemaire V, Taylor G, Daniel S, editors. Proceedings of ICML workshop on unsupervised and transfer learning. Proceedings of machine learning research, vol. 27. Bellevue, Washington, USA: PMLR; 2012. p. 17−36.

[11] Goodfellow I, Pouget-Abadie J, Mehdi M, et al. Generative adversarial nets. In: Ghahramani Z, Welling M, Cortes C, Lawrence ND, Weinberger KQ, editors. Advances in neural information processing systems. Curran Associates, Inc.; 2014. p. 2672−80.

[12] Gehring J, Auli M, Grangier D, Yarats D, Dauphin YN. Convolutional sequence to sequence learning. In: Proceedings international conference on machine learning ICML'17. JMLR.org; 2017. p. 1243−52.

[13] Hochreiter S, Schmidhuber Jürgen. Long short-term memory 1997;9:1735−80.

[14] Greff K, Srivastava RK, Jan Koutník, Steunebrink Bas R, Schmidhuber Jürgen. LSTM: a search space odyssey. In: Computing research repository (CoRR); 2015. abs/1503.04069.

[15] Cho K, Merrienboer B, Gulcehre C, et al. Learning phrase representations using RNN encoder-decoder for statistical machine translation. In: Proceedings of conference on empirical methods in natural language processing (EMNLP); 2014. p. 1724–34.

[16] Wu Y, Schuster M, Chen Z, et al. Google's neural machine translation system: bridging the gap between human and machine translation. CoRR; 2016. abs/1609.08144.

[17] Mnih V., Kavukcuoglu K., Silver D., et al. Playing Atari with deep reinforcement learning. In: NIPS deep learning workshop.

[18] Silver D, Huang A, Maddison C, et al. Mastering the game of go with deep neural networks and tree search. Nature 2016;529:484–9.

[19] Papineni K, Roukos S, Ward T, Zhu W. BLEU: a method for automatic evaluation of machine translation. In: Proceedings of association for computational linguistics; 2002. p. 311–8.

Complexity in the use of artificial intelligence in anatomic pathology

Stanley Cohen, MD [1,2,3]

[1]*Emeritus Chair of Pathology & Emeritus Founding Director, Center for Biophysical Pathology, Rutgers-New Jersey Medical School, Newark, NJ, United States;* [2]*Adjunct Professor of Pathology, Perelman Medical School, University of Pennsylvania, Philadelphia, PA, United States;* [3]*Adjunct Professor of Pathology, Kimmel School of Medicine, Jefferson University, Philadelphia, PA, United States*

Introduction

The previous chapters were designed to demystify the machine learning strategies that are at the core of artificial intelligence (AI) by describing its algorithmic building blocks in detail, while avoiding mathematical formulation or computer code. As we have seen, the underlying theme of machine learning is classification, which essentially boils down to identifying similarities and differences among things. From this one can progress to understanding relationships among data for prediction and inference. In anatomic pathology, AI can be used to determine if a lesion is cancerous, evaluate the degree of malignancy from subtle morphological differences, predict clinical behavior, and suggest therapeutic strategies.

AI is beginning to be a robust tool at academic centers. For this reason, commercial ventures to exploit it for pathology are proliferating. A major step forward for practical applications has been the approval of whole slide imaging for diagnostic purposes (as digital images are essential for machine learning). However, for anatomic pathology, there are a number of bottlenecks that must be addressed. Some that clearly stand out are (a) the huge databases required for training (true of neural networks in general, and not just in pathology), (b) image complexity, i.e., the large number of features needed to define the samples (instances) within the dataset, and (c) the topological complexity of the data. An example of this complexity is an image dataset, where each sample may contain normal as well as abnormal tissue and abnormal regions may vary in morphology in important ways.

In addition to the above, relationships are important, such as the distribution and location of vasculature, lymphatics, inflammation, mitosis, necrosis, and their spatial relationship to the areas of pathology on the slide. Complicating these factors is the need for the integration of morphological, genetic, and various "-omics," for various predictive analytics. Omic analysis in itself requires identification of relationships

Artificial Intelligence and Deep Learning in Pathology. https://doi.org/10.1016/B978-0-323-67538-3.00004-X

within the data such as clustering and activation patterns, thus making its integration with morphologic information difficult. Combining omic and morphological data presents a daunting challenge, and translationally relevant work in this area has only just begun.

These kinds of complexity issues are not unique to pathology; a good example involves autonomous driving algorithms where all of the above come into play. Interestingly, autonomous driving algorithms are developed by data scientists and computer learning experts, with relatively minor input from professional drivers. For the development of AI in pathology, there must be a close interaction between the pathologists (as content providers, content annotators, and ground truth arbiters for training) and the computer scientists who devise the appropriate machine learning algorithms for use. The purpose of this chapter is to expand on previous chapters describing the basics of machine learning and some advanced deep learning strategies for pathologists to bridge that gap, as well as real-world examples of the principles that are involved.

In this chapter, we will first discuss how images can be segmented into regions of interest, using mitosis detection as an example, and then explore various ways of dealing with petascale datasets through weak supervision and possibilities for so-called one-shot learning. Other topics include the choice of an algorithm for a given task and the problem of parameter tuning within that algorithm. This is not designed to be a comprehensive review; subsequent chapters will provide detailed descriptions of state-of-the-art work being done in a number of pioneering laboratories. It will be apparent that the basic strategies for image interpretation can be used across a wide spectrum of other topics of interest to pathologists, including natural language processing and analysis and prediction from genetic arrays, proteomics, transcriptomes, microbiomes, etc.

Life before machine learning

Before proceeding it is important to note that there were many approaches toward the solution of these problems before the widespread use of machine learning. Many of these involve the extraction of important and measurable features from samples and the use of clustering. In image analysis, mathematical operations have been used to distinguish pixel areas on the basis of intensity, color, texture, shape, and geometric relationship. Blobs (connected areas in an image), edges, and boundaries are important to identify in these tasks. One example of a mathematical operation used is the Hough transform, which can be utilized to isolate features of a particular shape within an image. While these techniques could locate nuclei, glands, and other structural elements within the image for the pathologist, they could not generalize from a constellation of these features to an overall classification or diagnosis of the tissue under study. Machine learning facilitated the transition from image analysis to image interpretation.

Multilabel classification

When we think of the use of AI in analyzing images, we tend to think of deep learning structures that can recognize differences between normal and malignant tissues, provide reliable and accurate estimates of degree of malignancy (grading), and provide information regarding prognosis and optimizing therapeutic choice. Often this is based upon overall pattern recognition and classification based on these patterns. However, if there are separate islands of tumor embedded within long stretches of normal stroma or tissue, the segmentation of those tumor fields will allow the program to treat the normal as a kind of background noise. Also, in addition to overall patterns, pathologists look for specific defining features within the image. These might include the presence of mitoses, degree of vascularization, the presence of tumor clusters within lymphatics or small vessels in the tumor, necrosis, and so on. Also important are spatial relationships among these features.

For all these reasons, in pathology, the need for massive datasets is magnified by the need for extensive annotation within each image. This problem is often addressed by decomposing the image into subsets (image patches or tiles) and trying to automate the process of finding regions of interest as much as possible. Dividing an image into subsets obviously increases the number of training instances needed. Moreover, within those regions of interest, there are often specific features we wish to identify as well as identifying and grading the lesion as a whole. We can use traditional segmentation, and object detection schemes embedded into deep neural networks, or alternatively, use a single suitably powerful network for all these tasks.

Multilabel classification is based on image segmentation into regions of interest. There are several kinds of image segmentation, as illustrated in Fig. 4.1, which illustrates segregation categories for scenes of cats and dogs as a simple example.

Semantic segregation is separation on the basis of classes within the image; in the illustration, the algorithm has separated classes corresponding to grass, cat, tree, and sky by color without information as to the relative importance of these classes to the

FIGURE 4.1

Categories of image segmentation. Creative Commons, public domain.

human observer (first panel). Object detection involves localizing and classifying the object of interest within the image and either highlighting it for human action or identifying it for further analysis, as shown in the second panel. One can detect multiple classes in the same image (third frame). Finally, there is instance segmentation, in which each of the dogs is individually (and uniquely) identified. In other words, in instance segmentation, we separately identify each instance within a given class, as compared to semantic segmentation, where we identify each class but not the individual elements of that class.

The final goal of this use of machine learning is thus to identify features of interest within the regions of interest and use these in conjunction with overall pattern recognition of the lesion. When dealing with problems involving multilabel classification, a number of machine learning algorithms may be used including multilabel K-nearest neighbor, multilabel decision trees, multilabel support vectors, and multilabel neural networks. A review of multiclassification methods before advent of deep learning can be found in Ref. [1], with more technical aspects in Ref. [2].

Single object detection

As is the case for AI in general, there is no one algorithm that is optimal for all problems. The use of machine learning for the identification of mitoses provides a good example of this principle and is discussed in detail in Ref. [3]. By way of introduction, it should be noted that detecting mitoses is a difficult problem because of issues relating to interobserver variability that impose constraints on ground truth and because the many papers that have been published make use of widely varying AI approaches. This has been studied in a systematic way. By way of background, for many tumors, prognostic factors related to tumor proliferation have proven to be very important. There are a number of histochemical markers for proliferation. Two examples are Ki67 and BRDU. Ki67 is a protein that increases in cells as they prepare to divide. BRDU is a marker that is incorporated into cellular DNA. However, simply counting mitotic figures in tumors by pathologists remains the most widely form of assessment of proliferation. Although time-consuming and subjective, direct morphological observation can, under ideal conditions, identify mitotic phases. Breast tumors are good examples of cases in which proliferation has prognostic significance. However, even in tumor types where proliferation does not correlate as well with behavior, the presence of morphologically abnormal mitosis can confirm the diagnosis of malignancy.

In 2013, the Assessment of Mitosis Algorithms (AMIDA13) Study was launched (as a competitive challenge, the results were analyzed by Veta et al. and summarized in Ref. [3]). The training data available to all participants consisted of image data accompanied by ground truth mitosis annotations (with due attention to correction for interobserver variability). Two months after the training dataset was released, a testing dataset was made available. This consisted only of image data; annotations were withheld by the challenge organizers to ensure independent evaluation. Results were uploaded to the challenge website for evaluation.

The learning strategies that were compared were computational neural networks, random forests, support vector machines, Bayesian methods, and various boosting strategies. Most of these methods involved a two-step object detection approach in which the first step identified candidate objects that were then classified in the second step as mitoses or nonmitoses. Two of the methods evaluated did not use candidate extraction but instead evaluated every pixel location to obtain a mitosis probability map for each image, from which mitoses were detected.

By measures of precision and recall, all of the models described in Ref. [3] gave good performance, with the best being the procedure with multiple alternating convolutional net and max-pooling layers. The F1 score (based on the ratio of the product of precision and recall divided by the sum of precision and recall) of this method was comparable to the interobserver agreement among pathologists. The worst performance, by these measures, made use of random forest classifiers. Interestingly, experiments with combining results from the different methods by majority voting or intersection of the better performing methods showed no performance gain over the best individual method.

Multiple objects

Image segmentation, multilabel classification, and multiple-instance learning (MIL) (see weakly supervised learning section) all have features in common. For example, in the case of histopathologic material, only a small part of the image may be useful for processing and analysis. Thus, a prior step is localization, in which we identify areas of interest. In many applications, this is done by breaking the image up into small contiguous patches and either identifying the "regions of interest" through prior annotation of the training set or by strategies within the algorithm itself. This is similar to the methods used for MIL to be discussed in a subsequent section.

As aforementioned, object detection is based on the use of a classification label for the objects of interest within the sample images, rather than simply for the sample as a whole. Various machine learning strategies led to the simultaneous identification and classification of multiple labels within images. As is the case for image analysis in general, neural networks have transformed this field. Typically, one extends a convolutional neural network (CNN) to multilabel classification by transforming it into multiple single-label classification sets. These treat the labels independently and so have difficulty in modeling dependency between labels. Object detection is not limited to neural network analysis. Many of the machine learning strategies can be applied to this task as well. There have been only a few comparative studies of these using standardized datasets. One example has already been described in detail [3]. Bjednordi et al. have compared 32 algorithms for detecting lymph node metastases [4]. Twenty-five were based on deep convolutional networks, while the remainder utilized support vector machines or random forests and statistical and structural texture features. The tasks included both metastasis identification and whole slide image classification. All the algorithms performed well, and several were better than the best performing pathologists in the comparison panel.

Advances in multilabel classification

At this point, it is helpful to compare this image analysis problem to issues that arise in autonomous driving. The algorithms must be able to identify human beings, other cars, road markers, traffic signs, and their specific locations within a scene and thus make use of multilabel classification strategies. As driving is a dynamic process, there needs to be a way of dealing with sequential data, and for this purpose, recurrent neural networks (RNNs) are an obvious choice as they capture temporal relationships. Recently, there have been several advances in the use of visual attention or RNNs combined with CNNs for this purpose. Recall from the previous chapter that whole CNNs are good for dealing with spatially related data and RNNs are good at handling temporally related data. Previously, RNNs have been used for signal analysis, sequential images (video), and natural language processing (where the temporal sequence of words in a sentence matters). They can also be used for static image analysis. Here, an RNN processes inputs sequentially, dealing with locations within the images one at a time, and incrementally combines information so obtained to create the internal representation.

For example, Wang et al. [5] described a model inspired by the way humans analyze images by continuously moving and their attention from one discriminative object to the next when performing image-labeling tasks. As usual, the CNN extracts the deep feature representations, and the RNN (in this case a long term short term memory (LSTM) network) iteratively locates class-related regions and predicts label scores for these. LSTM networks are explained in Chapter 3. This model also appears to allow for class redundancies in labeling. For example, for many purposes, labels such as "baby cat" and "kitten" have pretty much the same meaning. Although this study did not involve histopathological materials, more recently, Alom et al. performed similar studies combining residual and recurrent networks [6]. This sophisticated model was applied to blood vessel segmentation, skin cancer segmentation, and lung lesion segmentation. This model yielded state-of-the-art performance in all three tasks.

The possibility of exploiting reinforcement learning for image recognition tasks in pathology is especially interesting. In the case of autonomous driving, reinforcement learning has been applied to dynamic sensory input, but reinforcement learning has only begun to be exploited for tasks involving static image analysis. Mathe et al. [7] have described sequential search strategies that accumulate evidence from a set of image locations utilizing reinforcement learning concepts such as exploration and reward. Basically, traditional object detection is based upon an exhaustive spatial search and is brute force in nature whereas reinforcement learning involves moving toward a defined goal in a stepwise manner. Chen et al. [8] have combined attentional models with reinforcement learning where the "reward" is classification correctness.

Interestingly, biological neural networks such as brains utilize reinforcement learning in visual pattern recognition. They also learn to recognize sequences of patterns. Thus, it appears likely that approaches such as these will be fruitful in pathology as well.

Graphical neural networks

Sophisticated implementations such as those above capture relationships among the objects in an image in addition to classifying them. However, there are a number of modern approaches that deal explicitly with such relationships. The majority of these fall into the category of graph neural networks. In mathematical terminology, a graph is a collection of distinct objects (vertices or nodes) and lines (edges) connecting them (Fig. 4.2).

Both neural networks and decision trees are graphs, as are connecting flight maps and highway maps connecting cities. In the case of a neural network, the nodes are the simulated neurons and the edges show the direction in which weighted information flows toward the next layer of nodes. Edges can be unidirectional or bidirectional. As an example, network analysis, which is a branch of graph theory, is used to understand relationships and patterns within transcriptomes.

If data can be expressed as a network, then it is possible to analyze not only the relationship of a test sample to the classes defined by the training set but also the relationship between the attributes that define that sample. A graphical network

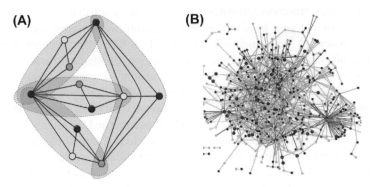

FIGURE 4.2

(A) Sample graph showing nodes and edges connecting them, as well as apparent clustering into four subgroups. *Reprinted from Wikipedia commons, public domain.* (B) Actual protein expression network of a treponeme.

Reprinted from Wikipedia commons, with attribution: Hauser, et al., The syphilis spirochete, PLoS One 2008; 3(5):e2292. https://doi.org/10.1371/journal.pone.0002292.

operates at this level. To do so, there must be a way of quantitating the relationships among the nodes. The connections can be described by what is known as an adjacency matrix. The elements of the matrix indicate whether pairs of vertices are adjacent (the element at the intersection of row and column is a one, if there is a connection between them, and otherwise zero). In other words, the adjacency matrix represents the adjacency of vertices. There is another form of representation of a graph that is known as an incidence matrix that, as its name suggests, represents the incidence of vertices and edges. These matrices are constructed from the graph in visual form. Conversely, it is possible to recreate a pictorial diagram of a graph from its matrices (or one functionally identical or isomorphic to that diagram). As neural networks are based on linear algebra, the graph as defined by its matrix is now amenable to computation by the network. The effective implementation of a graphical network is a topic of active investigation. The models are quite complex and beyond the scope of this discussion. However, for the mathematically sophisticated, Zhou et al. [9] have recently published a review of methods and applications involving graphical neural networks.

It is possible to analyze graphical relationships from CNN output without an explicit use of a graphical neural network. For example, newly published work by Jung et al. [10] has demonstrated the power of integrating traditional deep learning with the mathematics of graph theory for the analysis of histopathologic images involving collagen deposition in immunostained images in relation to HIV Infection. A CNN is first used for segmentation of the whole slide image. Parallel processing is applied to convert segmented collagen fibrils into a relational graph and graph theory is used to extract topological and relational information from the collagenous framework.

In brief, graphical networks are designed to deal with relationships among its nodes which may represent attributes, attribute sets, or attribute patterns. Conventional CNNs are not very good at this. When dealing with images, there is another area of weakness. A neural network can identify a face from representations that define overall shape, shape, number, and position of elements within the face (two eyes, one nose, one mouth). A model capable of good generalization will have no trouble with different shapes such as round or oval eyes, broad or narrow noses, and so on. They can also handle translational, rotational, and scaling relationships of the elements. To a CNN, a face in which one eye and the mouth are switched may appear to be similar because they are constructed of similar elements, yet they are quite different to a human observer. The internal data representation of a CNN simply does not take into account important spatial hierarchies between simple and complex objects and thus their meaningful relationships to each other.

Capsule networks

Another newly emerging idea is that of the capsule network, in which the output of each artificial neuron is not a scalar, but rather a vector that encodes both a probability of detection of a feature (length) and its state (orientation). Thus, neuronal activities are directly associated not only with feature detection but also the orientation of that feature. Hinton's group [11] recently described the basic architecture and the process of dynamic routing between capsules.

Capsule networks are relatively new and, in their current form, are difficult to train and not very accurate. Thus, it is still too early to assess their ultimate utility.

Weakly supervised learning

There have been many attempts to achieve unsupervised learning, i.e., to obtain predictive representations from unlabeled data. Although human beings can do this, it has proven very difficult to implement this strategy in a robust way for practical AI. As described in Chapter 2, clustering algorithms such as K-means and principle component analysis are two ways of finding relationships and/or identifying critical features in a database containing unlabeled examples and in that sense are unsupervised. Much current research involves employing these and related strategies within the context of deep learning via hybrid strategies. However, for the most part, current efforts in pathology are devoted to weakly supervised rather than unsupervised classification. Weak supervision may be thought of in a simplistic way as the obverse of multilabel classification. In multilabel classification, complexity is introduced by the need to simultaneous identify complex subimages or patterns within each example from a well-defined dataset. In the case of weakly supervised learning, the classifications need not be complex but are based upon an incompletely labeled dataset itself. In both cases, the task is to abstract information that is much more complicated than simply assigning a class label to an unknown sample.

There are three basic types of weak supervision. In incomplete supervision, only a small subset of training data has labels. This is typically the case for image analysis. Huge datasets may be available, but usually only a small subset of these is annotated. In the case of inexact supervision, some supervision information is given, but it is not as exact as desired. For example, a dataset may consist of breast cancer images, but only the diagnosis is known for the slides. These are coarse labels. Fine-grained information, such as that obtained by annotation by trained pathologists, may only be available for a small subset of these slides. Inaccurate supervision refers to situations in which the label information may not be perfect ground truth. In pathology, this is sometimes due to interobserver variability and sometimes due to the presence of noise, as for example, difficulty in distinguishing between a mitotic and a pyknotic nucleus. For a good general survey of these concepts and approaches, see Ref. [12].

With this as background, it is relatively straightforward to understand the concepts behind weakly supervised learning. For incomplete supervision, we can try to make do with the small labeled subset that is available. Recall that a neural network learns by developing increasing complex (and lower dimensional) representations of the data at each hidden layer within the network. This process is implemented by adjusting the weights of the connections between layers by comparing the output of the network with its input and minimizing a loss or error function. The starting point involves random weights across the connections, and these are then adjusted via backpropagation. In the previous chapter, several methods for obtaining representational information in the early layers of a neural network using only limited subsets of the data were described. These include autoencoders and generative adversarial networks (GAN). In both of these cases, the initial stages are unsupervised in that the program creates an internal representation by reconstructing an input as its output. This gives rise to internal representations of the data that may then be used as the starting points for a conventional neural network such as a CNN. The initial stages of a GAN or autoencoder thus learn a set of weights that can be used as the starting points of the CNN instead of beginning with a set of random weights. This reduces the size of the training set, and so only a subset of the training set needs be labeled.

Also, as it was pointed out previously, as early representations may have similar properties across different but similar datasets, it is possible to pretrain a new model by using the early layers of the model previously fully trained on a similar problem, and using the weights in those layers as starting points rather than the usual beginning random weights (see Chapter 3). This is known as transfer learning.

In all these cases, a limited set of annotated data is used as for the beginning steps in the training of the algorithm. These are some of the most effective ways of dealing with incomplete supervision. Examples of the use of autoencoders, GANs, and transfer learning, respectively, are found in Refs. [13,14]. It is also possible to bootstrap learning by using labels assigned to unknown examples by the network with limited labeled data available to it and using these new examples to expand the labeled training set. This is closely related to strategies used to generate synthetic data when there is class imbalance, as will be discussed in the next section.

For inexact supervision, there are a number of multiple-instance approaches (MIL). In these, the focus is shifted from discrimination of the samples themselves to discrimination of "bags," i.e., breaking up the images into tiles or patches (Fig. 4.3).

It should be noted that the MIL approach is not confined to deep learning (neural network) algorithms. It has been applied to support vector machines [15] and in combination with feature clustering [16]. Campanella et al. [17] apply an MIL to a residual neural network in a highly sophisticated manner to the study of prostate, basal cell, and breast cancer at the terabyte scale (discussed in detail in a subsequent chapter).

The above examples all represent semisupervised learning. There are fully unsupervised learning strategies as well. A classic example is the K-means algorithm described in Chapter 2. This and related clustering algorithms require no information about the labels of the sample but instead find clusters in the data based upon geometric closeness in an n-dimensional space. However, to be useful in a diagnostic/predictive setting, the clusters must ultimately be given a label. However, it is not necessary to label every sample in a given cluster individually; one can use the same class label for each element of that cluster. Clustering can be the basis

Bag

Feature Vector
(Instance)

MIL
Classifier

+1: Diseased

-1 : Normal

FIGURE 4.3

Multiple-instance learning (MIL) for image analysis. The diagnostic image is first split into rectangular patches. A set of features are extracted from each patch, and an instance is formed by the resultant feature vector. Patches belonging to the same diagnostic image are grouped into a bag. The bag is then classified into diseased or healthy by an MIL method.

Reprinted from Kandemirand M, Hamprecht FA, Computer-aided diagnosis from weak supervision: a benchmarking study, Computerized Medical Imaging and Graphics *2015;42:44–50.*

of an unsupervised network for image classification (CUnet) [18] or can be combined with other strategies such as MILs.

For inaccurate supervision, the goal is to both increase the accuracy of ground truth through the use of multiple trained observers and reduce "noise" by statistically based data preprocessing.

Previous chapters have discussed the concept of ensemble learning. In all of the above examples, weakly supervised learning strategies attempt to achieve strong generalizations (performance) from limited amounts of labeled (annotated) data. In contrast, ensemble learning attempts to achieve strong generalizations from the use of multiple learners. While addressing different aspects, these two approaches may be synergistic with each other [19].

Synthetic data

Weakly supervised methods are needed when there are large datasets available, but a limited number of annotated examples within that dataset. There are a number of other situations in which the dataset is well annotated, but there is class imbalance in that set. For example, there are usually many examples of normal tissue but limited examples of specific kinds of neoplasms of that tissue. Clearly, this creates a situation where there are not enough examples of each class for successful training. In addition, it can lead to a spurious kind of accuracy. As an example, suppose we are studying a neoplasm that has an incidence of 1%. Our training set consists of 10,000 entries of which 100 are positive and the remainder negative. We can easily generate an algorithm with an accuracy of 99% by simply calling every sample negative. Thus, every AI strategy that generates 99% accuracy is suspect. We can guard against this by calculating metrics such as precision and recall as described above.

We can expand the number of samples by the use of so-called synthetic data. Synthetic data are created rather than obtained from real-world samples. A typical example is a dataset in which some entries are missing one or more attributes. One can fill in those blanks by approximations based upon a statistical analysis of the collective data attributes in the set. Another method of generating synthetic data is to create a physical model that explains the observations and then reproduce random data using that model, because in many cases observed features of a complex system can often emerge from simple rules. Patki et al. [20] have described a system that builds machine learning models out of real datasets to create such artificial data, the Synthetic Data Vault. This model captures correlations among the multiple features. In their study, the investigators found no significant performance difference when using synthetic data as compared with using only real-world data.

For the case of image analysis, we can create synthetic data by taking real samples and manipulating them in some controlled way to create randomized new examples that share properties of the real data. There are a number of available programs such as GANpaint Studio that allows the creation of realistic images of faces or scenes (available as a free demo from the internet). Such programs have been used to generate so-called "deepfake" images for nefarious purposes, but such algorithms can be used to create synthetic images from real ones for use as supplemental in machine learning protocols. Hou et al. [21] have used GANs to generate histopathology images that model the distribution of real data.

N-shot learning

When performing tasks such as classification using AI, large datasets are used to create internal representations for each class that can be used to generalize to new unlabeled examples. Humans do not learn in this fashion. For example, show an infant a banana a few times and the child will recognize that banana. It is true that complex patterns require more learning; however, it is well known that one can "train" second-year medical students to distinguish between normal, benign, and malignant examples with much less than 100 samples. In general, humans can classify based on limited examples if they have adequate information about their appearance, properties, and in some cases their functionality. This may be a general capability of suitably complex biological brains. Levenson et al. [22] have demonstrated that it is possible to train pigeons to accomplish cancer diagnostic tasks with high degrees of precision in less than 200 trials! An ensemble of 16 pigeons was able to achieve performance approaching that of a trained CNN.

A "shot" is defined as a single example available for training. In one-shot training, we only have a single example of each class. In N-shot learning, there are N examples. The task is to classify any test image into a class using that constraint. One way of doing this is by the use of "prototypical networks." Unlike the usual deep learning architecture, prototypical networks do not classify the images directly. They learn the mapping of the image into metric space. This means that images of the same class are placed in close proximity to each other, while different classes are placed at further differences. When a new example is presented, the network just checks for the nearest cluster to it. These models are essentially sophisticated forms of the K-means clustering algorithm and are based on CNNs. Models in this category are known as "Image2Vector" models. More sophisticated models involve neural networks augmented with memory via a neural attention mechanism. These can be complicated to describe, but a good example is seen in Ref. [23]. Although "one-shot learning" should be used to describe the case where N = 1, that term is also used more generally when N is very small.

The method for N-shot learning with the greatest potential for one-shot learning currently appears to be the Siamese network. Instead of a model that learns to classify its inputs, the neural network learns to differentiate between two inputs. A typical Siamese network consists of two identical neural networks, each taking one of the two images. Identical means that they have the same configuration with the same parameters and weights. The last layers of the two networks are jointly fed into a contrastive loss function that calculates the degree of similarity between the two images. An example from natural language processing involves scoring an exam question. Here one input is the question sentence and the other input is the answer. The output is how relevant the answer is to the question. This is not a simple classification task in that we do not have a database consisting of all possible answers that are judged "correct" and examples that are judged "wrong." Nevertheless, a Siamese network can extract similarity or a connection between question and answer.

Very often the term one-shot learning is used whenever n is a small number. In any event, Siamese Networks have achieved state-of-the-art performance in one-shot image recognition tasks (Koch et al. [24]). In this study, each of the two networks was a standard CNN. The final convolutional layer output was flattened into a single vector, which was then fed into a fully connected layer, and then to an additional layer that computes the distance metric between the outputs of each Siamese twin.

There are relatively few examples of one-shot learning involving pathology subject matter. Within the past few months, Yarlagadda et al. [25] demonstrated the use of a one-shot learning model for cervical cancer cell classification in histopathological images.

One-class learning

It is important to distinguish between one-shot learning and one-class learning. Closely related to N-shot learning is the concept of one-class learning. The object of one-class classification is to recognize instances of a class by only using examples of that class. All other classes are lumped together and are known as alien classes. In other words, the difference between one-class and binary classification is due to the absence of training data from a second class. While this approach has received a great deal of attention for simple datasets, it has proven difficult to obtain good results in real-world datasets. Recently, Perera and Patel [26] have achieved impressive results using a CNN model and two novel loss functions (compactness loss and descriptiveness loss) as compared to typical squared difference and/or entropic loss functions used in other deep learning algorithms. They achieved results better than those obtained by competing methods including graphical, K-nearest neighbor, and support vector models. Decision tree—based models were not considered.

One-class learning can be useful for outlier detection, and as it only involves a single class, it is essentially unsupervised. There have been previous approaches to anomaly detection using one-class support vector machines, directly, or hybrid methods combining feature extraction via deep learning with support vector machines [2]. More recently, R. Chalapathy et al. [27] have described a one-class neural network that uses a novel loss function. Here the specific features of the hidden layers are constructed for the specific task of anomaly detection. This is in contrast to the generic feature extraction methods used in previous approaches. It is possible to treat cancer as a tissue anomaly. Most such studies have involved classifying tumor transcriptomes as compared to normal (for example [28]). However, it is easy to envision a training protocol in which only normal tissue images are used, and a metastatic focus is then treated as an outlier. As of the date of the preparation of this manuscript no examples of work in this area were found. However, industrial techniques involving the detection of anomalies in images of surfaces suggest that this is a feasible avenue to explore.

Risk analysis

The purpose of all the methods discussed here is to go beyond simple classification (with grading based on overall morphological appearance) by examining specific and often quantifiable subfeatures of the images mimicking the real-world approach by pathologists. An ultimate goal is to learn how to do this using limited information, rather than training sets consisting of thousands of images for each specific classification/diagnostic task. A variety of AI strategies have been explored in this chapter; in most cases morphologic information is analyzed directly. While strictly not within the purview of this review, it is important to note that a number of studies have appeared that involve a computational approach for learning patient outcomes from digital pathology images by combining traditional deep learning algorithms with a standard risk hazard model. For a number of reasons, including computational ease and the ability to deal with nonlinearity, logarithmic models are used, and in particular, the Cox proportional hazard model. We will discuss two approaches: DeepConvSurv [29] and Survival Convolutional Neural Networks [30]. Both look at image patches from regions of interest within the biopsy specimen. DeepConvSurv is basically a CNN except that it uses a Cox function as the loss function that is used to train the network. In DeepConvSurv, a large number of semirandomly collected image patches undergo dimensional reduction using K-means clustering. Aggregated clusters are then run through the connected neural network with boosting via the Cox's negative log function. Finally, the aggregated patch risk data are equated to patient risk. This, however, is only a loose approximation because patient risk also includes size and location of tumor, all modified by age, sex, and comorbidity, and in modern medicine, genomic and proteomic features.

SCCN is more sophisticated, in that it explicitly utilizes genomic data as well as image morphology. It requires annotation of the image dataset which is then run through a full CNN. The genomic data are inputted directly into the fully connected layers, bypassing the convolutional layers. The network is trained in the usual fashion with a standard loss function, except that the outputs are then entered into a final Cox approximation layer. In effect, SCCN is taking advantage of the universal approximation theorem, namely that a single layer with an appropriate activation factor can approximate any arbitrary function. Here the function is the Cox partial hazard function. By providing a risk-based heat map overlying histological features in their publication, the authors documented that the algorithm is detecting meaningful risk elements.

Looking ahead, it is likely that deep learning algorithms will become better able to integrate morphological data with the whole spectrum of available patient information, allowing optimal tailoring of therapy to the specific disease as manifested in a specific patient, thus enabling truly personalized precision medicine.

General considerations

In this chapter, the examples chosen for illustration made use of a variety of machine learning strategies, and in some cases hybrid networks were utilized as well. An important practical question involves the choice of an algorithm to solve a given problem. Unfortunately, there is no correct answer. In this context, it is important to reflect upon the so-called "no free lunch" theorem of Wolpert and Macready [31], which states "for any algorithm, any elevated performance over one class of problems is offset by performance over another class."

Simply stated, there is no one model that works best for every problem. However, each method may be best aligned with a particular class of problems. This means that it is not possible to generalize that the best performing algorithm in a given study is the best strategy for other machine learning tasks. Thus, it is important to choose the appropriate model for a given problem. Unfortunately, there is no theoretical basis upon which to choose. This must be done empirically through trial and error. The algorithm assessment study [3] provided a good specific example of this general principle.

Regardless of the choice, every model has tunable parameters or hyperparameters. For example, in the case of neural networks, the tunable parameters include the number of nodes in each layer and the number of layers. Backpropagation involves choices of momentum and learning rate. For a CNN, decisions must be made about the size of the convolution matrix. Initial weights must be randomized, but there most random numbers are generated by computer starting with a "seed" number. That seed is also a parameter. This list is by no means exhaustive. For random forests, the number of trees, the number of branches, the tree depth, and so on are parameters that must be chosen. For k-means, one must choose the number of clusters, as well as the k random number seeds that start the iterative process of defining clusters. Tunable parameters are a fact of life for the artificial intelligentsia.

The other consideration in selecting a model is the implicit bias of that model. This does not refer to external biases such as those that arise from choices of the elements of the training set, or a value-based assessment of the feature or class labels, but rather to the assumptions baked into each model. For example, K-means assumes roughly spherical clusters similar in size to each other (although there are better models that do not have these constrains). Naïve Bayes assumes that the attributes describing the feature vector are independent of each other. Assumptions about data distributions are at the heart of almost every machine learning algorithm. It is important to understand the nature of the dataset in sufficient detail to allow choosing the algorithm whose constraints are least critical for that dataset. Unfortunately, the use of the term "bias" tends to anthropomorphize the AI program and obscures the issues involved.

The detection of implicit bias in a deep learning network is made difficult in that we have no true understanding of how that network is processing its inputs to arrive at the correct outputs. In other words, there are problems with explainability and interpretability. Interpretability is the ability to predict the effect of a change in input or algorithmic (tunable) parameters. Explainability is the ability to understand the basis upon which the algorithm is drawing its conclusion. For example, it might be reassuring to be able to explain to a surgeon the basis upon which the AI came up with a diagnosis of a high grade malignancy, or how it differentiated between two morphologically similar but biologically different tumors. It is interesting that if one questions a reference level, high-trained pathologist as to how he or she arrived at a diagnosis, they will often refer to the "years of experience" that led to the diagnosis. When pressed for more specific criteria, they may make them up, but it is often on an ad hoc basis, to justify the decision already intuitively made. For this reason, the black box nature of neural networks while disquieting to some does not bother others of the artificial intelligentsia.

There are ways of gaining some insight as to what is happening behind the scenes so that we can raise the curtain to see the wizard at work. For example, saliency maps create a visualization of the pixels in an image that contributes most to the predictions by the model. By calculating the change in predicted class by applying small adjustments to pixel values, we can measure the relative importance of each pixel to the ultimate output value. This is discussed in Ref. [32]. Other approaches involve trying to determine the activity of neurons in the hidden layers as backpropagation proceeds, and additionally to obtain visual representations of the increasingly complex outputs of the hidden layers by mapping characteristics of these such as intensity, orientations, color, and shapes.

These approaches may provide some insight as to how the neural network is discriminating among classes, but still do not "explain" what is going on in human terms. When an AI makes an unexpected and startling chess move that has no obvious strategic importance to a human observer, and that move initiates a winning sequence, these internal measures provide no clue as to how the program created the move that, in retrospect, turned out to be "brilliant." Thus, they do not create a true learning experience for the human observer. On the other hand, this occasionally happens when human observers watch a human Grand Master at play. Nevertheless, knowledge about the internal decision-making process of a machine learning algorithm may inform the development of better algorithms, so there is something to be said for insisting on AI explainability while accepting our occasional inability to understand human genius.

In spite of all these caveats, studies using different "shallow" learning AI strategies on the same dataset often get similar results. The arrival of deep learning led to a great improvement in machine learning over most, if not all, alternate approaches. When dealing with complex, multidimensional feature sets, neural networks substantially outperform other kinds of machine learning. Even here, when papers dealing with the same dataset but using variations of network models are compared, the improvements claimed by each tend to be incremental. While some are better than others, they all seem to converge around results that achieve greater than 90%–95% accuracy (with similar results for the other evaluation metrics). This, however, may be merely because of the fact that careful attention has been made to optimize the program of choice in each. There are also differences in computational power that must be considered. For this latter reason, performance speed should never be used in comparing one algorithm to another unless they are running on exactly the same platform. Another reason is that often the training sets are simplified and carefully curated versions of data that are found in the wild. This raises the possibility that in less structured situations, greater differences may be observed. Finally, results obtained by a given algorithm in one setting may not always correspond to results using the same algorithm in a different setting. In other words, past performance is not guarantee of future results.

Because of considerations such as these, various ensemble methods have been used, as well as hybrid models involving combining two or more different algorithms sequentially or in parallel. Examples have been presented above for both multilabel detection and weak supervision.

Summary and conclusions

Although we have not discussed the use of AI for clinical laboratory data, natural language processing, or (with one exception) genetic, expression, and protein "-omics," considerations similar to those discussed hold for all these applications. With respect to image recognition and analysis, we are far beyond merely identifying a lesion and predicting outcomes based upon morphological patterns. Our images are complex, and both abnormal structures and the relationship of the normal elements to these must be analyzed. Simultaneously, specific features within the lesion that provides diagnostic or predictive information must be identified and, where possible, quantified. Some of the tools for accomplishing these tasks have been presented in this chapter, and specific references that illustrate their use in real-world settings have been provided. Important caveats have also been noted. The field is growing at an exponential pace; a number of the references chosen did not exist at the beginning of this project. A major consideration for all of these involves the need for huge datasets. As shown, there are a number of approaches to make the generation of training sets more efficient and hopefully to reduce the size of these sets.

To be useful across laboratories, all these approaches are dependent on standardization of each stage of the process from whole slide imaging to final diagnostic output. It will also require consensus regarding annotation standards. However, given that this is rapidly coming to pass, the future is bright for AI as an augmenter and enhancer of human capability in pathology.

References

[1] Devkar R, Shiravale S. A survey of multi-classification for images. International Journal of Computer Application 2017;162:39—42.

[2] Zhang M, Zhou Z. A review on multi-labeling algorithms. IEEE Transactions on Knowledge and Data Engineering 2014;26:1819.

[3] Veta M, et al. Assessment of algorithms for mitosis detection in breast cancer histopathology images. 2014. arXiv:1411.5825v1.

[4] Bejnordi BE, et al. Diagnostic assessment of deep learning algorithms for detection of lymph node metastases in women with breast cancer. JAMA 2017:2199—210.

[5] Wang Z, et al. Multi-label image recognition by recurrently discovering attentional regions. 2017. arXiv:1711.02816v1 [cs.CV].

[6] Alom MZ, Hasan M, Asari VK. Recurrent residual convolutional neural network based on R2U-Net for medical image segmentaion. 2018. arXiv:1802.06955v5.

[7] Mathe AP, Sminchisescu C. Reinforcement learning for visual object detection. 2016. https://doi.org/10.1109/CVPR.2016.316.

[8] T.Chen, et al. Recurrent attentional reinforcement learning for multi-label image recognition. In *32nd AAAI conference on artificial intelligence (AAAI-18)*, https://www.aaai.org/ocs/index.php/AAAI/AAAI18/paper/download/16654/16255.

[9] Zhou J, et al. Graph neural networks: a review of methods and applications. 2019. arX1v:1812.08434v3.

[10] Jung H, et al. Integration of deep learning and graph theory for analyzing histopathology whole-slide images. In: IEEE imagery pattern recognition workshop; 2018. https://doi.org/10.1109/AIPR.2018.8707424.

[11] Sabour S, Frosst N, Hinton GE. Dynamic routing between capsules. In: 31st conference on neural information processing systems (NIPS), Long Beach, CA; 2017. p. 1—8.

[12] Zhou Z-H. A Brief introduction to weakly supervised learning. National Science Review 2017;5:44—53. https://doi.org/10.1093/nsr/nwx106.

[13] LeHou, et al. Improving prostate cancer detection with breast histopathology images. 2019. arXiv:1903.05769v1 [cs.LG].

[14] Fischer, et al. Sparse coding of pathology slides compared to transfer learning with deep neural networks. In: BMC informatics 19, supplement 18; computational approaches for cancer; 2018. p. 109−17. art. 489.

[15] Andrews S, et al. Support vector machines for multiple-instance learning. Advances in Neural Information Processing Systems 2002;15:561−8.

[16] Xu Y, et al. Multiple clustered instance learning for histopathology cancer image classification, segmentation and clustering. In: IEEE Conference on computer vision and pattern recognition; 2012. https://doi.org/10.1109/CVPR.2012.6247772.

[17] Campanella G, et al. Clinical-grade computational pathology using weakly supervised deep learning on whole slide images. Nature Medicine 2019;25:1301−9.

[18] Dong L, et al. A compact unsupervised network for image classification. IEEE Transactions on Multimedia 2016. arXiv:11607.01577v1 [cs.CV].

[19] Zou Z-H, et al. When semi-supervised learning meets ensemble learning. Front Range Electrical Engineering 2010;5. https://doi.org/10.1007/s11704-009-0000-0.

[20] Patki N, Wedge R, Veeramachaneni K. The synthetic data vault. In: 2016 IEEE 3rd internationaa conference of data science and advanced analytics, vol. 1; 2016. p. 399−420. https://doi.org/10.1109/DSAA.2016.49.

[21] Hou L, et al. Unsupervised histopathology image synthesis. 2017. arXiv:712.05021v1.

[22] Levenson RM, et al. Pigeons as trainable observers of pathology and radiology breast cancer images. PloS One 2015;10(11). doi:1371/journal.pone.0141357.

[23] Vinyals O, et al. Matching networks for one shot learning. 2017. arX1v:1606.04080v2 [cs.LG].

[24] Koch G, Zemel R, Salakhutdinov R. Siamese neural networks for one—shot image recognition. In: Proceedings of the 32nd International Conference on Machine Learning, vol 37; 2015. Liile, France.

[25] Yarlagadda, et al. System for one-shot learning of cervical cancer cell classification in histopathology images. In: Presented at 2019 SPIE medical imaging conference, San Diego, CA; 2019. https://doi.org/10.1117/12.2512963.

[26] Perera P, Patel VM. Learning deep features for one-class classification. 2019. p. 1−15. arXiv:1801.05365v2 [cs.CV].

[27] Chalapathy R, Menon AK, Chawla S. Anomaly detection using one-class neural networks. 2018. arX1v:1802.06360v1 [cs.LG].

[28] Quinn TP, et al. Cancer as a tissue anomaly: classifying tumor transcriptomes based only healthy data. Frontiers in Genetics 2019;10:599. https://doi.org/10.3389/fgene.2019.00599.

[29] Zhu X, et al. WISA: making survival prediction from whole slide histopathological images. IEEE Conference on Computer Vision and Pattern Recognition 2018:7234−42.

[30] D. Mobadersany P, et al. Predicting cancer outcomes from histology and genomics using convolutional networks. 2018. www.pnas.org/cgi/doi/10.1o73/pnas.1717139115.

[31] Wolpert DH, Mcready WG. No free lunch theorems for optimization. IEEE Transactions on Evolutionary Computation 1997;1:67−82.

[32] Simonyan K, Vedaldi A, Zisserman A. Deep inside convolutional networks: visualizing image classification models and saliency maps. 2014. arXiv:1312.6034v2 [cs.CV].

Dealing with data: strategies of preprocessing data

5

Stanley Cohen, MD [1,2,3]

[1]*Emeritus Chair of Pathology & Emeritus Founding Director Center for Biophysical Pathology, Rutgers-New Jersey Medical School, Newark, NJ, United States;* [2]*Adjunct Professor of Pathology, Perelman Medical School, University of Pennsylvania, Philadelphia, PA, United States;* [3]*Adjunct Professor of Pathology, Kimmel School of Medicine, Jefferson University, Philadelphia, PA, United States*

Introduction

Most of the applications of artificial intelligence algorithms are dependent upon the use of large labeled datasets (supervised learning). Although there has been great progress in the use of weakly or sparsely supervised learning, for the most part, applications to pathology have not yet exploited these in a systematic way. Similarly, while reinforcement learning makes use of reward strategies rather than loss or cost functions derived from comparison of label to prediction, these have not been typically applied to the topics of interest to pathologists. Recently, however, sophisticated algorithms have been developed using reinforcement learning for image classification [1–3]; so this is likely to change in the near future.

Because of the current dependence of these artificial intelligence algorithms on "large data," it becomes important to make sure that data are in an optimal form for input into the chosen algorithm. At the very least, good data are at least as important as a good algorithm, and often they may be more important. In fact, the majority of data science work involves getting data into the format needed for the model to use and in its most compact and informative form. The reason for this is that the corollary of "garbage in, garbage out" is "better data beat fancier algorithms." Real-life data are messy and unruly; it has to be beaten into submission. It is often incomplete or inconsistent and may contain errors. We must make sure that our samples are representative of the various classes we are trying to predict from sample attributes, we must make sure that the samples themselves are relevant, and we must deal with missing attributes among the samples and determine whether outliers are significant or artifacts. Where there is class imbalance, we must try to correct this either by reducing part of the dataset or constructing synthetic data. These tasks can be broadly categorized as feature engineering and involve feature selection, feature standardization and normalization, feature extraction, and feature correction. These terms are simply descriptions of various aspects of the same process rather than a distinct set of procedures, and they overlap to some extent. Collectively, they fall

Artificial Intelligence and Deep Learning in Pathology. https://doi.org/10.1016/B978-0-323-67538-3.00005-1

under the general category of data preprocessing. Other terms used in the literature for this process are data preparation, data cleaning, and data scrubbing. There are both straightforward and commonsense approaches to analyzing the data as well as highly sophisticated mathematical approaches. The former will be discussed first.

Overview of preprocessing

The initial step in working with data is the choice of the most relevant features. This determination depends entirely on the information you are trying to obtain from the data. For example, consider a database for vehicles that includes the following information:

> number of wheels, cargo capacity, height, length, brand, acceleration, road-holding, number of passengers, and type of navigation system. To determine the distribution of truck versus cars, brand, acceleration, and number of passengers are not as important as height, length, and cargo capacity. For determining the brand, whether the vehicle is a car or a truck may be irrelevant. For identifying a sports car, acceleration and roadholding may provide important information. The presence or absence of a navigation system and what kind it is are not likely to be helpful for any of these potential uses of the data but could be important in another context. In other words, it is important to understand what the data will be used for to determine the appropriate sample attributes to be used.
> There is another aspect to preprocessing based upon the so-called "curse of dimensionality."

At first glance, it would seem that the larger the dimensionality of the feature vector (the larger the number of attributes), the easier it would be to distinguish among different classes of the data. However, when we have too many features, observations actually become harder to cluster. While we can think of a feature as a point in some higher dimensional space, it is easy to visualize that as the number of dimensions grows, the further apart each specific observation gets, and no meaningful clusters of the data can be found. At the extreme, each sample will be sufficiently separate from the other, so that it becomes a separate class. Effectively, the algorithm memorizes the data, and while it can thus achieve a perfect score on the test data, it has no basis on which to generalize to new data. This is what is meant as the "curse of dimensionality" and is closely related to the problem of overfitting in machine learning.

As the number of features increases, we need to increase the number of samples proportionally to have all combinations of feature values well-represented in the samples, and in the real world, this is often hard to accomplish. This problem is of special importance in neural network—based machine leaning models because of the intrinsic need, in most cases, for large amounts of labeled multiattribute data even under optimal conditions.

Feature selection, extraction, and correction

These are best discussed in the context of a specific example, related to the sinking of the Titanic based on Kaggle data. Kaggle is an online resource for users to find, publish, explore, and enter competitions and maintains many useful databases for these purposes. In particular, it contains a public domain 60 KB data source (train.csv) of the Titanic manifold for its final voyage [4]. This provides information on a large number of attributes for the passengers, and based on these, the Kaggle challenge is to predict if an arbitrary passenger on the Titanic would survive its sinking. A sample of the data from the manifest is shown in Fig. 5.1.

To summarize, the categories of available information are the following:

Passenger ID	PClass	Name
Sex	Age	SibSp(sibling or spouse)
Ticket	Fare	Parch (parent and child)
Cabin no.	Embarked from	Survival information

If we consider survived and not survived as the two classes, then each sample has 11 attributes.

We cannot directly plug this dataset into a machine learning algorithm because of inconsistencies, omissions, and redundancies. Excellent summaries of the issues involved are found in Refs. [5,6]. To summarize, 687 of the 891

	PassengerId	Survived	Pclass	Name	Sex	Age	SibSp	Parch	Ticket	Fare	Cabin	Embarked
0	1	0	3	Braund, Mr. Owen Harris	male	22.0	1	0	A/5 21171	7.2500	NaN	S
1	2	1	1	Cumings, Mrs. John Bradley (Florence Briggs Th...	female	38.0	1	0	PC 17599	71.2833	C85	C
2	3	1	3	Heikkinen, Miss. Laina	female	26.0	0	0	STON/O2. 3101282	7.9250	NaN	S
3	4	1	1	Futrelle, Mrs. Jacques Heath (Lily May Peel)	female	35.0	1	0	113803	53.1000	C123	S
4	5	0	3	Allen, Mr. William Henry	male	35.0	0	0	373450	8.0500	NaN	S
5	6	0	3	Moran, Mr. James	male	NaN	0	0	330877	8.4583	NaN	Q
6	7	0	1	McCarthy, Mr. Timothy J	male	54.0	0	0	17463	51.8625	E46	S
7	8	0	3	Palsson, Master. Gosta Leonard	male	2.0	3	1	349909	21.0750	NaN	S
8	9	1	3	Johnson, Mrs. Oscar W (Elisabeth Vilhelmina Berg)	female	27.0	0	2	347742	11.1333	NaN	S

FIGURE 5.1

Sample of data obtained from manifest of Titanic for final voyage in 1912. Kaggle Repository.

passengers in the dataset have no cabin information, so it is best to simply eliminate this attribute. In contrast, there are only 2 empty embarked values, so these samples can simply be dropped. There is no information for 177 passengers. We can create pseudodata for these entries by finding some statistical measures. For example, we can impute an age based on the mean of all those who resided in a given passenger class or some other attribute that appears reasonable. In doing so, it would be helpful to look at the actual distributions involved to see whether they appear to fit a normal distribution. Another approach, where the data may not be amenable to this kind of statistical analysis, is to simply label missing categorical data as "missing" and missing numerical data as "0" just to meet the technical requirement for no missing variables. Using this technique is essentially allowing the algorithm to estimate the optimal value instead of just filling it in with the mean.

The next step is to decide which features are likely to be useful and which are not. While a bit counterintuitive, keeping the entire attribute set may actually harm the predictive accuracy of the algorithm. Passenger ID and passenger name are redundant, so we can eliminate the passenger name column before inputting the data. However, before this step, that information might be useful in uncovering errors. For example, in 1912, if a male and female cabinmate had different surnames, not only are they unlikely to be an unmarried couple but also they were unlikely to be married to each other. This may simply be a listing error. However, there are some other possibilities, such as a grandparent—child combination or siblings of opposite sex (although this latter might have also have been an issue in 1912). This may be useful information in checking the accuracy of SibSp data, for example. One can also cross-check SibSp and Parch data for discrepancies. Age may give clues as well. A 13-year-old is unlikely to have a spouse. An 80-year-old is unlikely to have a parent on board. Erroneous data can be treated as missing data.

In reducing the attribute set, it is important to look for dependencies. For example, fare for a given embarkation point might correlate with passenger class, and if so, one of these might be dropped. Cabin also is likely to correlate with fare and class, but this gives additional information, such as location in relation to deck level and proximity to stairs. These choices involve informed guesses, so different data scientists could wind up with different attribute subsets. For example, in the example used in Ref. [6], the attributes chosen were age, Sibsp, Parch, Fare, Sex, Passenger Class, and Embarked.

For the next step, it is important to consider the metric for each. While there are only two possible values for "Sex" (this is 1912) and three possible values for class, there are seven distinct values of SibSp and 8 distinct values for Parch in the dataset. There are, however, 281 distinct fares, and it is not likely that fine distinctions would help the model, so it possible to group the fare values into a smaller number of range categories.

These examples demonstrate that raw data are merely the tip of the iceberg!

Feature transformation, standardization, and normalization

As data are either numeric or coded in numeric form for input to a computer, it may be important for each attribute to fall into a similar numeric range, so that one feature does not contribute disproportionally. Normalization usually refers to scaling a variable to have a value between zero and one. Standardization, on the other hand, usually means rescaling the database to a mean of zero and a standard deviation of 1 [7]. Proper scaling can often lead to a boost in algorithmic accuracy even after all its hyperparameters are optimally tuned.

Feature engineering

Feature engineering is the process of using domain knowledge of the data to create features that optimize machine learning algorithms that use those features as input. In other words, feature engineering is about creating new input features from existing ones. This improves computation efficiency and, in some cases, accuracy by reducing the feature set to a more manageable size. It makes use of your domain expertize. The simplest form of feature engineering is to combine features. For example, if two attributes are "weight" and "volume," and absolute size is not necessary, then the single value "density" may be more appropriate. If some of the attributes are not well-represented in the dataset, it may be possible to combine them. In the vehicle example in the previous section, we might combine data on "acceleration" and "roadholding" into a single variable "performance." This may sometimes be helpful for sparse classes as well, for example, the category of non—small cell lung carcinoma, instead of separating these into individual morphologic variants. Finally, categorical or text values may be replaced by binary variables. Brick, wood, vinyl, and stone may be able to be replaced by "brick" and "nonbrick" or zero and one, respectively. Many of these techniques lead to dimensional reduction. In the next section, we will describe some formal, mathematically based techniques for data reduction.

The most sophisticated form of feature engineering is the creation of new relevant features rather than merely combination or replacement. Features useful for face recognition include distances between various facial features, overall size and shape, and so on. All these are quantifiable and become a feature set rather than the raw pixels of the image. Similarly, there are mathematical techniques such as Hough transforms and "blob" analysis that allow the quantification of density contrasts and the detection of edges. These can also be used to create additional features. All these steps involve transforming the data. The use of the data in a machine learning algorithm is merely the final (although admittedly the most sophisticated and mathematically intensive) step. This process is illustrated in Fig. 5.2.

The power of deep learning systems such as neural networks is that they can implicitly learn to do feature engineering all on their own. The algorithms can automatically create higher level features from the raw input. The more representation

FIGURE 5.2

The flow of preprocessing for training and evaluation. The attributes for new and unknown examples must be processed in the same way as those of the training and validation sets.

Copyright © 2018 Andrew Glassner under MIT license.

power an algorithm has, the more it is able to derive good features. This is approximately based on the number of layers present and the number of artificial neurons in each layer. Creation of an implicit feature set can be done for all forms of highly dimensional data and not just images. Images are a special case because of magnitude, density, and interrelationships of the data they encode, and as has been described in previous chapters, it took the invention of convolutional neural networks to deal with this effectively. However, even in the case of deep learning, feature selection, processing, and human feature engineering are helpful in optimizing algorithmic function.

The above steps in data preprocessing are summarized in Fig. 5.2.

Mathematical approaches to dimensional reduction

As described above, there are a number of straightforward approaches to reducing the size of the feature set by taking advantage of dependencies among attributes, eliminating redundant or minimally contributory features, and so on. We can take this a step further by determining which of the features contribute most and which contribute least to classification. This is the basis of a number of approaches to feature dimensional reduction. We will primarily discuss principal component analysis (PCA) as it is one of the most highly used procedures. PCA was first invented at the beginning of the 20th century as a statistical technique and thus precedes the advent of machine learning by half a century. It has become an important tool for data preprocessing across many fields and especially in machine learning. PCA is used to identify those features that provide the most information in regard to distinguishing among examples for the purpose of classification and to remove the others. This is done by transforming the data based upon their contribution to the variance of that data. Another way of thinking about PCA is to note that our data usually contain many variables, some of which may be correlated. This leads to a redundancy in the information in the dataset. In essence, PCA transforms the original variables to linear combinations of these variables that are independent. PCA can be a difficult topic to understand, so we will approach it in two ways, first a more or less intuitive approach and then a more precise explanation of the underlying mathematical principles.

A good intuitive account of this is found in Ref. [8]. The article begins by noting that variance is a measure of how far a set of numbers is spread out. It describes how much a variable differs from its expected value. If each feature had the same value in all samples, the model using it would have no predictive value because each sample would be identical. Thus, variance is useful as a feature variable in the model. If we define the target as the value to be predicted, then we want features that have nonzero variances with respect to the target. Mathematically, variance is the mean squared difference between the predicted and true values. While variance describes how multiple instances of a single variable vary, covariance is a measure of how much two or more random variables vary together.

As noted above, PCA automates data reduction and does so in an unsupervised manner. It does so on the basis of variance. It begins by finding the direction of maximum variance in the data. This is basically the direction along which the data are most spread out. In analogy with linear regression, we can find a line such that the mean squared difference between the original data points and the nearest point of the line is minimized. This line gives the first principal component. The next principal component will be the line that minimizes loss of information while also being perpendicular to the component already found (Fig. 5.3). This process can be repeated until there are as many components as the original data had dimensions. As will be seen below, these operations represent linear transformations of the data and can be reversed to reconstruct the original data. Thus, both represent equivalent information about the dataset.

At this point, there is no dimensional reduction. However, each component contributes less and less information, as we have started out with the direction in which the data are most spread out. This means that we can discard some of the later components without doing much damage. This will make the component-based dataset dimensionally smaller than the original dataset. The trick is to determine how much bathwater can be discarded while retaining the baby. This is usually by plotting variance as a function of component number and looking for a cutoff point beyond which there is little variance. Fig. 5.4 provides a good illustration of this. This is

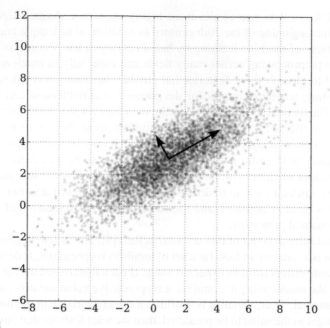

FIGURE 5.3

The longer arrows show the direction of the first component and the shorter arrow shows the direction of the second arrow. As the data in this example are two-dimensional, there are only two principal components. Each represents an axis along which variance is calculated. Wikipedia commons.

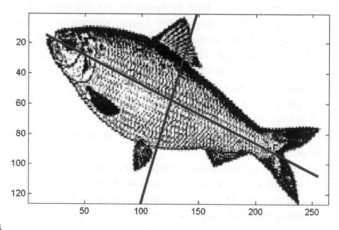

FIGURE 5.4

We can easily identify this as a fish without seeing it head-on. The set of data points that define the fish has less variance in the Z direction than in the X and Y directions. Wikipedia commons.

a 2D sketch of a fish, and it can easily be recognized as a fish. To classify different kinds of fish, we would need enough samples with sufficient variation among the respective attributes to provide enough information to define a generalized set of fish classes, and we can then determine in which class an unknown fish belongs. The interesting thing is that we do not need to see the fish head-on to perform this task. Most fish are not very thick and therefore there is less of a contribution to variation in that third dimension.

For a more general example, consider an ellipsoid of data points in three-dimensional (3D) space. If the ellipsoid is very flat in one direction, we can recover most of the data structure while ignoring that flat region. If we had samples with **n** attributes rather than just three, then the data are **n**-dimensional, and we can derive principal components along each of the **n** dimensions. We can then construct a "scree plot," which is a simple line segment plot that shows the fraction of total variance in the data with respect to the principal components. Typically, a scree plot shows variance dropping steeply with component number until a point where further changes are minimal. Discarding those later components therefore reduces the dimensionality with only minimal effect of the overall variance in the set of attributes. This is seen in Fig. 5.5.

Here, the amount of variance contributed by a principle component is plotted against component number. The ordinate in Fig. 5.5 is labeled both in terms of

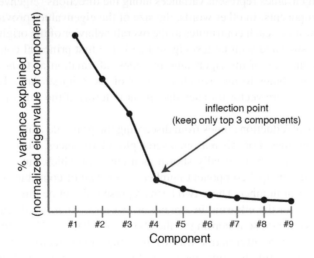

FIGURE 5.5

A typical scree plot. The curve has a steep fall off until the point where changes in eigenvalue are minimal. That point is chosen as the cutoff. By eliminating the principal components that contribute least, we are reducing the dimensionality of the feature vector by that amount while minimizing the effect on the data. In this example, the first three components are kept.

With permission, from A. Williams. Everything you did and didn't know about PCA. http://alexhwilliams.info/ itsneuronalblog/2016/03/27/pca/.

variance and "eigenvalues." As shown below, the eigenvalues are calculated from a covariance matrix in PCA, the eigenvalues represent variance, and so the terms can be used interchangeability for graphical analysis. Most scree plots have a point of inflection, and when this occurs, it defines the cutoff for discussing later components. In Fig. 5.5, we would keep the first three components and discard the rest.

This is a very oversimplified explanation of PCA. To understand the actual implementation of PCA, a bit of mathematical detail is necessary [9]. What we are actually doing is using linear algebra to transform a feature set into a new set based on variance. We do this by finding linear combinations of variables that best explain the covariance structure of the variables. We implement this task by first constructing a covariance matrix from the raw data matrix (in some applications, a correlation matrix is used; for the purposes of this discussion, we can ignore this distinction). A covariance matrix is a matrix whose element in the i,j position is the covariance between the ith and jth elements of the original vector. The eigenvalues and eigenvectors of this matrix are then calculated. Eigenvectors are vectors that describe a fixed direction under a given linear transformation and eigenvalues are scaling factors for these vectors. The most intuitive explanation, I have come across, is that the eigenvalues of a linear mapping provide a measure of the distortion induced by the transformation and the eigenvectors tell you how the distortion is oriented. In PCA, the matrix is constructed in terms of covariances in the original data, and so the eigenvalues represent variances along the directions (eigenvectors) of the principal components. In other words, the size of the eigenvalues provides information as to how much each contributes to the overall behavior of the original data. The eigenvector associated with largest eigenvalue is the first principal component, and so on. Thus, the size of the eigenvalue provides information as to how much that eigenvalue contributes to the overall behavior of the original data. The final step is to write the feature vector for each data point in terms of the sum of the principal components.

Dimensional reduction comes from discarding the principle components with the smallest eigenvalues. For this reason, a scree plot of variances, such as the one that was shown in Fig. 5.5, is usually shown as a curve in which the eigenvalues are plotted against principal component number rather than of contribution to variance versus component number. These two terms represent the same thing. To put this in concrete terms, for the ellipsoid in a previous example, when we discard the direction of flatness, we do so according to the above calculations. The scree plot would have shown how little information was lost in going from a 3D to 2D representation.

PCA is a powerful statistical technique that predates machine learning. It has turned out to be useful in virtually all forms of machine learning. Not only does PCA reduce the curse of dimensionality by stripping out less important features in the data, but also it provides a means by which the data can be better visualized in graphical form, as it is usually hard to represent more than three or four dimensions. PCA is not the only technique for doing this. Some others are embedding single value decomposition, linear discriminant analysis, and factor analysis. There are also nonlinear dimensionality reduction methods. These are based on the concept of a manifold. A manifold is a topological space that locally resembles flat Euclidean space near each point. For example, if you think of a linear space as a flat sheet of paper, then a rolled-up sheet of paper is a nonlinear manifold, as each point has a small region near it that is linear. Some nonlinear reduction methods include multidimensional scaling, isometric feature mapping, local linear embedding, and spectral embedding, among others. There are also probabilistic approaches for nonlinear reduction such as t-distributed stochastic neighbor embedding. This technique computes the probability that pairs of data points in the high dimensional space are related and then finds a low-dimensional embedding that produces a similar distribution. Although beyond the range of this discussion, a good summary can be found in Ref. [9].

Dimensional reduction in deep learning

Neural network—based algorithms provide many ways of performing unsupervised dimensionality reduction. Recall that within the neural network, a representation of the details is developed at increasing levels of complexity. Each of the derived features of the representation is built up from many original features in the dataset and therefore is of lower dimensionality. A convolutional neural network is a good example. The initial feature set may consist of millions of pixels. The convolutional and max pooling layers reduce this to a small number of features that encode the important data in the image. Other ways of generating such representations include autoencoders and generative adversarial networks, as described in Chapter 4. There is an interesting connection between autoencoders and PCA. Autoencoders develop a dimensionally reduced encoding (representation) of the input data by compressing it via convolution and then confirming its accuracy by deconvoluting it and comparing the result to the original input. Although this seems to bear no relationship to PCA, it turns out that if we were to run the data through an autoencoder without internal activation functions, then the mathematics of the resulting network is the same as running it through a PCA algorithm. However, if we include activation functions in the autoencoder, as is typically the case, then the system becomes much more powerful than PCA [10].

Imperfect class separation in the training set

In the above discussion and throughout the book, we have assumed the existence of a labeled training set in which the class of each instance in the dataset is accurately known and distinct from each other. However, there is sometimes a spillover in that one class is contaminated by a small but unknown number of samples from another either because of imperfect annotation or because of errors in constructing the training set. Fortunately, there are some sophisticated ways of dealing with this. The simplest case is the situation of training a binary classifier to reliably separate a positive and a negative class, for example, cancer versus normal. Here, we consider the situation in which the positive set is known, but the negative set is unknown in that it contains both positive and negative examples. In other words, we have to isolate a set of so-called "reliable negatives" for training purposes. Techniques for doing this are known as PU (positive-unlabeled) learning algorithms. The trick is to begin by treating all the negatives as truly negative and train the classifier. Next, using the classifier, score the unknown class and eliminate those for whom the classification is least reliable. Retrain with the positives against that truncated negative set, and repeat as necessary until some stopping condition is met [11,12]. Another approach involves bagging the unknown into distinct subsets and evaluating each subset for training [13].

In problems such as this, we assume that the positive set is large enough for effective training. However, often the available positive set is smaller than the negative set, and ways of dealing with this such as the creation of synthetic data have been discussed in previous chapters. It is interesting to note that PU learning itself can be used for classification problems, where there is only a small positive training set available. This involves augmenting the set of labeled positive examples with a set of unlabeled samples that includes both positive and negative examples. In the example of PU learning described above, we assume a sufficiently large set of positive training examples and that the positive samples were drawn from the same distribution as the contaminating positives in the negative set. In this new scenario, in addition to finding a set of reliable negatives, we wish to identify reliable positives hidden within the negative set. An interesting variant of PU using this strategy is known as "learning from probabilistically labeled positives" (LPLP). LPLP has been described for document classification [14] but has obvious applications for image interpretation as well.

Fairness and bias in machine learning

There are two kinds of bias in machine learning: coding or model bias and data bias. Coding bias is important for understanding the validity of a given algorithm for the problem it is addressing, but it is not analogous to human forms of bias. Instead, it refers to assumptions made in constructing the model. For example, in the K-means clustering model, it is assumed that the clusters are of similar size and essentially globular. In naïve Bayes, it is assumed that the feature attributes are independent variables. In neural network backpropagation, it is assumed that local minima can serve as surrogates for the global minimum. Model bias is not a fault; it is basic to the simplifying assumptions that are made in constructing useable models that are computationally efficient while retaining the ability to provide useful and meaningful outputs. Such built-in assumptions are also often necessary simply to allow the problem to be solved within the current state of the art. In any event, it is important to understand the limitations of the algorithm that is being used.

Data bias is much more insidious than coding bias. Most clinicians in general, and pathologists in particular, will be users, rather than creators, of machine learning models, so minimizing coding bias may be outside our domain of expertise. However, we will serve as content providers and annotation experts for the training set data. Thus, we are the first line of defense in scrutinizing the data itself for unintended bias.

We can define bias as unfair prejudice in favor or against one thing, person, or group compared with another. For humans, bias can be defined as a particular tendency, trend, inclination, feeling, or opinion, usually preconceived or unreasoned. Bias may be unconscious in that we may have attitudes or stereotypes without conscious awareness of them (implicit bias). As machines lack inclinations or opinions, or as far as we know, awareness, fairness in machine learning can be represented as the relationships between a sensitive attribute (race, gender, nationality, etc.) and the output of the model. In case of both human and machine, the output is incorrectly classified based upon an attribute that, in point of fact, has no causal relationship to that output. In the case of human bias, the result is often judgmental; in the case of the machine, it can lead to false judgments by humans.

There are many ways that bias can arise in machine learning. Sample bias is where the data used to train the model do not accurately reflect the domain of the problem. For example, the data may be restricted or poorly collated, or where there may be a marked imbalance in the training sets. An example of the former would be a training set in which all cats were placed on red rugs and dogs on brown rugs. An unknown sample of a dog on a red rug might be classified as a cat. Another would be a set of head shots of men and women, where the women all had long hair. An unknown woman with a pixie cut might be classified as a man. Note that these examples do not exhibit prejudice, and they are merely wrong because of "faulty" assumptions about properties of a population. These are relatively harmless examples. However, imagine a training set for distinguishing cocker spaniels from Doberman pinchers, in which the spaniels were all shown biting their owners, while the Dobermans' were shown cuddling. While both breeds can be docile or aggressive, this would paint an unfair picture of the relative temperaments of these two breeds and could lead to an unfair prejudice against cocker spaniels.

Set imbalance can contribute to machine bias in a much more insidious and problematic way. For example, in 2015, Google developed an algorithm to identify faces as humans, rhesus monkeys, baboons, gorillas, and other primates. The algorithm classified African Americans as gorillas! This was not neo-Nazi programming but rather related to a limited set of African Americans in the training set and large numbers of Caucasian examples, as well as large numbers of the various nonhuman primates. Google did not do this intentionally; it worked with the images at hand and did not notice the imbalance in the numbers of people of different races or ethnicity in their database. The neural network had learned skin color as a discriminant between humans and apes! The obvious fix would have been to expand the database, but Google's initial fix was simply to block the algorithm from identifying gorillas altogether.

Data bias can also lead to poor medical care on a population basis. Recently, Obermeyer et al. [15] examined a commercial algorithm used for healthcare decision-making and found that at a given risk score, black patients are considerably sicker than white patients. Remedying this disparity would increase the percentage of black patients receiving additional help from 17.7% to 56.5%. The bias was not because of judgmental issues but rather because of the underlying data structure. The algorithm used healthcare costs as a surrogate variable for degree of illness, on the apparently reasonable notion that the sicker you are, the more you spend on medical care. However, this equivalence rests on the assumption of equal access to healthcare. However, unequal access to healthcare and/or socioeconomic factors means that we spend less money caring for black patients. In this case, the fix is simpler; look at more appropriate measures of illness (or better still, having identified the societal problem, fix it).

These results should be contrasted to another study published by the same author in 2003 [16]. In this study, a large bank of fictitious job resumes was created. He also used fictitious names such as Emily and Greg versus Lakisha and Jamal and assigned them randomly to these resumes. The resumes were then sent to employers who posted job advertisements in the media of the day. White sounding names received 50% more callbacks for interviews than black sounding names. Applicants living in better neighborhoods received more callbacks, but this parameter was unaffected by perceived race. The amount of discrimination was uniform across occupations and industries. These results suggested that racial discrimination was still a prominent feature of the labor market in 2015.

It is instructive to note the differences in the causes of bias in these two examples. In the latter, which is much more pernicious, it is presumably based on unfair stereotyping. In the former, it is because of an error in the choice of attribute (cost vs. actual illness) rather than an unfair generalization. Nevertheless, both can lead to significant negative consequences.

Issues relating to understanding the features used for analysis are not confined to machine learning but are also problematic in traditional statistical analysis. In Ref. [17], Smith describes a study that, using statistical analysis, found that patients with sepsis with high pH levels are more likely to be readmitted to the hospital after discharge than patients with low pH. This implied that having a low pH is a good thing. This was surprising as it is well-known that acidosis in sepsis is associated with more severe disease. Analysis of the data revealed that the data included patients who had died during their hospital stay. The patients least likely to be readmitted are the ones discharged to the mortuary!

It can be very difficult to evaluate fairness in machine learning models. We initially defined fairness in machine learning in terms of the relationships between a sensitive attribute (race, gender, nationality, etc.) and the output of the model. However, it is obvious from the above examples that one cannot evaluate fairness in this context without considering the data generation strategies for the model and the causal relationships embedded within the data. For example, differences in disease prevalence based on genetic makeup may not reflect unfair bias in the data. On the other hand, differences in disease prevalence because of environmental or socioeconomic factors may reflect an underlying unfair bias. Recently, scientists at Google's DeepMind have used a technique known as causal Bayesian network analysis to explore these issues in an attempt to build fairer learning systems [18,19].

Summary

Good performance of a machine learning model requires a large set of features to allow classification and prediction from the data. There is an optimal point for this. Increasing the attribute number beyond that point can degrade performance. This can usually be overcome by increasing the complexity of the network, in terms of both layer width and layer depth. However, the downside here is that the network may lose its ability to generalize from the known examples to novel ones. In addition, irrelevant features can degrade performance by the network focusing on these rather than the ones that are truly important. For all these reasons, there must be a balance between algorithmic power and the structure of the data. A data scientist must pay as much attention to data preprocessing as to the choice of a machine learning model. There are also ethical considerations with respect to data such as restricted or poorly constructed datasets leading to implicit biases on the part of the model as well as privacy issues. These are very important and have come under increasing study as artificial intelligence is becoming more and more ubiquitous in society. For all these reasons, understanding the data as well as the algorithms is essential to address these issues properly.

References

[1] Chen T, et al. Recurrent attentional reinforcement learning for multi-label image recognition. arXiv; 2017. 1712.07465c1 [cs.CV].

[2] Wang Z, Sarcar S. Outline objects using deep reinforcement learing. arXiv; 2018. 1804.04603v2 [cs.CV].

[3] Mathe S, Pirinem A, Sminchisescu C. Reinforcement learning for visual object detection. IEEE Conference on Computer Vision 2016. https://doi.org/10.1109/CVPR.2016.316.

[4] https://www.kaggle.com/hesh97/titanicdataset-traincsv.

[5] https://towardsdatascience.com/a-beginners-guide-to-kaggle-s-titanic-problem-3193cb56f6ca.

[6] https://medium.com/@andrewadelson/testing-different-models-for-the-titanic-dataset-be5f725b7ec0.

[7] S Raschka. Feature Normalization and Scaling and the Effect of Standardization for Machine Learning Algorithms. https://sebastianraschka.com/Articles/2014_about_feature_scaling.html.

[8] T Yiu. Understanding Principal Component Analysis. https://towardsdatascience.com/understanding-pca-fae3e243731d.

[9] J.T. Raj. A Beginner's guide to dimensionality reduction in machine learning. https://towardsdatascience.com/dimensionality-reduction-for-machine-learning-80a46c2ebb7e.

[10] Glassner A. Chapter 25:autoencoders. In: Deep learning: from basics to practice; 2018. p. 1414.

[11] Liu B, Dai Y, Li X, et al. Building text classifiers using positive and unlabeled examples. In: Third IEEE international conference on data mining; 2003. p. 179–86.

[12] Fusilier DH, Montes-y-Gómez M, Rosso P, Guzmán Cabrera R. Detecting positive and negative deceptive opinions using PU-learning. Information Processing and Management 2015;51:433–43. https://doi.org/10.1016/j.ipm.2014.11.001.

[13] Mordelet F, Vert J-P. A bagging SVM to learn from positive and unlabeled examples. Pattern Recognition Letters 2014;37:201–9. https://doi.org/10.1016/j.patrec.2013.06.010.

[14] Li X-L, Liu B, Ng S-K. Dealing with data: strategies of preprocessing data. In: Kpketal JN, editor. Machine learning: ECML 2007: 18th European conference on machine learning. Springer-Verlag; 2007. p. 201–13.

[15] Obermayer Z, et al. Dissecting racial bias in an algorithm used to manage the health of populations. Science 2019;366:447–53. https://doi.org/10.1126/science.aax2342.

[16] Bertrand M, Mullainathan S. Are Emily and Greg more employable than Lakisha and Jamal? A field experiment on labor market discrimination. National Bureau of Economic Labor Studies Program; 2003. NBER Research Working Paper No. (9873).

[17] Smith G, Cordes J. Using bad data. In: Smith G, Cordes J, editors. The nine pitfalls of data science. Oxford University Press; 2019.

[18] Chiappa S, Isaac WS. A causal bayesian networks viewpoint on fairness. arXiv; 2019. 1907.06430v1 [stat.ML].

[19] Chiappa S, Gilliam PS. Path-specific counterfactual fairness. 2018. arXiv:1802.018139v1 [stat.ML].

Digital pathology as a platform for primary diagnosis and augmentation via deep learning

Anil V. Parwani, MD, PhD, MBA

Professor, Pathology and Biomedical Informatics, The Ohio State University, Columbus, OH,
United States

Introduction

The field of pathology is entering into an exciting time with the more widespread use of digital imaging in pathology. Pathologists have been using images for a long time, but only in the last 20 years, there has been an increased effort to digitize the workflow [1,2]. The electronic communication of digitized images, digital pathology, and the ability to transfer a microscopic image between one pathologist and another physician or member of the health care team has applications today in the national as well as global pathology community to be used for primary diagnosis, education, peer-review, intraoperative consultation, second opinion consultations, and quality reviews [1,3—15].

The most exciting aspect of digital pathology is the development and widespread use of whole slide imaging (WSI) technology [6,16]. WSI allows the scanning of entire glass slides, with an outputting of an image file that is a digitized reproduction of the glass slide with images that boast diagnostic quality standards [2,5,17,18]. The College of American Pathologists has published recommendations for validation of WSI scanners for clinical use [16,19—21]. In the last 2 years, the US Food and Drug Administration (FDA) has approved two WSI vendors to market devices for primary diagnosis, which have been major milestones in the journey toward adopting and implementing digital pathology systems [22,23]. A new set of regulatory pathways are now potentially going to be implemented as tools like deep learning (DL) and artificial intelligence (AI) start their way from research labs and clinical labs [14,24—30].

WSI scanners and the infrastructure surrounding the use and storage of digital images have advanced significantly since the description of the first one in 1997 by Ferreira et al. [31,32]. In the last decade, innovations and significant technical advancements in WSI have contributed to the ability of clinical laboratories to image

Artificial Intelligence and Deep Learning in Pathology. https://doi.org/10.1016/B978-0-323-67538-3.00006-3

large numbers of slides automatically, rapidly, and at high resolution [6]. The ability to routinely digitize entire slides not only allows pathologists to better apply computer power and network connectivity to the study of histomorphology but also has significantly improved the quality and accessibility of biospecimen repositories [33], particularly large image datasets that can be used for research in the areas of DL and AI [34–40]. The tools have also paved the way toward creating remote networks of digital pathology scanning centers to enable rapid sharing of clinical cases [41]. The latter inventions and innovations in the field of AI are paving the way to augment the clinical diagnostic workflow and primary diagnosis in pathology [28,42]. This chapter will focus on providing an overview of digital pathology and particularly WSI as a unique platform for clinical applications such as primary diagnosis and the potential to augment this diagnosis via DL and AI [11,20,26,43,44].

Digital imaging in pathology

Imaging plays a critical role in modern pathology practice and is a driving technology to enhance workflows within the clinical laboratory. Pathology images are unique in the healthcare environment and present significant challenges in labeling, storage, and management. Imaging workstations can be thought of as PCs with image-specific software and the appropriate hardware peripherals needed to handle digital images [32,45–47].

With improved computing power and infrastructure increasingly supporting more powerful computers, more robust networking, and cheaper storage, this is a perfect time when pathologists are able to review large images rapidly and easily as they can now manage text. Many of the laboratory information system (LIS) vendors are now able to provide integration with WSI systems [18]. In recent years, we are witnessing a vast improvement in capture, storage, and retrieval of images handled by the LIS [48]. Digital images continue to be used for teaching, quality assurance studies, and even consultation. The basic ability to capture the digital image faithfully must be validated before further applications can be developed [49–51].

Imaging software comes in many flavors and serves many functions. Software for image processing allows the adjustment of brightness, contrast, hue, and resolution and is therefore extremely useful for providing pathologic images for academic use [52]. Many laboratories have implemented image acquisition and management systems that acquire images during all stages of the specimen workflow (requisition scanning, gross and microscopic examination) and store them into either customized home-grown systems or commercial systems [52–54]. These images are linked to the surgical accession numbers, which in turn are linked to the electronic medical record and the LISs [49]. The most critical aspect of this workflow is the ability to integrate with the LIS and have images readily available for patient care [46,51].

Several laboratories have utilized image-embedded reports to improve the care of patients by providing additional information and can also include annotations, tables, graphs, and diagrams. Such reports can in addition provide the clinician with added insight to the practice of pathology, facilitating greater understanding between disciplines. Image-embedded reports also serve as a powerful marketing tool for expanding the outreach capabilities of the laboratory [55,56]. The advent of AI tools will pave the way in the future to automate many of the tasks of "choosing" the right image based on clinical data and other relevant information. There are also significant advances occurring in parallel in the field of molecular pathology, which together with digital pathology and AI will provide the next generation of powerful and advanced diagnostic tools [53].

Digital images in pathology originate from several sources including autopsy, gross room, cameras mounted on microscopes or scanned using scanners. There are numerous situations where digital imaging in pathology has provided useful solutions to pathologists including their deployment in pathology reports, conferences, presentations, quality assurance studies, and creation of teaching sets of rare and archival material. These images may be published as a collection of archived images on the Internet or local intranet for teaching. Digital images are also acquired for legal situations [54,57,58].

Telepathology

Telepathology technologies allow light microscopic examination and diagnosis from a distance. These systems may be combined with DL algorithms to assist the pathologist to screen a remote case for consultation or extract features from these images for assisted diagnosis. Telepathology use cases include primary diagnosis, teleconsultation, intraoperative consultation, telecytology, telemicrobiology, quality assurance, and teleeducation [59−61]. There are three general approaches to telepathology. These include dynamic, static, and hybrid systems [32,62−67].

Dynamic systems are remote-controlled microscopes that provide the pathologist with a "live" view of the distant microscopic image while allowing them to control the stage, focus, and change the magnification, remotely. An advantage of the dynamic systems is that they give the remote pathologist control and [68] flexibility in viewing any region of the entire slide and do so at any power. These systems tend to be more expensive with proprietary software requirements [69−71].

The second method of telepathology is "store-and-forward" telepathology in which digital images are first captured via cameras or acquired via WSI systems for transmission to the consultant. These images can be captured in standard file formats and can be viewed via a remote viewer. In the future, this mode of telepathology may be used to send images to the cloud, where image analysis may be performed or DL algorithms may be run to prescreen for rare event detection or for diagnosis or grading of cancer or for identifying microorganisms [69,72−74].

The third method of telepathology is the use of hybrid systems which can combine features of both "store-and-forward" and dynamic systems. Hybrid telepathology systems can provide a "live" view using robotic-controlled microscopy with high-resolution still image capture and retrieval. This dual functionality makes them valuable. Some of the hybrid systems in the market today have capabilities for WSI as well [2].

Future developments in telepathology are likely to focus on three areas. The first is the adoption of standards that will help with interoperability. The second area will be to improve the integration with the LIS and electronic medical record to facilitate image viewing, reporting, and billing capabilities. The third area is the development of WSI for use in clinical practice. The latter will open up the area of applying DL and AI algorithms for remote locations [2,4,35,39,69].

Whole slide imaging

Much like the evolution of efficiency and effectiveness in radiology, the pressure on pathologists to reduce time to diagnosis and develop more efficient workflows is trending toward digitalization, and WSI is turning out to be a technology to enable this digital workflow [16,75–77]. WSI scanning robots provide the ability to digitize an entire glass slide which can be viewed as a digital file, providing capability similar to a radiology workflow including the use of picture archiving communication system (PACS) [78]. In other words, WSI technology allows the glass slides to be treated like digital files and shared at multiple locations simultaneously, providing means to collaborate, make a diagnosis remotely, and potentially apply DL algorithms either before viewing the image or after signing out to check for errors and diagnostic quality. Robust infrastructure and the reduction in costs for network, storage, and computing power have made the use of WSI even more feasible. There are large implications for the practice of pathology with the potential for major efficiency and quality gains [6,11,79,80].

A WSI scanner is basically a microscope that is under full robotic control, attached to highly specialized cameras which contain high-performance photosensors. There are two main approaches to create WSI files including the use of tile-based imaging, in which a square photosensor is used to capture multiple "tiles" adjacent to each other, or a line scan–based imaging, in which an oblong photosensor is used to continually capture strips of image data as it sweeps through the slide. Once the slides are digitized and converted to millions of pixels, we now have massive pixel pipelines which allow pathologists to remotely view the images and share them [6,81].

In addition, and more notably, these images can now be standardized and analyzed using DL and AI tools to look for specific features such as the number of mitotic figures, presence of infectious agents such as acid-fast bacilli, or even grade cancer. With the ease of availability of cloud computing, powerful processors, and robust infrastructure today, it is possible to create a pixel pipeline–based workflow which allows for creating AI-based prognostic or diagnostic algorithms [26,82–84].

WSI scanners have changed through several generations since the first commercially available scanner in 2001. In the last decade, there have been several vendors who are focusing on producing automated, high-speed WSI scanners with an emphasis on scanning speed, image quality, and high-throughput capabilities. A modern WSI scanner today can run in batch mode and can capture and compress an image of a slide with a 1.5 × 1.5 cm tissue section in under a minute with spatial sampling as low as 0.25 microns/pixel. These scanners have now also implemented cutting-edge optics, illumination, and sensors which allow for high-speed image capture [31,32].

WSI scanners of the future still have many chances to improve many aspects of the mechanics and performance such as speed, point spread function, scan to view timing latency, and other methods of captures such as Z-stacking, immunofluorescence, and phase contrast. These enhancements should result in substantial improvements in speed, throughput, and resolution in the future. Z-stacking is an especially important consideration for organizations and/or laboratories that will be scanning cytology specimens and/or blood smears.

Many recent studies have demonstrated the utility of WSI in teaching and assessment [7,85,86]. The high-speed WSI robot industry is becoming highly diverse with a wide range of optics, detectors, slide handling devices, and software resulting in an increasing range of capabilities and costs. The quality of the images produced is generally of diagnostic quality, and with the viewing software, it is possible to have annotations and clinical metadata presented with the image, resulting in a virtual microscope with all the clinical information needed to sign out the case [8,9,87,88].

The quality of focusing is limited by multiple optical and mechanical constraints, notably numerical aperture (NA) of the objective and movement resolution on the vertical (z) axis. Newer devices are implementing nontraditional optics, illumination, and sensors designed specifically for very high-speed image capture, resulting in significant improvements in speed, throughput, and resolution. Several scanners come with automatic algorithms to determine the optimal focus throughout the slide, but most scanners only have the capacity to image one level of the z-axis at a time.

The ability of a WSI system to create sharp, well-focused digital images in true color is determined by a combination of several components of the system's optical setup, including platform stability, optics, camera, adapter, and condenser setup. In general, the resolution feature represents an objective comparison measurement of the capability of an optical-based system to represent fine details in an image, usually represented as μm/pixel. Resolution correlates to the combined NA of the objective lens and condenser. Higher NA values result in higher image resolutions [6,89—91].

Increasing resolution also presents compromises to the overall scanner performance, including increased scanning time and decreased depth of field of focus, resulting in more frequent focus adjustments. The increased operational and algorithmic performance needs, coupled with lower sensitivity to histological preparation artifacts, may result in higher rescan rates. However, higher resolution is critical for interpretation of digital images of certain tissue types/applications such as transplant kidney biopsies [36]. For example, a scanning resolution approaching 0.15 μm/pixel enables the pathologist to determine the presence of clinically important subtle details within the digital side that are typically visible while utilizing a traditional optical microscope [89].

The main component of the optical microscope is the objective lens. High NA objectives are typically used in optical microscopes provided within a WSI system [92]. NA affects image resolution; scanning conducted with higher NA objectives creates sharper images. Lenses are typically nonpropriety to the WSI manufacturer. Vendors are beginning to incorporate multiple objective lens configurations within a single device. Majority of WSI systems are supplied with a 20× objective lens for scanning purposes, as the 20× objective lens configuration provides the best match of field size and resolution [93]. However, interpretation of specific pathology tissue types such as neuropathology or transplantation pathology may require higher resolutions that are obtained using higher magnification lens and configurations [93].

The scanning resolution offered by currently marketed WSI systems using a bright-field light source with a 20× magnification objective configuration ranges from 0.22 to 0.5 μm/pixel, and when using a 40× magnification objective configuration, it is about 0.25 μm/pixel.

The balance between image resolution and magnification and the resulting digital image display on a computer monitor are important points to consider in selecting and configuring a WSI system. It is difficult to match a WSI image to an image obtained using a traditional microscope. The design of a bright field optical system is composed of multiple stages or planes from where light is collected and focused on the specimen, through the objective and connected tube lens/camera adaptor to reach the camera chip sensor, and ultimately to the human eye via monitor display. To understand and optimize the resulting image quality on a monitor display, it is important to relate the resolution of the various components of this system [94,95].

Innovations in illumination are being utilized by WSI vendors; the traditional bright field halogen lighting, although still currently used in many scanners, is being replaced with newer light-emitting diode (LED)—based modules, to provide improved color consistency. New techniques in illumination also include LED "strobing" or flash illumination instead of constant illumination, as this minimizes motion artifact enabling faster acquisition [92]. Automated multichannel fluorescent WSI is now readily available by some of the vendors [96,97].

Whole slide image viewers

All WSI systems are provided with software that supports viewing of WSI image files (digital slides) at the scanner control computer workstation. Imaging viewing software allows viewing of digital slides on a computer screen in a manner similar to the viewing of glass slides using a traditional optical microscope [98]. Most vendors provide feature-rich image viewing software solutions, offering many functions for image navigation, panning and zooming movements, image manipulation/editing with an enhanced ability to add annotations, and microscopic image measurements [6,78].

Image viewer software, unique to each vendor, is often installed on the local user's computer and may require administrative rights or the equivalent for deployment. However, to support the frequent need for remote image viewing, vendors often provide a web-based version of the viewing software. The latter usually offers slightly less functionality in terms of image modification, annotation, and measurement but allows for off-site viewing using protocols built off standard web technologies to facilitate ease of deployment.

The image viewer provided with each WSI system typically enables the viewing of WSI image files saved using a proprietary image format unique to their WSI system and does not support viewing of images created by other WSI scanner systems. However, several companies offer image viewers that currently support viewing of differently formatted files. The native, vendor-provided image viewing software and/or applications and their coupling to the corresponding vendor-specific pathology workflow software may offer several advantages over "generic" or viewing systems [78].

The main advantage of vendor-unique viewers includes access to specific vendor-encoded features such as user comments and/or annotations. Other advantages may include access to data while using third-party solutions such as viewing multichannel fluorescence data, as limited access to such solutions is available while using "generic" viewers. To support comparison of different slides, multiple slide viewing and navigation options are provided by various vendor-specific image viewers [58,98,99].

This feature is used to compare different biomarkers for a single case. Digital slide viewers allow the pathologist to see a virtual slide on a screen in a similar fashion as they would by looking through a traditional microscope. With these viewers, pathologists are able to view virtual slides at different magnifications. Furthermore, some of these viewers provide additional functionality like viewing of virtual slides at different magnifications in two windows or tools to annotate. Some viewers may also be linked to LISs, leading to a true digital workflow experience for the pathologist [98,100].

Whole slide image data and workflow management

Image and data management databases and tools are typically available as supporting software programs included with the majority of WSI systems intended for clinical or research use [50,101]. Nearly all WSI systems offer a choice of visualization and workflow/data management packages that include support for WSI file formats. Such software packages allow pathologists and histology technicians to view, manage, and analyze the digital slides and the associated clinical data [102].

Image and information management is an important benefit of creating a digital workflow for enabling the pathologist an access to the relevant patient information in a digital cockpit or workstation [11,14,18,103]. By providing rapid access to this information, time is saved and quality of the information is enabled. Once this information and images are managed in the workstation, the second important aspect of the value pyramid can become available which is the ability of "image sharing" [6]. This image sharing can be for access to experts for consultation, showing cases to a colleague for clinical and treatment decisions or for quality assurance or for "workload balancing." As these applications of image sharing are rapidly used, the value of digital pathology workflow will make an enormous impact on the care of the cancer patient. These benefits are not nearly as powerful as the third and yet not fully developed and exploited value of digital pathology, which is the field of image analysis and computer-aided diagnosis. Advances in the area of image analysis will provide the pathologists with powerful tools or "helper" applications to enable the pathologists to do manual and labor-intensive tasks more automated including detecting "rare events" such as finding tumor mets within a lymph node or accurately quantitating the volume of tumor in specimen or grading nuclei as a part of histological assessment [6,14,44,104].

Vendors provide a variety of anatomic pathology workflow solutions, from simple image management (e.g., tagging images with basic metadata for searching) to advanced integration with the LIS. Specific evaluation of these features should be based on the particular user or institutional requirements. However, the ability to integrate vendor-provided web-based viewers into third party applications is becoming commonplace. This eliminates the need to conform a customer workflow to specific vendor functions and gives total control of any needed customization, provided the customer can provide the necessary IT and software development expertise.

The vast majority of high-throughput scanners commercially available today possess automated slide matching/distribution/tracking capabilities. Image management software can support anatomic pathology workflow by supporting the automation process, matching slides to cases and permitting distribution of cases to the appropriate pathologist. Such systems can also improve case tracking abilities and provide immediate access to prior cases. Many WSI vendors provide dedicated workflow support solutions. Interoperability between the anatomical pathology laboratory information system (APLIS) and the whole slide imaging system (WSS) can automate data exchange between the systems and leads to an improved anatomical pathology workflow. Interoperability challenges remain with respect to integrating multiple vendor WSI systems into a unified laboratory workflow solution. This is mainly because of the various advanced imaging features available across WSI platforms and the optimized way in which these data are encoded per vendor. For example, many WSI systems allow scanning and encoding of multiple focal planes that can later be revisited "digitally" upon digital slide viewing [102].

In pathology, international standardization initiatives such as digital imaging and communications (DICOM) have helped to create an imaging standard so that pathology images too can be incorporated into PACS [102,105−107]. The DICOM supplements 122 and 145 provide flexible object information definitions dedicated, respectively, to pathology specimen description and WSI acquisition, storage, and display [106]. According to these recommendations, large multiresolution and multiplanar WSI can be stored by mapping subregions from each layer into a DICOM series. With such a tiled organization, images are stored in squares or rectangular tiles and subsequently arranged in two-dimensional arrays. Multiple resolutions are stored in this manner with the highest resolution forming the base of a pyramid [108].

Selection criteria for a whole slide scanner

Today, much progress has occurred in the industry, and there are multiple WSI scanners on the market in the United States and globally. These devices have all of the following basic features: automated tissue identification, autofocus, autoscanning, automated image compression, and automated barcode reading. Some of the key features that need to be considered when evaluating a new WSI scanner are listed in Table 6.1.

Table 6.1 Key features to consider when evaluating a new whole slide scanner.

✔ **Physical/general**
- Scanner dimensions
- Scanner weight
- Environmental tolerance
- Service support

✔ **Glass slide handling**
- Slide size
- Slide capacity
- Slide handling robotics

✔ **Image acquisition**
- Objective lens
- Bright-field illumination source
- Scanning resolution
- Camera features

✔ **Image digitization**
- Scanning method
- Scanning speed and time
- Tissue detection method
- Scanning region size
- Color calibration
- Z-stacking scanning capabilities
- Fluorescence scanning capabilities

✔ **Workflow**
- Laboratory information system integration
- Bar code support

Evolution of whole slide imaging systems

Early generation WSI systems were mostly built on a robotic compound microscope frame and often utilized the "stop–start" imaging methods to produce an initial low-resolution overview or thumbnail image of the glass slide for tissue detection [76,78,109]. Once tissue was located, each field of view was individually focused and captured, repeating this process until all present tissue areas were captured. The resultant image was then represented in full color (typically 24 bits per pixel) with a dimension of many thousands of pixels in both width and height. Image fields were captured with an overlap to provide context for a "stitching" process used to join the images together at a later step in the process. Because of their large data sizes, these images were represented as a pyramid-like structure organized into multiple layers, each layer containing a different resolution. This stratification of data by resolution allowed for more efficient viewing via specialized vendor-supplied software [76].

Second-generation WSI systems minimized image acquisition time by utilizing alternate camera technologies such as line scanning [6]. These techniques allowed slide movement at a near-constant velocity or speed and thereby eliminated start/stop delays, as well as minimized the amount of algorithmic image "stitching" required to create the final digital slide image. Focus detection algorithms were also improved to allow for interpolated focus adjustment during the scanning process. Expanded imaging methods enabled capture and digital revisiting of multiple focal planes. Camera speed improvements led to additional optical configuration options, including higher NA objectives (higher resolution imaging) and oil immersion modalities. In addition, more fail-safe mechanisms of slide loading mechanisms were developed, and WSI system slide loading capacity was increased [41].

The current generation of scanners has slide loaders with slide capacities up to 1000 slides per run, with the added ability to support various, nonstandard histology glass sizes such as whole mounts (e.g. "2 × 3" slides). Lastly, the availability of more economical data storage options in recent years has enhanced workflow making archival and remote web-based image viewing possible for routine daily workloads [6]. The newer scanners not only have faster processing and camera performance (measured by frames per second) but also have implemented enhancements to the continuous scanning techniques used by second-generation scanners by adopting illumination methods such as high-intensity LED strobes to eliminate delay in image capture because of motion artifact. Focus mapping, also known as predictive autofocusing, has remained a viable technique as it gives a priori information about focus position, but multiple tissue scans are required, thus decreasing scanning efficiency. An alternative technique, termed "frequency"-based sampling, saves time by incorporating the concept of focus maps with real-time continuous focus adjustments, whereby the system performs an autofocus for every number (N) of imaging fields scanned. Nonetheless, optimal focus is difficult to maintain at higher NAs without increasing autofocus frequency (i.e., reducing N), requiring increased time for each complete scan performed at higher magnification. Newer

WSI systems also offer advanced imaging functionality such as an epifluorescence (fluorescence) capability in addition to oil-immersion microscopy, thereby providing additional flexibility regarding potential uses of the WSI to support the anatomic pathology lab operations and needs. Over time, image capture time has decreased and image quality has improved, and the overall utility of the WSI has moved steadily toward a recognized increase in core value to both clinical and research imaging operations [6,29,41,110,111].

Infrastructure requirements and checklist for rolling out high-throughput whole slide imaging workflow solution

Step 1: Deploy scanners and initiate validation of anatomical pathology slides [112−114].

1. Depending on the volume of slides to be scanned, first step is to begin installing the desired number of scanners in a designated digital scan lab facility, ensuring that each scanning appliance is afforded a 10 Gbit link to the WSI Server Cluster, via a private unshared channel. These facilities should ideally be in the histology lab or in close proximity to the histology lab [112].

2. The WSI scanner needs to be installed along with the associated server in a secure, clinical grade, data center with networking to the scan facilities and collective scanning appliances using multiple dedicated 10 G bit channels.

3. The next step is to install, in sequenced fashion, the cohort of designated pathology workstation solutions in various locations, with each having an independent 1 G bit channel back to the server. This will enable the remote viewing of the WSI images by the pathologists in their work areas.

4. The next milestone is to establish connectivity between respective integration engines, such that patient demographics, case data, and other clinically relevant data as deemed necessary in support of primary case sign out, which can be populated into the digital pathology cockpit. This is accomplished by a bidirectional HL7 interface engine interface between scanners and the laboratory information.

5. This unified bidirectional HL7 interface will provide support for admissions, discharges, and transfers (ADT) and demographic updates, accession logs, specimen/block/slide logs and barcode IDs, internal histology orders, case history, slide archive inventory, and case narrative texts [115].

6. Finally, the pathologist workstation or cockpit will be ready for routine intramural case sign out capability. Moreover, this capability serves as the foundational work needed for subsequent optimization in support of full case volume sign out, upon the availability of use of digital pathology solutions for primary case sign out, utilizing FDA-approved devices.

7. The LIS serves as a single source of truth for preserved overall hospital-level referential integrity of data [114].

8. All pathologist sign out workstations/cockpits have to be passed with certification protocols, and all digital pathology workstation locations need to have the availability of full bandwidth under maximal concurrency conditions [115].

9. Routine pathology slides are scanned before sending out to pathologists, and images will be available in the pathology cockpit for digital sign out [18].

10. After a digital sign out is achieved, the next step is to build or buy prognostic and predictive biomarker assays using DL and AI methods.

Whole slide imaging and primary diagnosis

The first WSI scanner was approved by the FDA in 2017 and the second one in 2019, paving the way for using WSI as a primary diagnostic tool [22,116]. Before this, most of the financial gain from implementing WSI system was for remote consultations, frozen sections [117], education [118], and research. Utilizing WSI for primary diagnostics is helping labs with increased productivity and cost mitigation by increasing patient safety by providing pathology images for easy sharing for expert consultation, which in turn will lead to reduction in overcalls and undercalls in pathology diagnosis. One of the impacts of improved access to images and sharing images is also in the rapid inpatient review of cases and potential to decrease the number of hospital days of care and facilitate earlier discharge of patients where delay in pathology diagnosis may be resulting in discharge decisions. In a study published by the *Journal of Pathology Informatics*, a group from the University of Pittsburgh studied the positive effects of implementing digital pathology [119]. Workflow improvement benefits as a result of employing digital pathology included the support of lab automation (e.g., bar coding and tracking of assets and bidirectional interfaces with the scanners) and the potential to increase an individual pathologist's productivity by at least 13% because of improved organization and racking of surgical pathology cases [119]. Other possible areas for financial gains will be to increase number of pathology consults coming to a facility and indirectly by recognition of these new technologies creating a band recognition, more patients will come to a facility for surgery and treatment [119].

WSI technology has several advantages over conventional microscopy, such as portability, ease of sharing and retrieval of archival images, and the ability to make use of computer-aided diagnostic tools such as image algorithms and 3D reconstruction used to convert poorly oriented specimens into well-oriented ones. WSI has also created new business models in pathology [120]. One such example is the virtual immunohistochemistry service provided by large national laboratories. After the remote reference laboratory performs technical staining and slide scanning services, the referring pathologist is provided with full access to these immunostained slides for their interpretation or referral to a teleconsultant. This has allowed some pathology practices to recapture a portion of the reimbursement for professional interpretation services. Finally, some issues that still need to be satisfactorily addressed to truly accommodate the use of WSI for making primary diagnoses relate to regulations (e.g., FDA and validation guidelines), malpractice and liability issues, and reimbursement for technical services [22,121−123].

More recently, digital pathology association (DPA) has worked with FDA to downgrade the risk of WSI scanner. Under certain circumstances, manufacturers can opt to submit a de novo application for a moderate- or low-risk device, which has not yet been classified and for which there is no predicate device. The DPAs discuss with the FDA on the notion that manufacturers submit a de novo application. FDA indicated the WSI for primary diagnosis is, rather than a premarket approval (PMA), a candidate for de novo applications as a class II device. Once a de novo application receives marketing authorization, other companies will then be able to submit 510(k) for WSI. The first device was approved for primary diagnosis in 2017 and the second device was approved in 2019.

The practice of histopathology evaluation by benchtop optical microscopes remains the gold standard for pathology review. However, as the workflow of related specimen information transitions to fully digital systems including the use of whole slide image scanners, there has been an emerging need to incorporate the traditional glass slide histopathology findings as digital images to move toward a complete sideless and seamless digital workflow [11,50,87,124,125]. This need has been increasingly met over the past decade by the development of robotic telepathology systems and evolved to whole slide digitization technology and associated software for visualization and data management [113,126]. The selection of systems available in the marketplace ranges from offering broad-based anatomic pathology workflow solutions to those with feature sets suited to specific areas of pathology. Hospital administrators and C-suite executives are taking closer look at the cost-to-benefit analysis of WSI systems and deployments continue to increase steadily around the world [119].

Some of the lessons learned from early "validation" studies highlight the need for diagnostic standards and better design of study conditions for a direct comparison of light and WSI modalities [9,126−134]. Some important considerations are to look at intraobserver discrepancies and identify the causes [105,135,136]. Many times, these discrepancies are not image quality related but because of other factors. These discrepancies may be because subject pathologists sign out cases they are accustomed to signing out while general pathologists sign out general cases, whereas subspecialized pathologists sign out subspecialty cases only. Other factors which may result in discrepancies may be because of preanalytical factors such as different cutting and staining protocols as well as using scanners with special functions such as Z-stacking [21,22,137,138].

Whole slide imaging and image analysis

One of the major advantages of digitizing slides is the ability to use computer algorithms to conduct reproductive and accurate measurements, quantify immunohistochemical stain intensity, and provide accurate measurements (e.g., cell counting) [139–141]. Many WSI vendors have engaged in cooperation with companies developing computer-assisted diagnosis and providing quantitative image analysis by providing a selection of solutions from specific defined assays (e.g., HER2/neu) to rule-based image segmentation [142,143]. These application packages can interoperate with WSI formats, either via vendor-supplied interfaces or via provided programming interfaces. Several vendors, but not all, include image analysis software packages with a WSI system [144,145].

FDA-approved quantitative algorithms for diagnostic use are available for a limited number of vendors. Approved tests include breast cancer biomarkers—progesterone receptor, estrogen receptor, human epidermal growth factor receptor 2 (HER2/neu), the cell proliferation index marker Ki67, micrometastases in bone marrow, and p53 [146].

Whole slide imaging and deep learning

As more laboratories adopt digital pathology and digital images are incorporated into the diagnostic pathology workflow, there will be better case management and resulting of cases because of overall improvement in the information management surrounding a patient case [99]. Digital pathology workflow will help improve the efficiency of reading the cases [147–155]. AI tools can now be applied before signing out of the case to help collate and integrate the information that is needed for case review, but ultimately the pathologist will review the case and make a diagnosis [14,79,84,156,157].

Advances in digital imaging and ability to rapidly digitize glass slides have now paved the ways to start using these images in DL/machine learning (ML) algorithms leading to potentially novel and innovative diagnostic tools [158]. The use of DL and AI tools combined with digital pathology images can extend the value of digital pathology far beyond what is possible today and quantified above. This is the true value of digital pathology and the AI tools that have been developed and are being developed today will help transform diagnostic pathology [14,159].

As anatomical pathologists implement digital pathology, they now will have the capability to start using the smart DL tools in daily practice [28,158]. This is easy to illustrate by considering a specific area in surgical pathology, prostate cancer diagnosis, and grading. Adenocarcinoma of the prostate is one of the most common cancers diagnosed in men worldwide, second only to lung cancer. The increase in diagnosis stems from the increase in screening for prostate cancer, and it has led to unnecessary testing and overtreatment [160,161]. Prostate cancer has an excellent five-year survival rate of greater than 98% [147–155]. For this reason, it is important to determine if treatment will have an added benefit to the patient or simply decrease his quality of life. Current standards utilize Gleason scoring to determine if prostate cancer prognosis is from biopsy specimens [161].

Nagpal et al. (2019) have published a study on the development and validation of a DL algorithm for improving Gleason scoring of prostate cancer [162]. This study aimed to address the issue of grading variability, improve prognostication, and optimize patient management. A two-stage deep learning system (DLS) was developed to perform Gleason scoring and quantitation on prostatectomy specimens. The first stage was a deep convolutional neural network—based regional Gleason pattern classification. It was trained using 912 slides with 112 million pathologist-annotated image patches. About 1159 slide-level pathologist classifications were used for the second stage of training. A reference standard was created from the independent reviews of three pathologists as well as a genitourinary specialist pathologist on a dataset of 331 slides from 331 patients from 3 independent sources [162].

Twenty-nine additional pathologists reviewed the validation dataset as a comparison to the performance of the DLS. The mean accuracy of the 29 pathologists was 0.61 compared with an accuracy of 0.70 for the DLS ($P = .002$). Gleason Grade decision thresholds were also investigated with the DLS achieving area under the receiver operating characteristic curves between 0.95 and 0.96 at each threshold. At a Gleason Grade $\geq$4, the largest difference was seen, and the DLS showed greater sensitivity and specificity than 9 out of 10 pathologists [162].

Because of its clinical significance, Gleason pattern quantitation was compared among the groups; DLS had 4%—6% lower mean absolute error than the average pathologist, and the DLS predicted the same pattern as the pathologist 97% of the time. Lastly, the DLS was able to predict a more gradual transition from well to poorly differentiated by utilizing "fine-grained Gleason patterns," such as 3.3 or 3.7 instead of the traditional methods of Gleason scoring [162].

Bulten et al. (2020) reported on a DL method for the automated Gleason grading of prostate biopsies. The purpose of this latter study was to create a DLS that was fully automated for detecting cancer and performing Gleason grading without the need for training with manual pixel-level annotations. This was accomplished using previously developed epithelium and prostate cancer segmentation algorithms with slide-level Gleason grades from the original pathology reports of 5209 biopsies from the Radboud University Medical Center. The U-Net architecture was utilized in two stages: (1) Segmentation of the whole biopsy was done by assigning Gleason growth patterns to tumorous regions, and the normalization ratio of epithelial tissue was calculated. (2) The normalized volume percentages of each growth pattern were used to determine the grade group. The neural network was deepened to contain six levels with more skip connections in each layer block and upsampling operations in the expansion path. A test set of 535 biopsies that were not included in the training set was reviewed by three uropathologists, each with greater than 20 years of experience. A consensus score and Gleason Grade were determined by these expert pathologists, and this became the reference set [163].

This DLS attained a quadratic kappa agreement of 0.918 with the reference set. Misclassification occurred at the decision boundaries of grade groups 2 and 3 as well as groups 4 and 5. Determining benign versus malignant biopsies resulted in an area under the receiver operating characteristic curve of 0.990 with a specificity of 82%. In a subset of 100 cases assessed by an external panel of 15 pathologists, the median interrater agreement kappa value was 0.819, compared with the system kappa value of 0.854 [163].

Additional analyses showed that the DLS performs better than pathologists with less than 15 years of experience ($P = .036$) and is not significantly different to those with greater than 15 years of experience ($P = .955$). No significant difference was found between the DLS and the panel of pathologists for detection of benign and malignant specimens ($P = .704$). Lastly, the DLS was applied to an external data set of 641 cores that were annotated by two pathologists independently, and quadratic kappa values were 0.711 and 0.639. These values fall within the range of interobserver variability but are lower than those achieved by the reference set [163].

Both studies above showed that DLSs can achieve pathologist-level performance [162,163]. This is important in the field of pathology with increasing demand and not enough physicians going into pathology to keep up. The first study developed a DLS that was more accurate than several general pathologists in the quantitation of Gleason patterns. In addition, it created a system that could discriminate these patterns at a finer level. The second study created a DLS using an automated training system that did not require extensive additional pathologist work hours and thus saved valuable resources. It used a straightforward and easily interpretable system that is similar to the method pathologists currently use in clinical practice, which allows simple communication between the DLS and clinicians. Both studies created systems that can not only detect the presence of a tumor but accurately grade the aggressiveness of the tumor utilizing Gleason scoring [162].

There are important limitations to both studies that would need to be addressed before the implementation of these tools into clinical practice [162,163]. The first study employed a time-consuming and expensive method to train the DLS with 112 million pathologist-annotated image patches requiring almost 900 pathologist hours. The purpose of creating the DLS becomes obsolete if pathologists have to spend exuberant amounts of time training them. This study used prostatectomy specimens to determine the Gleason Grade. This means the grade obtained can only inform postoperative treatment decisions, instead of whether a prostatectomy was recommended to begin with [162]. The second study solved this issue by using biopsy specimens to determine Gleason Grade but only obtained data from a single center. This caused the DLS performance to be lower for the external test set [163]. Both studies utilized digital slide review, which is not universally accepted by all pathologists. They also did not show that either DLS could stage or review the slides for unusual pathology, other tumor types, or foreign tissue that could be present in prostate biopsies.

Overall, there have been promising advances in DLS for the automated Gleason grading of prostate cancer. Both of the studies discussed above were conducted at approximately the same time in slightly different manners. They used different training methods for each DLS as well as different types of specimens. It appears that semiautomatic labeling for training the DLS of the second study paired with the multicenter data retrieval of the first study could produce even more generalizable results. The ability to further classify regions into "fine-grained Gleason patterns" could increase classification accuracy and agreement within the DLS. Utilizing the Gleason Grade of biopsy specimens instead of prostatectomy specimens is essential in providing insight for determining the next steps in clinical care for patients with prostate adenocarcinoma. Other investigators have also developed and built algorithms for the diagnosis and detection as well as grading of prostate cancer [164—167], and it is expected that similar methods and tools will continue to flourish as digitization of pathology workflow continues to increase with increasing adoption of these tools.

Conclusions

Significant technologic gains have led to the adoption of innovative digital imaging solutions in pathology. WSI, which refers to scanning of conventional glass slides to produce digital slides, is the most recent imaging modality being employed by pathology departments worldwide. WSI continues to gain traction among pathologists for diagnostic, educational, and research purposes. The quality of the images produced is of diagnostic quality, and with the viewing software, it is possible to have annotations and clinical metadata presented with the image, resulting in a virtual microscope with all the clinical information needed to sign out the case [11]. Many recent studies have demonstrated the utility of WSI in teaching, quality assurance assessment, frozens, consultation, telepathology, image analysis, and research use [159,168,169]. Some of the advantages of using digital pathology, particularly WSI, has been the ability to help address several problems with conventional light microscopy, including eliminating the inefficiencies of "snapshot" imaging or taking images of regions of interest for meetings and conferences. Digital pathology has now paved the way to facilitate the sharing of cases/slides across distances. Now, we can have access to experts, irrespective of patient location. Digital workflow also contributes to our ability to share cases with multiple colleagues simultaneously. We can start creating more smart worklists particularly aiming in the prioritization of caseloads and workload balancing. It is now possible to reallocate cases across a network, which in turn enables the experts doing expert work and generalists doing general pathology. There are access-archived images, which in turn reduce and may be eliminate physical, more expensive, movement of glass slides.

Applications of AI and ML techniques such as deep neural networks may be trained to not only recognize specific patterns on a whole slide image of an H&E slide but also AI tools may help in the interpretation of features in the tissue that are predictive and/or prognostic. With DL software deployment, pathologists will gain in the three areas of pathology workflow: information management, image sharing, and image analysis [14,26,170,171].

References

[1] Evans AJ, et al. Implementation of whole slide imaging for clinical purposes: issues to consider from the perspective of early adopters. Archives of Pathology and Laboratory Medicine 2017;141(7):944−59.

[2] Farris AB, et al. Whole slide imaging for analytical anatomic pathology and telepathology: practical applications today, promises, and perils. Archives of Pathology and Laboratory Medicine 2017;141(4):542−50.

[3] Bauer TW, Slaw RJ. Validating whole-slide imaging for consultation diagnoses in surgical pathology. Archives of Pathology and Laboratory Medicine 2014;138(11):1459−65.

[4] Dangott B, Parwani A. Whole slide imaging for teleconsultation and clinical use. Journal of Pathology Informatics 2010;1.

[5] Cornish TC, Swapp RE, Kaplan KJ. Whole-slide imaging: routine pathologic diagnosis. Advances in Anatomic Pathology 2012;19(3):152−9.

[6] Zarella MD, et al. A practical guide to whole slide imaging: a white paper from the digital pathology association. Archives of Pathology and Laboratory Medicine 2019; 143(2):222−34.

[7] Pantanowitz L, et al. Whole slide imaging for educational purposes. Journal of Pathology Informatics 2012;3:46.

[8] Mukhopadhyay S, et al. Whole slide imaging versus microscopy for primary diagnosis in surgical pathology: a multicenter blinded randomized noninferiority study of 1992 cases (Pivotal study). The American Journal of Surgical Pathology 2018;42(1):39−52.

[9] Amin S, Mori T, Itoh T. A validation study of whole slide imaging for primary diagnosis of lymphoma. Pathology International 2019;69(6):341−9.

[10] Cohen S, Furie MB. Artificial intelligence and pathobiology join forces in the American Journal of Pathology. American Journal of Pathology 2019;189(1):4−5.

[11] Hanna MG, et al. Whole slide imaging equivalency and efficiency study: experience at a large academic center. Modern Pathology 2019;32(7):916−28.

[12] Malarkey DE, et al. Utilizing whole slide images for pathology peer review and working groups. Toxicologic Pathology 2015;43(8):1149−57.

[13] Romero Lauro G, et al. Digital pathology consultations-a new era in digital imaging, challenges and practical applications. Journal of Digital Imaging 2013;26(4):668−77.

[14] Parwani AV. Next generation diagnostic pathology: use of digital pathology and artificial intelligence tools to augment a pathological diagnosis. Diagnostic Pathology 2019;14(1):138.

[15] Farahani N, Parwani AV, Pantanowitz L. Whole slide imaging in pathology: advantages, limitations, and emerging perspectives. Pathology and Laboratory Medicine International 2015;7:23−33.

[16] Amin W, Srintrapun SJ, Parwani AV. Automated whole slide imaging. Expert Opinion on Medical Diagnostics 2008;2(10):1173−81.

[17] Pantanowitz L, et al. Review of the current state of whole slide imaging in pathology. Journal of Pathology Informatics 2011;2:36.

[18] Park Y, et al. Whole slide scanner and anatomic pathology laboratory information system integration with HL7 interface to support digital pathology sign-out workflow. Modern Pathology 2019;32.

[19] Pantanowitz L, et al. Validating whole slide imaging for diagnostic purposes in pathology: guideline from the College of American Pathologists Pathology and Laboratory Quality Center. Archives of Pathology and Laboratory Medicine 2013;137(12): 1710−22.

[20] Parwani AV, et al. Regulatory barriers surrounding the use of whole slide imaging in the United States of America. Journal of Pathology Informatics 2014;5(1):38.

[21] Saco A, et al. Validation of whole-slide imaging in the primary diagnosis of liver biopsies in a University Hospital. Digestive and Liver Disease 2017;49(11):1240—6.

[22] Evans AJ, et al. US Food and Drug administration approval of whole slide imaging for primary diagnosis: a key milestone is reached and new questions are raised. Archives of Pathology and Laboratory Medicine 2018;142(11):1383—7.

[23] Boyce BF. Whole slide imaging: uses and limitations for surgical pathology and teaching. Biotechnic and Histochemistry 2015;90(5):321—30.

[24] Allen TC. Regulating artificial intelligence for a successful pathology future. Archives of Pathology and Laboratory Medicine 2019;143(10):1175—9.

[25] Chang HY, et al. Artificial intelligence in pathology. Journal of Pathology and Translational Medicine 2019;53(1):1—12.

[26] Colling R, et al. Artificial intelligence in digital pathology: a roadmap to routine use in clinical practice. The Journal of Pathology 2019;249(2):143—50.

[27] Harmon SA, et al. Artificial intelligence at the intersection of pathology and radiology in prostate cancer. Diagnostic and Interventional Radiology 2019;25(3):183—8.

[28] Niazi MKK, Parwani AV, Gurcan MN. Digital pathology and artificial intelligence. The Lancet Oncology 2019;20(5):e253—61.

[29] Acs B, Hartman J. Next generation pathology: artificial intelligence enhances histopathology practice. The Journal of Pathology 2020;250(1):7—8.

[30] Abels E, Pantanowitz L. Current state of the regulatory trajectory for whole slide imaging devices in the USA. Journal of Pathology Informatics 2017;8:23.

[31] Ferreira R, et al. The virtual microscope. Proceedings of the AMIA Annual Fall Symposium 1997:449—53.

[32] Park S, et al. The history of pathology informatics: a global perspective. Journal of Pathology Informatics 2013;4:7.

[33] Amin W, et al. Use of whole slide imaging for tissue microarrays: the cooperative prostate cancer tissue resource model. Modern Pathology 2009;22:379a.

[34] Niazi MKK, et al. Advancing clinicopathologic diagnosis of high-risk neuroblastoma using computerized image analysis and proteomic profiling. Pediatric and Developmental Pathology 2017;20(5):394—402.

[35] LeCun Y, Bengio Y, Hinton G. Deep learning. Nature 2015;521(7553):436—44.

[36] Barisoni L, et al. Digital pathology imaging as a novel platform for standardization and globalization of quantitative nephropathology. Clinical Kidney Journal 2017;10(2):176—87.

[37] Khalid Khan Niazi M, Yazgan E, Lee C, Parwani A, Gurcan MN. Identifying bladder layers from H and E images using U-Net image segmentation, Proc. SPIE 11320, Medical Imaging 2020: Digital Pathology, 1132006, 2020: https://doi.org/10.1117/12.2549608.

[38] Wong STC. Is pathology prepared for the adoption of artificial intelligence? Cancer Cytopathology 2018;126(6):373—5.

[39] Wang S, et al. Artificial intelligence in lung cancer pathology image analysis. Cancers (Basel) 2019;11(11).

[40] Reyes C, et al. Intra-observer reproducibility of whole slide imaging for the primary diagnosis of breast needle biopsies. Journal of Pathology Informatics 2014;5(1):5.

[41] Saylor C, et al. Evaluation of whole slide imaging systems prior to establishing a model digital pathology network for the air force medical service: methods and selection criteria. Modern Pathology 2013;26:382a.

[42] Tizhoosh HR, Pantanowitz L. Artificial intelligence and digital pathology: challenges and opportunities. Journal of Pathology Informatics 2018;9:38.

[43] Aeffner F, et al. Whole-slide imaging: the future is here. Veterinary Pathology Online 2018;55(4):488—9.

[44] Salto-Tellez M, Maxwell P, Hamilton P. Artificial intelligence-the third revolution in pathology. Histopathology 2019;74(3):372—6.

[45] Aeffner F, et al. Digital microscopy, image analysis, and virtual slide repository. ILAR Journal 2018;59(1):66—79.

[46] Furness PN. The use of digital images in pathology. The Journal of Pathology 1997; 183(3):253—63.

[47] Yagi Y, Gilbertson JR. Digital imaging in pathology: the case for standardization. Journal of Telemedicine and Telecare 2005;11(3):109—16.

[48] Leong FJ, Leong AS. Digital imaging applications in anatomic pathology. Advances in Anatomic Pathology 2003;10(2):88—95.

[49] Park S, Pantanowitz L, Parwani AV. Digital imaging in pathology. Clinics in Laboratory Medicine 2012;32(4):557—84.

[50] Park S, et al. Workflow organization in pathology. Clinics in Laboratory Medicine 2012;32(4):601—22.

[51] Park SL, et al. Anatomic pathology laboratory information systems: a review. Advances in Anatomic Pathology 2012;19(2):81—96.

[52] Marchevsky AM, et al. Storage and distribution of pathology digital images using integrated web-based viewing systems. Archives of Pathology and Laboratory Medicine 2002;126(5):533—9.

[53] Brachtel E, Yagi Y. Digital imaging in pathology—current applications and challenges. Journal of Biophotonics 2012;5(4):327—35.

[54] Amin M, et al. Integration of digital gross pathology images for enterprise-wide access. Journal of Pathology Informatics 2012;3:10.

[55] Cross S. Websites review-pathology images. Histopathology 2001;38(4):376.

[56] Mai KT, et al. Creating digital images of pathology specimens by using a flatbed scanner. Histopathology 2001;39(3):323—5.

[57] Fung KM, et al. Whole slide images and digital media in pathology education, testing, and practice: the Oklahoma experience. Analytical Cellular Pathology 2012;35(1): 37—40.

[58] Camparo P, et al. Utility of whole slide imaging and virtual microscopy in prostate pathology. Acta Pathologica, Microbiologica et Immunologica Scandinavica 2012; 120(4):298—304.

[59] Monaco SE, et al. A "virtual slide box" using whole slide imaging for reproductive pathology education for medical students. Laboratory Investigation 2011;91:132a.

[60] Park S, et al. Whole slide image teaching sets to support graduate medical and pathology education. Histopathology 2012;61:44.

[61] Cucoranu IC, Parwani AV, Pantanowitz L. Digital whole slide imaging in cytology. Archives of Pathology and Laboratory Medicine 2014;138(3):300.

[62] Weinstein RS. Telepathology: practicing pathology in two places at once. Clinical Laboratory Management Review 1992;6(2):171—3. discussion 174—5.

[63] Evans AJ, Kiehl TR, Croul S. Frequently asked questions concerning the use of whole-slide imaging telepathology for neuropathology frozen sections. Seminars in Diagnostic Pathology 2010;27(3):160—6.

[64] Dietz RL, Hartman DJ, Pantanowitz L. Systematic review of the use of telepathology during intraoperative consultation. American Journal of Clinical Pathology 2020; 153(2):198−209.

[65] Chong T, et al. The California telepathology service: UCLA's experience in deploying a regional digital pathology subspecialty consultation network. Journal of Pathology Informatics 2019;10:31.

[66] Laurent-Bellue A, et al. Telepathology for intra-operative frozen sections. Annales de Pathologie 2019;39(2):113−8.

[67] Girolami I, et al. Diagnostic concordance between whole slide imaging and conventional light microscopy in cytopathology: a systematic review. Cancer Cytopathology 2020;128(1):17−28.

[68] Weinstein RS, Holcomb MJ, Krupinski EA. Invention and early history of telepathology (1985−2000). Journal of Pathology Informatics 2019;10:1.

[69] Weinstein RS, et al. Overview of telepathology, virtual microscopy, and whole slide imaging: prospects for the future. Human Pathology 2009;40(8):1057−69.

[70] Weinstein RS, et al. Telepathology overview: from concept to implementation. Human Pathology 2001;32(12):1283−99.

[71] Fritz P, et al. Experience with telepathology in combination with diagnostic assistance systems in countries with restricted resources. Journal of Telemedicine and Telecare 2019;25(3). 1357633X19840475.

[72] Oberholzer M, et al. Modern telepathology: a distributed system with open standards. Current Problems in Dermatology 2003;32:102−14.

[73] Wang S, et al. Computational staining of pathology images to study the tumor microenvironment in lung cancer. Cancer Research 2020. https://doi.org/10.1158/0008-5472.CAN-19-1629.

[74] Niazi MKK, Parwani AV, Gurcan MN. Computer-assisted bladder cancer grading: α-shapes for color space decomposition. In: SPIE medical imaging. International Society for Optics and Photonics; 2016.

[75] Henricks WH. Evaluation of whole slide imaging for routine surgical pathology: looking through a broader scope. Journal of Pathology Informatics 2012;3:39.

[76] Ghaznavi F, et al. Digital imaging in pathology: whole-slide imaging and beyond. Annual Review of Pathology: Mechanisms of Disease 2013;8:331−59.

[77] Amin M, et al. Implementation of a pathology teaching website with integrated whole slide imaging for greater compatibility with tablets/smartphones. Laboratory Investigation 2013;93:375a−6a.

[78] Ho J, et al. Use of whole slide imaging in surgical pathology quality assurance: design and pilot validation studies. Human Pathology 2006;37(3):322−31.

[79] Feldman MD. Beyond morphology: whole slide imaging, computer-aided detection, and other techniques. Archives of Pathology and Laboratory Medicine 2008;132(5):758−63.

[80] Velez N, Jukic D, Ho J. Evaluation of 2 whole-slide imaging applications in dermatopathology. Human Pathology 2008;39(9):1341−9.

[81] Wilbur DC, et al. Whole-slide imaging digital pathology as a platform for teleconsultation: a pilot study using paired subspecialist correlations. Archives of Pathology and Laboratory Medicine 2009;133(12):1949−53.

[82] Xing F, Yang L. Robust nucleus/cell detection and segmentation in digital pathology and microscopy images: a comprehensive review. IEEE Reviews in Biomedical Engineering 2016;9:234−63.

[83] Gurcan MN, et al. Histopathological image analysis: a review. IEEE Reviews in Biomedical Engineering 2009;2:147−71.

[84] Cruz-Roa A, et al. High-throughput adaptive sampling for whole-slide histopathology image analysis (HASHI) via convolutional neural networks: application to invasive breast cancer detection. PloS One 2018;13(5):e0196828.

[85] Foster K. Medical education in the digital age: digital whole slide imaging as an e-learning tool. Journal of Pathology Informatics 2010;1.

[86] Dziegielewski M, Velan GM, Kumar RK. Teaching pathology using 'hotspotted' digital images. Medical Education 2003;37(11):1047−8.

[87] McClintock DS, Lee RE, Gilbertson JR. Using computerized workflow simulations to assess the feasibility of whole slide imaging full adoption in a high-volume histology laboratory. Analytical Cellular Pathology 2012;35(1):57−64.

[88] Gilbertson JR PA, Yagi Y. Clinical slide digitization - whole slide imaging in clinical practice. In: Ogilvie RW, Gu J, editors. Virtual microscopy and virtual slides in teaching, diagnosis and research. Boca Raton: Taylor and Francis; 2005.

[89] Sellaro TL, et al. Relationship between magnification and resolution in digital pathology systems. Journal of Pathology Informatics 2013;4:21.

[90] Shrestha P, Hulsken B. Color accuracy and reproducibility in whole slide imaging scanners. Journal of Medical Imaging 2014;1(2):027501.

[91] Yagi Y. Color standardization and optimization in whole slide imaging. Diagnostic Pathology 2011;6(Suppl. 1):S15.

[92] Varga VS, Molnar B, Virag T. Automated high throughput whole slide imaging using area sensors, flash light illumination and solid state light engine. Studies in Health Technology and Informatics 2012;179:187−202.

[93] Rojo MG, et al. Critical comparison of 31 commercially available digital slide systems in pathology. International Journal of Surgical Pathology 2006;14(4):285−305.

[94] Rojo MG, Bueno G. Analysis of the impact of high-resolution monitors in digital pathology. Journal of Pathology Informatics 2015;6:57.

[95] D'Haene N, et al. Comparison study of five different display modalities for whole slide images in surgical pathology and cytopathology in Europe. Medical Imaging 2013: Digital Pathology 2013:8676.

[96] Varga VS, et al. Automated multichannel fluorescent whole slide imaging and its application for cytometry. Cytometry, Part A 2009;75(12):1020−30.

[97] Rojo MG, Daniel C, Schrader T. Standardization efforts of digital pathology in Europe. Analytical Cellular Pathology 2012;35(1):19−23.

[98] Ameisen D, et al. Towards better digital pathology workflows: programming libraries for high-speed sharpness assessment of whole slide images. Diagnostic Pathology 2014;9(Suppl. 1):S3.

[99] Al-Janabi S, et al. Whole slide images for primary diagnostics of gastrointestinal tract pathology: a feasibility study. Human Pathology 2012;43(5):702−7.

[100] Lebre R, et al. Collaborative framework for a whole-slide image viewer. 2019 IEEE 32nd International Symposium on Computer-Based Medical Systems (Cbms) 2019: 221−4.

[101] Thorstenson S, Molin J, Lundstrom C. Implementation of large-scale routine diagnostics using whole slide imaging in Sweden: digital pathology experiences 2006−2013. Journal of Pathology Informatics 2014;5(1):14.

[102] Marques Godinho T, et al. An efficient architecture to support digital pathology in standard medical imaging repositories. Journal of Biomedical Informatics 2017;71: 190−7.

[103] Girolami I, et al. The landscape of digital pathology in transplantation: from the beginning to the virtual E-slide. Journal of Pathology Informatics 2019;10:21.

[104] Yeh FC, et al. Automated grading of renal cell carcinoma using whole slide imaging. Journal of Pathology Informatics 2014;5(1):23.

[105] Campbell WS, et al. Whole slide imaging diagnostic concordance with Light microscopy for breast needle biopsies. Human Pathology 2014;45(8):1713−21.

[106] Jodogne S, et al. Open implementation of DICOM for whole-slide microscopic imaging. Proceedings of the 12th International Joint Conference on Computer Vision, Imaging and Computer Graphics Theory and Applications (Visigrapp 2017) 2017;6: 81−7.

[107] Clunie D, et al. Digital imaging and communications in medicine whole slide imaging connectathon at digital pathology association pathology visions 2017. Journal of Pathology Informatics 2018;9:6.

[108] Lajara N, et al. Optimum web viewer application for DICOM whole slide image visualization in anatomical pathology. Computer Methods and Programs in Biomedicine 2019:179.

[109] Khvatkov V, Harris E. Pathology: the last digital frontier of biomedical imaging. Medical Laboratory Observer 2013;45(11):28−9.

[110] Déniz O, et al. Multi-stained whole slide image alignment in digital pathology. In: SPIE medical imaging. International Society for Optics and Photonics; 2015.

[111] Schonmeyer R, et al. Automated whole slide analysis of differently stained and Co-registered tissue sections. In: Bildverarbeitung Fur Die Medizin 2015: Algorithmen - systeme - Anwendungen; 2015. p. 407−12.

[112] Hartman DJ, et al. Enterprise implementation of digital pathology: feasibility, challenges, and opportunities. Journal of Digital Imaging 2017;30(5):555−60.

[113] Ho J, et al. Needs and workflow assessment prior to implementation of a digital pathology infrastructure for the US Air Force Medical Service. Journal of Pathology Informatics 2013;4:32.

[114] Lloyd M, et al. How to acquire over 500,000 whole slides images a year: creating a massive novel data modality to accelerate cancer research. Modern Pathology 2018; 31:592−3.

[115] Guo H, et al. Digital pathology and anatomic pathology laboratory information system integration to support digital pathology sign-out. Journal of Pathology Informatics 2016;7:23.

[116] Boyce BF. An update on the validation of whole slide imaging systems following FDA approval of a system for a routine pathology diagnostic service in the United States. Biotechnic and Histochemistry 2017;92(6):381−9.

[117] Pradhan D, et al. Evaluation of panoramic digital images using Panoptiq for frozen section diagnosis. Journal of Pathology Informatics 2016;7:26.

[118] Dangott B, Parwani AV. Implementation of a whole slide image database for pathology residency education. Modern Pathology 2010;23:124a.

[119] Ho J, et al. Can digital pathology result in cost savings? A financial projection for digital pathology implementation at a large integrated health care organization. Journal of Pathology Informatics 2014;5(1):33.

[120] Lloyd M, et al. Sectioning automation to improve quality and decrease costs for a high-throughput slide scanning facility. Laboratory Investigation 2019;99.

[121] Wack K, et al. A multisite validation of whole slide imaging for primary diagnosis using standardized data collection and analysis. Journal of Pathology Informatics 2016; 7:49.

[122] Evans JL, et al. A scalable, cloud-based, unsupervised deep learning system for identification, extraction, and summarization of potentially imperceptible patterns in whole-slide images of breast cancer tissue. Cancer Research 2019;79(13).

[123] Rojo MG, Castro AM, Goncalves L. COST Action "EuroTelepath": digital pathology integration in electronic health record, including primary care centres. Diagnostic Pathology 2011;6(Suppl. 1):S6.

[124] Natan M. Achieving simultaneous improvements in workflow and multiplexing in whole-slide tissue imaging. Cancer Research 2018;78(13).

[125] Sarwar S, et al. Physician perspectives on integration of artificial intelligence into diagnostic pathology. NPJ Digital Medicine 2019;2:28.

[126] Menter T, et al. Intraoperative frozen section consultation by remote whole-slide imaging analysis—validation and comparison to robotic remote microscopy. Journal of Clinical Pathology 2019;1—3. https://doi.org/10.1136/jclinpath-2019-206261. online only.

[127] Jukic DM, et al. Clinical examination and validation of primary diagnosis in anatomic pathology using whole slide digital images. Archives of Pathology and Laboratory Medicine 2011;135(3):372—8.

[128] Thrall MJ. Validation of two whole slide imaging scanners based on the draft guidelines of the College of American Pathologists. Laboratory Investigation 2013;93: 487a.

[129] Bongaerts O, et al. Conventional microscopical versus digital whole-slide imaging-based diagnosis of thin-layer cervical specimens: a validation study. Journal of Pathology Informatics 2018;9:29.

[130] Lee JJ, et al. Validation of digital pathology for primary histopathological diagnosis of routine, inflammatory dermatopathology cases. The American Journal of Dermatopathology 2018;40(1):17—23.

[131] Bonsembiante F, et al. Diagnostic validation of a whole-slide imaging scanner in cytological samples: diagnostic accuracy and comparison with light microscopy. Veterinary Pathology 2019;56(3):429—34.

[132] Tabata K, et al. Whole-slide imaging at primary pathological diagnosis: validation of whole-slide imaging-based primary pathological diagnosis at twelve Japanese academic institutes. Pathology International 2017;67(11):547—54.

[133] Evans AJ, Asa SL. Whole slide imaging telepathology (WSITP) for primary diagnosis in surgical pathology: a comprehensive validation study at university health network (UHN). Laboratory Investigation 2012;92:391a.

[134] Pekmezei M, et al. Concordance between whole-slide imaging and light microscopy for surgical neuropathology. Laboratory Investigation 2014;94:509a.

[135] Ordi J, et al. Validation of whole slide imaging in the primary diagnosis of gynaecological pathology in a University Hospital. Journal of Clinical Pathology 2015;68(1): 33—9.

[136] Baidoshvili A, et al. Validation of a whole-slide image-based teleconsultation network. Histopathology 2018;73(5):777—83.

[137] Sturm B, et al. Validation of diagnosing melanocytic lesions on whole slide images-does z-stack scanning improve diagnostic accuracy? Virchows Archiv 2017;471: S15.

[138] Eze O, et al. Validation of multiple high-throughput whole slide imaging (WSI) systems for primary diagnoses and clinical applications at a large academic institution. Laboratory Investigation 2019;99.

[139] Robertson S, et al. Digital image analysis in breast pathology-from image processing techniques to artificial intelligence. Translational Research 2018;194:19—35.

[140] Dimitriou N, Arandjelovic O, Caie PD. Deep learning for whole slide image analysis: an overview. Frontiers in Medicine 2019;6.

[141] Aeffner F, et al. Introduction to digital image analysis in whole-slide imaging: a white paper from the digital pathology association. Journal of Pathology Informatics 2019; 10:9.

[142] Kong H, Gurcan M, Belkacem-Boussaid K. Partitioning histopathological images: an integrated framework for supervised color-texture segmentation and cell splitting. IEEE Transactions on Medical Imaging 2011;30(9):1661—77.

[143] Voelker F, Potts S. Whole-slide image analysis with smart tissue finding on common toxicological problems. Toxicologic Pathology 2009;37(1):146.

[144] Lin HJ, et al. Fast ScanNet: fast and dense analysis of multi-gigapixel whole-slide images for cancer metastasis detection. IEEE Transactions on Medical Imaging 2019; 38(8):1948—58.

[145] Niazi MKK, Downs-Kelly E, Gurcan MN. Hot spot detection for breast cancer in Ki-67 stained slides: image dependent filtering approach. In: SPIE medical imaging. International Society for Optics and Photonics; 2014.

[146] Strack M, Sandusky G, Rushing D. Digital whole slide quantitative image analysis of TOPO II and P53 in sarcomas evaluating both primary and lung metastatic tumors. Cancer Research 2016;76.

[147] Romo-Bucheli D, et al. Automated tubule nuclei quantification and correlation with oncotype DX risk categories in ER plus breast cancer whole slide images. Medical Imaging 2016: Digital Pathology 2016:9791.

[148] Shin H-C, et al. Deep convolutional neural networks for computer-aided detection: CNN architectures, dataset characteristics and transfer learning. IEEE Transactions on Medical Imaging 2016;35(5):1285—98.

[149] Sirinukunwattana K, et al. Locality sensitive deep learning for detection and classification of nuclei in routine colon cancer histology images. IEEE Transactions on Medical Imaging 2016;35(5):1196—206.

[150] Bejnordi BE, et al. Context-aware stacked convolutional neural networks for classification of breast carcinomas in whole-slide histopathology images. Journal of Medical Imaging 2017;4(4).

[151] Chen M, et al. Automated segmentation of the choroid in EDI-OCT images with retinal pathology using convolution neural networks. Fetal Infant Ophthalmic Medical Image Analysis (2017) 2017;10554:177—84.

[152] Cruz-Roa A, et al. Accurate and reproducible invasive breast cancer detection in whole-slide images: a Deep Learning approach for quantifying tumor extent. Scientific Reports 2017;7.

[153] Jamaluddin MF, Fauzi MFA, Abas FS. Tumor detection and whole slide classification of H&E lymph node images using convolutional neural network. 2017 IEEE International Conference on Signal and Image Processing Applications (Icsipa) 2017:90—5.

[154] Korbar B, et al. Looking under the hood: deep neural network visualization to interpret whole-slide image analysis outcomes for colorectal polyps. 2017 IEEE Conference on Computer Vision and Pattern Recognition Workshops (Cvprw) 2017:821—7.

[155] Nirschl J, et al. Deep learning classifier to predict cardiac failure from whole slide H&E images. Modern Pathology 2017;30:532a—3a.

[156] Gurcan MN, et al. Image analysis for neuroblastoma classification: segmentation of cell nuclei. In: 28th Annual international conference of the IEEE engineering in medicine and biology society. IEEE; 2006.

[157] Di Cataldo S, et al. Automated segmentation of tissue images for computerized IHC analysis. Computer Methods and Programs in Biomedicine 2010;100(1):1—15.

[158] Chen CM, et al. A computer-aided diagnosis system for differentiation and delineation of malignant regions on whole-slide prostate histopathology image using spatial statistics and multidimensional DenseNet. Medical Physics 2020;47(3):1021—33. https://doi.org/10.1002/mp.13964.

[159] Volynskaya Z, Evans AJ, Asa SL. Clinical applications of whole-slide imaging in anatomic pathology. Advances in Anatomic Pathology 2017;24(4):215—21.

[160] Epstein JI. Is there enough support for a new prostate grading system factoring in intraductal carcinoma and cribriform cancer? European Urology 2020;77(2):199—200.

[161] Gandhi JS, et al. Reporting practices and resource utilization in the era of intraductal carcinoma of the prostate: a survey of genitourinary subspecialists. The American Journal of Surgical Pathology 2019. https://doi.org/10.1097/PAS.0000000000001417. online only.

[162] Nagpal K, et al. Development and validation of a deep learning algorithm for improving Gleason scoring of prostate cancer. NPJ Digital Medicine 2019;2:48.

[163] Bulten W, et al. Automated deep-learning system for Gleason grading of prostate cancer using biopsies: a diagnostic study. The Lancet Oncology 2020;21(2):233—41.

[164] Zhou NY, Gao Y. Optimized color decomposition of localized whole slide images and convolutional neural network for intermediate prostate cancer classification. Medical Imaging 2017: Digital Pathology 2017:10140.

[165] Campanella G, et al. Clinical-grade computational pathology using weakly supervised deep learning on whole slide images. Nature Medicine 2019;25(8):1301.

[166] Huang CH, Racoceanu D. Automated high-grade prostate cancer detection and ranking on whole slide images. Medical Imaging 2017: Digital Pathology 2017: 10140.

[167] Kyriazis AD, et al. An end-to-end system for automatic characterization of Iba1 immunopositive microglia in whole slide imaging. Neuroinformatics 2019;17(3):373—89.

[168] Parimi V, et al. Validation of whole frozen section slide image diagnosis in surgical pathology. Modern Pathology 2016;29:399a—400a.

[169] Fertig RM, et al. Whole slide imaging. The American Journal of Dermatopathology 2018;40(12):938—9.

[170] Ibrahim A, et al. Artificial intelligence in digital breast pathology: techniques and applications. Breast 2019;49:267—73.

[171] Stevenson CH, Hong SC, Ogbuehi KC. Development of an artificial intelligence system to classify pathology and clinical features on retinal fundus images. Clinical and Experimental Ophthalmology 2019;47(4):484—9.

Applications of artificial intelligence for image enhancement in pathology

Tanishq Abraham[1], Austin Todd[2], Daniel A. Orringer, MD[3], Richard Levenson, MD[4]

[1]*Department of Biomedical Engineering, University of California, Davis, CA, United States;* [2]*UT Health, San Antonio, TX, United States;* [3]*Associate Professor, Department of Surgery, NYU Langone Health, New York City, NY, United States;* [4]*Professor and Vice Chair, Pathology and Laboratory Medicine, UC Davis Health, Sacramento, CA, United States*

Introduction

This chapter will describe and discuss opportunity for artificial intelligence (AI) to contribute to image quality improvements and to simplify and accelerate imaging methods. There are two major goals for adding AI to imaging tasks. The first is direct image enhancement and conversion to different imaging modes (for example, autofluorescence to simulated H&E) for direct visual "consumption." The second is the eventual deployment of AI-based classification and quantitative approaches. We will concentrate on the former and give one example of the latter, which demonstrates the real-world application of AI in intraoperative surgical guidance in brain tumor surgery. This approach, which has already entered the clinic, accomplishes not only improved patient care via accelerated, high-quality tumor-site imaging but also can reintegrate pathology into surgical decision-making and reinforce collaborative relationships. This will be explored in detail in the latter section of this chapter.

The basic underpinning of all the approaches to be discussed below is that there is information content present in images that is hard to discern with direct (human) visual observation, but that can be elicited using AI tools that have been trained to associate image type 1 with image type 2. This requires some degree of image content stereotyping, in that the relationships have to be established within a context of a relatively limited spatial, textural, and biological variability. While transfer learning from "irrelevant" sources, such as images of cats and dogs, can prime a learning network to be sensitive to image primitives such as edges and textures, it will not do a good job predicting image content for histology specimens without specific and focused exemplars. To take this argument to the limit, the more random noise or extreme variation is present, the poorer AI predictive or conversion tools will perform. It is impossible to take an image consisting of pure noise, downsize it, and then predict via AI its true high-resolution content. Fortunately, histology does exhibit a limited repertoire—only so many colors are anticipated, nuclei

Artificial Intelligence and Deep Learning in Pathology. https://doi.org/10.1016/B978-0-323-67538-3.00007-5

have a reasonable degree of self-similarity, the background is often mostly white or mostly black, and so on.

Various image conversion tasks have been identified as worth pursuing in histology, and these are described below.

Common machine learning tasks

In histopathology, there are several tasks that can be assisted through the application of deep learning technologies. Most of these problems fall into four classes: classification, segmentation, image translation, and image style transfer. Here, we will briefly define these tasks and explain how problems in histopathology can be formulated as common machine learning tasks. In all cases, we focus on image tasks, as this is most relevant to histopathology.

Classification

Image classification refers to the task of assigning a label to an image. Much of the field of histopathology is comprised of various classification tasks. This is since histopathology is mainly focused on assigning a diagnosis based on review of slide-based microscopy. Automatic classification of tissue structures and subtypes can also be extremely useful to augment and improve the histopathology workflow.

As a central problem in computer vision and machine learning, the methodologies for solving classification problems have been broadly explored in both academic and well-funded commercial enterprises and considerable progress has been made. The leading algorithms for image classification are convolutional neural networks (CNNs), which have demonstrated better-than-human performance on various benchmark datasets [1–6], although their real-world performance across novel institutions and differently curated collections remains to be determined. We will briefly cover an example application of deep learning–based classification in histology used for intraoperative surgical guidance in Deep learning for computationally aided diagnosis in histopathology section.

Segmentation

Image segmentation refers to the task of assigning labels to specific regions of an image. It can also be seen as a pixel-level classification task. Segmentation of subcellular structures, such as nuclei and cytoplasm and membrane compartments, can be useful for automating common tasks such as cell enumeration (via nuclei counting), determination of intracellular locations of molecular markers, and is important for analysis of subcellular morphological features such as nuclear size, eccentricity and chromatin texture [7]. Automatic segmentation can also be used to help pathologists recognize tissue components by delineating different tissue types. While segmentation in pathology is not a focus of this chapter, some image microscopy problems can be reformulated as segmentation problems. More importantly, the most common deep learning architecture for segmentation, U-nets, is often utilized for image enhancement tasks, as we will see later.

Image translation and style transfer

Image translation refers to the conversion of one image representation to another image representation. The goal is to learn the transformation between the input and output images. This can be applied to a wide variety of applications, such as converting between night and day images, winter and summer images, or more useful tasks like converting satellite images to maps. In computational pathology, image-to-image translation has been explored for stain color normalization (Section Stain color normalization) and for converting between different image modalities (Section Mode switching). The most common models used for image translation tasks are generative adversarial networks or their variants (Section Generative adversarial networks and their variants). Most model architectures for image translation tasks require paired-image datasets. However, in some cases, obtaining paired datasets may be difficult or even impossible. For example, when converting between image modalities, it may be impossible to obtain pixel-scale paired images using different image modalities. Therefore, models like CycleGANs (Section Generative adversarial networks and their variants) have been developed to solve the problem of unpaired image-to-image translation.

Another task related to that is style transfer [8,9]. Style transfer focuses on transferring the style of a single reference image to the content of the input image in order to generate an output image. Style transfer can be thought of as a single-sample version of image-to-image translation. Style transfer also has potential applications in computational pathology, such as for stain-color normalization, the task being to convert an input image to have the color gamut and structural color assignments that mimic a target, reference image. This is demonstrated in Ref. [10].

Commonly used deep learning methodologies
Convolutional neural networks

A CNN belongs to a class of deep learning algorithms most commonly used for image tasks such as image classification (Fig. 7.1A). The building blocks of a CNN are learned convolutional kernels [11,12]. These convolutional kernels are applied to the image and their subsequent representations in the neural network in order to extract learned features. The convolutional kernels are developed during the training process, and updated through backpropagation. A key advantage of convolutional layers is their shift invariance [11]. As the convolutional kernel is applied over the entire image, shifts in the input shift the output in an equivalent manner. This is an especially useful property for microscopy. The stacking of convolutional layers and other layers such as fully connected layers and pooling layers are used to build CNNs.

FIGURE 7.1

(A) Convolutional neural networks take in images with an input layer, extract features with convolutional blocks in the hidden layers, and often output a label probability for classification tasks. (B) U-nets comprise a contracting feature-extraction path and an expanding up-sampling path, finally outputting a segmentation map. (C) Generative adversarial networks utilize both a generator and discriminator network. The generator network takes in an input and generates an image. The discriminator tries to classify between real and generated images. The discriminator tries to maximize correct classification in the form of a GAN loss, while generated images try to minimize it. (D) CycleGANs contain two sets of generators and discriminators to convert between two domains in both directions.

(A) Adapted with permission from Topol EJ. High-performance medicine: the convergence of human and artificial intelligence. Nature Medicine *2019;25(1):44–56. https://doi.org/10.1038/s41591-018-0300-7; Shaban MT, Baur C, Navab N, Albarqouni S. Staingan: stain style transfer for digital histological images. In: 2019 IEEE 16th international symposium on biomedical imaging (ISBI 2019); 2019. pp. 953–956. https://doi.org/10.1109/ ISBI.2019.8759152; (B) Adapted with permission from Ronneberger O, Fischer P, Brox T. U-net: convolutional networks for biomedical image segmentation. In: Medical image computing and computer-assisted intervention — MICCAI 2015, Cham; 2015. pp. 234–241. https://doi.org/10.1007/978-3-319-24574-4_28; (D) Adapted with permission from Zhu JY, Park T, Isola P, Efros AA. Unpaired image-to-image translation using cycle-consistent adversarial networks. In: 2017 IEEE international conference on computer vision (ICCV), Venice; 2017. pp. 2242–2251. https://doi.org/10.1109/ICCV.2017.244.*

A variety of CNN architectures have been developed, but some network architectures are more commonly used due to their generalizability and effectiveness over a wide variety of tasks. Some of the most common architectures include VGG nets [4], ResNets [5], and Inception nets [6].

For many computer vision tasks, there is little data available for successful training of CNNs from scratch. However, the knowledge of models trained on larger datasets can be transferred for application to learning cycles applied to a smaller, focused dataset [13]. This takes advantage of the fact that many of the convolutional layers derived from large-dataset-derived models serve to extract general, low-level features. Therefore, only some of the layers of models that were pretrained on larger datasets are subsequently retrained on the smaller dataset. This process is known as transfer learning.

U-nets

A wide variety of algorithms and deep learning architectures [14,15] are used for image segmentation, but undoubtedly the most common neural network architecture for image segmentation is the U-net [16] (Fig. 7.1B). Ronneberger et al. originally introduced U-nets specifically for biomedical segmentation, but this approach has now been used across a variety of segmentation problems. This work builds upon existing fully convolutional architectures [14] by adding up sampling operations with many feature channels to the contracting subnetworks. As a result, there is an expansive path that is symmetric to the contracting path, leading to a u-shaped architecture. This model was tested successfully across various cell and more complex tissue segmentation tasks [16].

While U-nets were originally developed for segmentation, they have been used for other paired image tasks such as achieving computational super-resolution [17], and are commonly employed as components in some generative adversarial networks (GANs) (described below). With some 10,000 citations already reported in Google Scholar, the U-net architecture is clearly one of the most influential deep learning architectures developed to date.

Generative adversarial networks and their variants

A generative adversarial network (GAN) is a deep learning method that was pioneered by Goodfellow et al. [18] and leverages multiple neural networks working "against" each other to transform images of different classes (Fig. 7.1C). The basic premise is that one neural network (the "generator") is trained to take images of one class and transform them into a second class, for example, taking zebras and turning them into horses. The second neural network (the "discriminator") is trained to discriminate real images of horses from fake images generated by the first network.

This is done cyclically until the images generated cannot be classified accurately as generated or real by the discriminator. The potential for this method has been continually explored and expanded since its original description in 2014; it has found many applications, such as in super-resolution [19] and artistic endeavors [20]. One of the early limitations of this general methodology was that the data had to be pixel-registered to facilitate training. In other words, the starting and target mode images needed to contain exactly the same scene. This is tractable in situations in which a slide is imaged under one condition, and then reimaged perhaps after additional staining steps. In this case, the scenes being viewed have intrinsically pixel-registered content. This requirement makes creation of large datasets for complex applications costly and time-consuming if it is possible at all. CycleGAN [21] is a variation of the traditional method that aimed to correct this problem by adding cyclic consistency between the conversions, allowing the training to be completely unsupervised with spatially unpaired (but contextually paired) images (Fig. 7.1D). This is accomplished by doubling the number of neural networks and training the network to not only convert from, for example, zebras to horses, but also from zebras to horses and then back to zebras. By forcing the reconstruction of the original image from the converted image the training is almost pseudo-supervised, permitting unpaired image training. Applications of this class of deep learning tools (mostly) in histopathology are described in more detail below.

Common training and testing practices
Dataset preparation and preprocessing

Often, when applying deep learning to microscopy, ground truth and input images are collected separately. For example, images of the same sample may be taken on separate microscopes with different imaging modalities. In this case, the images need to be aligned to obtain a paired-image dataset. Many image coregistration approaches have been developed for accurate image coregistration [24]. Often a global registration algorithm is used for rough coregistration of the image, while a subsequent local coregistration algorithm is used to account for local deformations. Often, accurate coregistration is essential for the performance of an algorithm on a paired dataset. Note that coregistration is not required for unpaired image translation tasks, however.

Not infrequently, datasets are quite small and only represent a small sample of the kinds of images a trained model could be applied to. A neural network model generalizes well across a diverse set of samples if there is a large and diverse training set. If the dataset is small, the model might perform well on the training set, but may not perform well on unseen data. This phenomenon is known as overfitting. In order to overcome this challenge, two methods are commonly used. Transfer learning, as discussed in the Convolutional neural networks section, can be used to decrease the amount of data required for training [13]. Additionally, data augmentation is a common approach for improving the utility of small datasets. This involves the creation of synthetic but representative examples for the dataset. More specifically, transformations like rotation, flipping, distorting, color variation, etc. are used to create new images and augment the original image dataset [25]. Data augmentation is therefore a useful technique for limiting overfitting.

Loss functions

In order to train a neural network, the weights (i.e., the trainable parameters of the network) of the neural network are adjusted to minimize a user-defined loss function that best represents the task that the neural network is required to solve. For classification tasks, the most commonly used loss function is a cross entropy loss. When comparing between predicted and ground-truth images in image-mapping tasks, the cost function is instead usually based on per-pixel differences, such as mean absolute error (L1 loss) or mean squared error (L2 loss). Other networks can also have specialized loss functions for training, such as GANs (adversarial loss) and cycleGANs (cyclic loss). Loss functions can also be augmented with regularization terms (e.g., weight decay, identity loss) in order to prevent overfitting. In many cases, careful selection of the loss function is critical in optimizing the performance of the neural network.

Metrics

Quantitative metrics are required in order to reliably evaluate the performance of a model. For classification tasks, the most common metrics includes accuracy and area under the curve of the receiver operating characteristic (AUC-ROC). For segmentation tasks, the most common metrics are intersection over union and Dice scores. However, for image translation and style transfer tasks, the most appropriate metric is often dependent on the application. For applications in microscopy, metrics such as structural similarity index (SSIM), peak signal-to-noise ratio (PSNR), and Pearson correlation coefficient are often used to compare the structural content between the predicted and ground truth images.

Deep learning for microscopy enhancement in histopathology

Stain color normalization

A major problem in the field of computational pathology and computer-aided diagnosis (CAD) is variability between individual stained whole-slide (WSI) microscopy images. Different scanners, staining procedures, and institutional environments can lead to wide variance in staining appearance. Image analysis methods find it difficult to cope with these variations in image appearance. In fact, a major contributor to CAD algorithm performance is proper deployment of a standardization algorithm [26]. Consequently, a significant body of work has been dedicated to methodologies intended to reduce variability between and within microscopy image datasets. Collectively, these algorithms are designated as stain color normalization methods (Fig. 7.2A).

One of the most popular algorithms is color deconvolution [27,28]. This algorithm attempts to determine a stain matrix, which describes how much each stain contributes to the final pixel color. However, these stain matrices do not generalize well to images from other labs and scanning platforms. Other common approaches use clustering-based algorithms. However, these require that clusters to be

FIGURE 7.2

(A) Stain color normalization is often formulated as trying to change the color of the input image to be similar to the reference image of desired H&E color. (B) The StaNoSA algorithm successfully adjusted the color distribution of the input image to match the reference image, with accurate coloring of subcellular structures. (C) An end-to-end neural network was developed with a two-path architecture. A feature extractor path utilizes a VGG19, while a transformer network utilizes feature-aware normalization units to transform the input image into a normalized image. (D) A GAN-based approach was used to successfully normalize H&E images and reduce interscanner variability. Additionally, using GAN-based normalization as preprocessing also improved classification results on a tumor dataset.

(A) Adapted with permission from Janowczyk A, Basavanhally A, Madabhushi A, Stain normalization using sparse AutoEncoders (StaNoSA): application to digital pathology, Computerized Medical Imaging and Graphics *2017; 57:50—61. https://doi.org/10.1016/j.compmedimag.2016.05.003; (B) Adapted from permission from Janowczyk A, Basavanhally A, Madabhushi A, Stain normalization using sparse AutoEncoders (StaNoSA): application to digital pathology,* Computerized Medical Imaging and Graphics *2017;57:50—61. https://doi.org/ 10.1016/j.compmedimag.2016.05.003; (C) Adapted with permission from Bug D, et al., Context-based normalization of histological stains using deep convolutional features. In:* Deep learning in medical image analysis and multimodal learning for clinical decision support, Cham; *2017. pp. 135—142. https://doi.org/10. 1007/978-3-319-67558-9_16; (D) Adapted with permission from Shaban MT, Baur C, Navab N, and Albar-qouni S, Staingan: stain style transfer for digital histological images. In* 2019 IEEE 16th international sympo-sium on biomedical imaging (ISBI 2019); *2019, pp. 953—956. https://doi.org/10.1109/ISBI.2019.8759152.*

proportionately represented in the images. Both of these approaches are color-based and do not incorporate spatial information. However, recent algorithms, especially those that employ deep learning, have begun to utilize contextual information to improve normalization.

Here, we will highlight a few studies that incorporate deep learning into new stain normalization algorithms. For a more thorough review on both traditional and deep learning—based stain color normalization algorithms, please refer to Ref. [29,30].

In Janowczyk et al. [27], an unsupervised deep learning approach termed Stain Normalization using Sparse AutoEncoders (StaNoSA) was developed to overcome some of the challenges with traditional stain color normalization methods (Fig. 7.2B). A sparse autoencoder is trained on the dataset, and the embeddings of the template were clustered with K-means clustering and the input image embeddings were assigned to the K clusters. Then a traditional histogram matching algorithm was applied per cluster. Three datasets were used to evaluate the StaNoSA algorithm. A breast biopsy slide dataset was used to study how StaNoSA could decrease intrascanner and interscanner variation. A gastrointestinal biopsy slide dataset was used to study how StaNoSA could decrease variability between sites, which was simulated with different staining protocols. The third dataset is a subset of the second with nuclei annotations to test how StaNoSA could improve object detection in pathology. StaNoSA was also compared with four state-of-the-art techniques. StaNoSA was demonstrated to bring the interscanner error to a similar range of the intrascanner error. It also decreased variability between staining protocols with better performance than other tested techniques. Finally, StaNoSA had the best Dice score for nuclei segmentation using a simple thresholding method.

While the previous study utilized a neural network to improve normalization, a neural network architecture can also be used for end-to-end normalization processes, as done in Bug et al. [31]. Their network utilized two parallel network paths: a main transformation path and a feature extractor path (Fig. 7.2C). The feature extractor path is based on a pretrained VGG-19 architecture. The transformation path is composed of novel network blocks termed Feature Aware Normalization (FAN) units, which are inspired by batch normalization and long short-term memory units (LSTMs). The features from each block in the feature extractor network were passed into the FAN unit to gradually rescale and shift the image (similar to batchnorm) through addition and multiplication gates (similar to LSTM). As there are no paired data from H&E images, noise is deliberately added to the reference image. The noise model is constructed using normal distribution data with variances defined based on principal component analysis. To train and test the model, the staining protocol was varied by either increasing or decreasing hematoxylin concentration, eosin concentration, and slice thickness. The changes in color deviation were measured with the sum of squared differences between the color histogram (SSDH). Influence on texture was measured with the structural dissimilarity index (SDSIM). The magnitude of perceivable colors (color volume) was measured by the product of the standard deviations of the LAB color-space channels. In terms of SSDH and color volume, the proposed method significantly outperformed previous approaches. When assessed using alternative metrics, other methods performed equally well. However, these other methods required similar tissue distributions in the input and reference images, and therefore also required careful selection of a reference image. The proposed method overcomes these challenges, while providing an end-to-end algorithm to perform stain normalization, with the caveat that introduction of contextual information in the conversion model did introduce some undesirable textural changes.

Generative models have also been applied for histopathological stain color normalization. Zanjani et al. [32] introduces fully unsupervised generative models for stain-color normalization. The GAN model includes a generator network, discriminatory network, and an auxiliary network. The images are converted to CIE-LAB color space, and the lightness channel is passed into the generator, and only the chromatic channels are generated by the GAN. The auxiliary network is based on the InfoGAN architecture [33] in order to maximize the information present in the generated image. The variational autoencoder (VAE) model [34] is inputted with the H&E image in the HSD color space, with the encoder being trained to segregate the input image into tissue channels. The parameters of the color distribution are computed per tissue class. The decoder network reconstructs the chromatic channels of the input image. The deep convolutional Gaussian mixture model (DCGMM) used by these authors was a fully convolutional network jointly optimized with the parameters of a Gaussian mixture model (GMM). The DCGMM fits the GMM to the pixel-color distribution while being conditioned on the tissue classes. The detection of the tissue classes is done by exploiting CNN embeddings, in similar fashion to the output of encoder of a VAE. The algorithms were evaluated with a normalized median intensity (NMI) measure to assess color constancy of the normalized images. Out of the three models, and compared with previous state-of-the-art results, the DCGMM had highest performance, with the lowest standard deviation and coefficient of variation. While these models do not make assumptions about H&E image content, they do rely on other assumptions such as various hard-coded thresholds and nuclei shape fitting that may not be applicable to other tissue types.

The stain color normalization problem can also be reformulated as an image translation task. For example, in Shaban et al. [23], a CycleGAN was trained to reduce interscanner variability (Fig. 7.2D). The stain normalization task was reformulated as image translation between images from two different scanners. The CycleGAN, termed StainGAN in this study, outperformed other methods in terms of SSIM, FSSIM, Pearson correlation coefficient, and PSNR. StainGAN was also applied as a preprocessing step for cancer classification on the Camelyon16 dataset. The StainGAN improved the AUC-ROC of classification when compared with no normalization and alternative normalization preprocessing steps. The use of a GAN also eliminates human error that can arise when an expert is called upon to manually select a reference slide for normalization. While this application was tasked to decrease interscanner variability, similar models could be used for interlaboratory variability as well.

Tellez et al. [35] also developed a network-based stain normalization algorithm by formulating it as an image translation problem. The authors trained a U-net architecture to reconstruct the original images from inputted augmented images. The model was trained on a multiorgan, multisite dataset. They also performed systematic multicenter evaluation of several other stain color augmentation and normalization algorithms. A total of four classification tasks spanning different centers were used to determine the effect of data augmentation and stain normalization on the performance of these tasks. These tasks are mitotic figure detection, tumor metastasis detection, prostate epithelium detection, and colorectal cancer tissue type detection. Basic, morphology-based, brightness and contrast, HSV-based, and H&E-to-DAB (HED)-based augmentation methods were tested. In terms of stain normalization, starting points of no transformation, grayscale transformation, and a chromatic distribution—based technique were tested. The augmentation and stain color normalization methods were used as preprocessing for a simple patch CNN classifier. A CNN classifier was trained for each combination of organ, color normalization, and data augmentation method studied. The performance of the classifier was evaluated with the AUC-ROC metric. A global ranking of the methods based on their AUC-ROC score for each task and organ was established. Based on these rankings, it was determined that stain color augmentation was crucial for the performance of the CNN classifier. The novel deep learning—based stain color normalization also improved the results. Importantly and somewhat surprisingly, using the deep learning normalization method did not alleviate the need for color augmentation. Utilizing stain color normalization alone is insufficient to achieve high classification accuracy.

Mode switching

Traditionally, microscopy with H&E (or related) staining or fluorescent labeling requires time-consuming and potentially variable labeling procedures. In addition, staining or labeling can typically only be used for ex vivo applications. Another major disadvantage is the damage to the sample that staining and/or labeling can induce. Additionally, the act of imaging itself can degrade the specimen via forms of photodamage.

Many novel microscopy techniques have been developed in order to overcome these challenges. However, the traditional H&E-stained histopathology images are most accessible to histopathologists. Additionally, the images obtained with these new techniques may be harder to interpret, as well as susceptible to varieties of artifacts, making these techniques more difficult for histopathologists to adopt. Therefore, converting novel modalities to resemble H&E-stained slides (or vice-versa) may allow for a wider adoption of these modalities. For example, Fig. 7.3A demonstrates how quantitative phase imaging is an imaging modality that is hard for the uninitiated to interpret, but still can be introduced in a histopathologist's workflow by utilizing neural networks to convert these images to H&E-like results. We will describe several reports of how deep learning techniques are used for such mode of conversion. Most of these reports utilize GAN architectures and their variants, discussed in Section 2.3.

Quantitative phase imaging (QPI) is a relatively recent label-free imaging technique with lower phototoxicity that can be deployed on various platforms (including portable platforms). In order to bridge the gap between QPI and standard histopathology, Rivenson et al. [36] used a GAN to convert phase-based microscopy images to histological images (Fig. 7.3A—B). Three models were

FIGURE 7.3

(A) Often, novel image modalities can be difficult to interpret. However, deep neural networks can be used to convert these images to H&E-like images for better interpretation. (B) Quantitative phase imaging is an example of a difficult-to-interpret imaging modality that has other benefits over H&E images, such as lower phototoxicity and portability. A GAN was trained to convert the QPI images to digital H&E stained images. (C) A fully convolutional neural network and pixel-based VGG classification was tested for converting multiphoton microscopy images to H&E-stained images. (D) Confocal laser endomicroscopy allows for in vivo real-time analysis of tissue but is difficult to interpret. Instead of using traditional image translation algorithms like GANs, neural style transfer was used to digitally stain CLE images. GAN, generative adversarial network; QPI, quantitative phase imaging; CLE, confocal laser endomicroscopy.

(A) Adapted with permission from Rivenson Y, Liu T., Wei Z., Zhang Y., de Haan K, and Ozcan A, PhaseStain: the digital staining of label-free quantitative phase microscopy images using deep learning, Light: Science & Applications 2019;8(1):1–11. https://doi.org/10.1038/s41377-019-0129-y (B) Adapted with permission from Rivenson Y, Liu T, Wei Z, Zhang Y, de Haan K, and Ozcan A, PhaseStain: the digital staining of label-free quantitative phase microscopy images using deep learning, Light: Science & Applications 2019;8(1):1–11. https://doi.org/10.1038/s41377-019-0129-y (C) Adapted with permission from Borhani N, Bower AJ, Boppart SA, and Psaltis D, Digital staining through the application of deep neural networks to multi-modal multi-photon microscopy, Biomedical Optics Express 2019;10(3):1339–1350.https://doi.org/10.1364/BOE.10.001339; (D) Adapted with permission from Izadyyazdanabadi M, et al., Fluorescence image histology pattern transformation using image style transfer, Frontiers in Oncology 2019;9. https://doi.org/10.3389/fonc.2019.00519

trained for H&E for skin tissue, Jones' stain for kidney tissue, and Masson's trichrome for liver tissue. The models were then applied to similar images that were not present in the training set. They utilize a custom global coregistration method and elastic image registration for local feature registration. A U-net architecture is used for the generator, with H&E images converted to YCbCr color space passed as the input. With fast inference time, and by removing the need for staining, this technology has the potential to reduce labor and time costs. While lens-free holographic microscopy was used, this algorithmic approach could be applied to other QPI techniques.

In Ref. [37], the authors sought to convert confocal microscopy images to virtually stained H&E images for easier interpretation by pathologists and surgeons. Confocal microscopy can be operated in both reflectance (RCM) and fluorescence (FCM) modes. Both types of confocal microscopy can be used to digitally generate images resembling H&E. First, a fully convolutional network is used to despeckle the RCM images. This network is trained with artificially contaminated single-channel H&E images, as appropriate despeckled RCM images are not available. The RCM and FCM images are linearly combined to form an RGB image, by assigning RCM images an eosinlike color, and FCM images a hematoxylin-like color. This naively converted image is then passed to the CycleGAN to improve the overall mode conversion. Importantly, it was demonstrated that despeckling is important for functional mode switching. Without it, the CycleGAN generated unwanted artifacts.

Another attractive microscopy modality with high potential applicability is multiphoton microscopy (MPM). MPM uses multiple near-infrared photons that arrive nearly simultaneously at excitable molecules to induce fluorescent, with a potential for less photodamage and deeper tissue observation than is provided by both one-photon excitation fluorescence, and even tissue staining. In addition, since there are many endogenous fluorophores, it also allows for in vivo tissue imaging, which is not typically possible with tissue staining. However, the high-dimensional data produced by MPM is hard for histopathologists to interpret.

Therefore, Borhani et al. [38] demonstrates techniques for deploying deep learning for mapping label-free MPM to H&E-stained brightfield images. First, a modal coregistration method applies an affine transformation to the H&E image to align the MPM and H&E images. This is done at a global and local level. Color reduction to 16 colors by k-means clustering was performed to decrease complexity of the required modal transfer DNN architectures. Two models were developed: a pixel-to-pixel classification model and an area-to-pixel classification model (Fig. 7.3C). The pixel-to-pixel model is a two-layer fully connected classifier, which maps one pixel from MPM to its respective H&E pixel. The area-to-pixel classification model uses a VGG network to map an image tile from MPM to the respective central pixel for H&E. These models performed well when trained and applied to rat liver samples. The area-to-pixel models performed better than pixel-to-pixel models as they consider spatial and structural information as well. Coregistration was also demonstrated to be important for accurate results. When the liver-trained model was applied to mouse ovary and rat mammary tumor tissues, the model performed poorly. This indicates that this model can only be applied to datasets similar to the source dataset and must be retrained for other tissue types. Nevertheless, this novel approach that does not require GAN architectures could increase accessibility for MPM microscopy.

In certain settings, staining procedures can result in irreversible modifications or damage; this is usually regarded as disadvantageous as it can preclude further analysis of the tissue. However, this is particularly true in the special case of sperm cell selection for in-vitro fertilization (IVF) due to the potential cytotoxicity of staining. Interferometric phase microscopy (IPM) is currently used for sperm evaluation, as it is compatible with available medical microscopes which are modified with an additional wavefront sensor to allow for holographic microscopy. This combination provides quantitative topological maps of the cells without the need for stains. However, morphological evaluation of cells is most effectively accomplished using chemical staining of cell organelles. A method, "HoloStain," was therefore developed to convert quantitative phase images and phase gradient images, which are extracted from the digital holograms, to virtually stain brightfield images using DCGANs [39]. For each cell, an ensemble of four images was used to train the model: stain-free quantitative phase image, two stain-free phase gradient images, and the target-stained brightfield image. An advantage of HoloStain is that cells that were out of focus could be virtually stained and refocused. This is possible since digital reconstruction of the holograms can be done such that unfocused cells can be brought into focus. In order to demonstrate the usefulness of the algorithm, sperm cells were classified by an embryologist using data from brightfield images (no staining), stain-free quantitative phase images, one of the stain-free gradient images, and HoloStain images. The HoloStain method had the highest F1 score compared with the alternative three methods.

While most research studies employ GANs, it is also possible to use image-style transfer algorithms as an alternative approach as demonstrated by Izadyyazdanabadi et al. [10]. In particular, the authors sought to convert confocal laser endomicroscopy (CLE) images to H&E. CLE is a real-time, in vivo interoperative imaging technique with high potential to assist neurosurgeons during surgery. The authors developed a transformation tool that can remove common CLE artifacts, add histological patterns, and avoid removing critical features or adding unreal features to images (Fig. 7.3D). Unfortunately, due to problems in exact colocalization and intrinsic tissue movements, it is difficult to obtain spatially registered H&E-CLE image pairs. Instead, the authors used an image-style transfer algorithm using a pretrained VGG19 architecture and a content and style loss. One advantage of style transfer is that it only requires a single image of the desired style (H&E). Five neurosurgeons independently judged the stylized CLE images as having a significantly higher diagnostic quality than the original CLE images.

The potential for these methods is quite high, as well as being quite close in terms of implementation, with multiple groups working on clinical trials. The quality of images acquired from these methods greatly exceeds the current gold standard for real-time pathology, frozen sections, which introduce artifacts that can render evaluation challenging. By converting images from fluorescence color scheme to one immediately familiar to the pathologist, the odds of adoption increase dramatically. These imaging modalities have the potential to become a new gold standard of real-time pathology in the near future; hence the widespread interest in accurate color mapping.

In silico labeling

Deep learning has supported the development of methods that can extract information from other image modalities in order to reconstruct brightfield stained images. However, can molecularly stained images, highlighting fluorescently labelled cellular structures be reconstructed from stain-free brightfield images (Fig. 7.4A)? Recent research has suggested these kinds of transformations are indeed possible. We refer to such work as in-silico labeling, as inspired by Ref. [40].

Rana et al. [41] demonstrated how it is possible to use cGANs to computationally stain images of unstained paraffin-embedded WSIs. Both staining and destaining models were trained, using traditional GAN and L1 loss functions, but also utilizing an additional regularization term based on Pearson's correlation coefficient in order to prevent tiling noise. The models could be used for further downstream tasks such as tumor diagnosis.

Rivenson et al. [42] instead utilized autofluorescence generated by exciting unstained histology sections using a DAPI excitation/emission filter set to reconstruct

FIGURE 7.4

(A) New research has demonstrated it is possible to convert unstained images to digitally stained images using deep learning. (B) A GAN-based model was successfully applied to convert unstained autofluorescence images to H&E virtually stained images. (C) A multitask model was trained to convert unlabeled transmitted-light images to fluorescently labeled images. GAN, generative adversarial network.

(A) Adapted with permission from Rana A, Yauney G, Lowe A, and Shah P, Computational histological staining and destaining of prostate core biopsy RGB images with generative adversarial neural networks, In 2018 17th IEEE international conference on machine learning and applications (ICMLA), Orlando, FL; 2018. pp. 828–834. https://doi.org/10.1109/ICMLA.2018.00133 (B) Adapted with permission from Rivenson Y, et al., Virtual histological staining of unlabelled tissue-autofluorescence images via deep learning, Nature Biomedical Engineering 2019;3(6):466–477. https://doi.org/10.1038/s41551-019-0362-y; (C) Adapted with permission from Christiansen EM, et al., In silico labeling: predicting fluorescent labels in unlabeled images, Cell 2018; 173(3):792–803. https://doi.org/10.1016/j.cell.2018.03.040.

stained images using GANs. They trained on salivary gland tissue stained with H&E, kidney tissue stained with Jones stain, and liver and lung stained with Masson's trichrome. The GAN model performed very well converting the images, with considerable detail generated and accurate histopathological features captured in the virtual images (Fig. 7.4B). The virtually stained images were also evaluated by pathologists, and no significant difference between the virtually stained and regular brightfield images was observed. This indicates the virtually stained images can provide similar diagnostic utility. The variation in the colorization of the virtually stained images is lower than that of the histologically stained images. Therefore, intrinsic staining standardization is an interesting positive by-product of this approach. The authors also demonstrated transfer learning by using it to rapidly train the model for application on thyroid tissue sections. This technology has the potential to be applied to non−slide-based methods, which would allow for impressive label free imaging without the need to retrain pathologists. The added ability to generate special stains increases the applicability, as many of these stains require hours of skilled technician time and expensive reagents.

While histochemically stained images can give useful information about the cellular and extracellular components, fluorescent labels can give even more detailed information about desired subcellular structures. Hence, there is tremendous interest in obtaining fluorescently labeled images in cell biology and pathology. Ounkomol et al. [43] developed a U-net architecture to convert 3D transmitting light and 2D electron microscopy (EM) to 3D fluorescence microscopy and 2D immunofluorescence (IF) microscopy. Importantly, the predictions for the different structure models can be combined into a 3D multichannel fluorescent image prediction from a single 3D TL image. Another application of image modality conversion is to facilitate automatic registration between images. EM and IF images of ultrathin brain sections are commonly collected as part of an array tomography protocol. However, as they are collected from two different microscopes, they are not inherently aligned, and manual registration is tedious and time-consuming. The authors trained a model on manually registered EM and immunofluorescence images labeled for myelin basic protein (MBP-IF). The MBP-IF prediction, and therefore the original EM image, was registered with the target MBP-IF image using traditional intensity-matching techniques. While EM is not routinely used for clinical diagnosis outside of renal biopsies, converting images to immunofluorescence stains has great utility as these stains are often expensive, cumbersome, and take hours to complete. While in its early stages with further validation and interest, this technology could be very useful for pathologists.

In Christiansen et al. [40], a more universal and flexible architecture was developed to address a similar problem. A multitask, multiscale deep neural network was trained on paired sets of fluorescently labeled 2D images and transmitted light z-stack images (Fig. 7.4C). These z-stack images include images from various focal planes, with the hypothesis that even out-of-focus planes contain information useful for accurately predicting the fluorescent labels. The images were obtained from various labs, samples, and even imaging modalities. This allows for the training of a generalizable network through multitask learning. When tasks are similar in multitask learning, common features can be learned to improve the performance of the model. The training set included human motor neurons derived from induced pluripotent stem cells, primary murine cortical cultures, and breast cancer cell lines. The fluorescent labels used were Hoechst and DAPI for labeling nuclei, propidium iodide (PI) for assessing cell viability, and CellMask for labeling plasma membrane. Some cells were also immunolabeled with antibodies against TuJ1 (labeling for neurons), the Islet1 protein (labeling for motor neurons), and for MAP2 (labeling dendrites). The deep neural network had multiscale input with five paths for each of these scales (Fig. 7.4D). The scale with finest detail stays at the same scale, while the other scales have contracting and upsampling convolution operations, inspired by a U-net architecture. The final network outputs a discrete probability distribution over 256 intensity values (all possible 8-bit pixel values) for all the pixels in the image. It reads z-stacks of either brightfield, phase-contrast, or differential interference contrast images.

The network was tested for various tasks. It was first used to predict Hoechst or DAPI fluorescence in order to label cell nuclei. Qualitatively, the *in silico* labels and the true fluorescent labels looked identical. The Pearson correlation coefficient between the true and predicted pixel intensities was 0.87, indicating the model accurately predicted the nuclear regions. Similar experiments were done to predict propidium iodide (PI) fluorescence, used to detect dead cells (since live cells can exclude the dye). The network also performed well-predicting immunolabels for TuJ1 protein, which labels neurons. The neural network was also able to successfully predict independent axon and dendrite labels, which was unexpected as it was unclear whether the transmitted-light images contained enough information to be able to distinguish whether a neurite extending from a cell was an axon or dendrite. In order to demonstrate the flexibility of the model, transfer learning was used to learn how to predict a different label from a different cell type from data from a single well. Specifically, transfer learning was used to predict CellMask (cell membrane label) fluorescence from differential interference contrast images from cancer cells. The model was trained from data from a single training well, but was regularized by simultaneously training on previous conditions. The network had a Pearson correlation score of 0.95. This suggests this model could continue to learn and be adapted for other tasks, when provided with more training examples.

While fluorescent microscopy is not commonly used in routine clinical pathology applications, deep learning techniques used for fluorescence microscopy could also be applied in histopathology. In particular, Christiansen et al. [40] suggested a way to solve a key problem in deep learning for mode conversion. Most mode conversion methods are limited by constraints imposed by differences in magnification, staining, modality, tissue types, and other factors. However, Christansen et al. used a multitask and multiscale network that was generalizable to various tissue types, magnification scales, and even various modalities. Using transfer learning, these universal models could also be further trained for more specific tasks with very additional little data. The development of similar models for conversion to H&E images could greatly facilitate the adoption of novel imaging modalities for use in histopathology.

Super-resolution, extended depth-of-field, and denoising

In order to generate high-quality WSIs, it has been necessary to use high-numerical-aperture lenses that can capture high-resolution images. The downside is that these lenses have restricted fields of view, which greatly increases the scanning time, as well as shallow depths of field (Fig. 7.5A). While used increasingly for improving the resolution of standard (macro) photography images [19], the application of deep learning methods to increase the resolution of microscope images is quite recent. Wang et al. [44] used a training set consisting of pixel-matched images taken with a 10×/0.4 NA lens paired with images taken with a 20×/0.75 NA lens. The use of paired data forces the GAN to concentrate on improving the resolution of the image and confers high-quality transformations with little artifacts or errors

FIGURE 7.5

(A) In traditional microscopy, there are key trade-offs between exposure, resolution, and speed. However, application of deep learning can augment this design space and diminish these trade-offs. (B) A GAN-based approach was successfully applied to convert diffraction-limited fluorescence images to super-resolved images. (C) A U-net architecture was successfully utilized for image denoising of fluorescent microscopy images. (D) Even with grayscale cameras, deep learning can be used to determine the color of emitters, as the point spread function is determined by the wavelength. GAN, generative adversarial network.

(A) Adapted with permission from Weigert M, et al., Content-aware image restoration: pushing the limits of fluorescence microscopy. Nature Methods *2018;15(12):1090—1097. https://doi.org/10.1038/s41592-018-0216-7; (B) Adapted with permission from Wang H, et al., Deep learning enables cross-modality super-resolution in fluorescence microscopy.* Nature Methods *2019;16(1):103—110. https://doi.org/10.1038/s41592-018-0239-0; (C) Adapted with permission from Weigert M, et al., Content-aware image restoration: pushing the limits of fluorescence microscopy.* Nature Methods *2018;15(12):1090—1097. https://doi.org/10.1038/s41592-018-0216-7; (D) Adapted with permission from Hershko E, Weiss LE, Michaeli T, Shechtman Y, Multicolor localization microscopy and point-spread-function engineering by deep learning.* Optics Express *2019;27(5):6158—6183. https://doi.org/10.1364/OE.27.006158.*

(Fig. 7.5B). The benefit is a field of view that is four times larger, while allowing for a similar reduction in scanning time. This has major implications not only for speeding up scanning but also for allowing larger fields of view in time-lapse studies, allowing for more data to be collected from a single experiment. Another benefit is that the depth of field of the $10\times$ lens is greater, so the focus and sharpness of the generated images can actually be better than the ground truth images themselves, meaning that they are not only equivalent but superior in terms of quality. This is not limited to brightfield as the group has also published similar deep learning algorithms to convert brightfield images from a $40\times$ lens to those better than a $100\times$ oil immersion lens even though the latter was used as the target for the transformation [45]. All the same benefits apply from the previous fluorescent paper with the added benefit that a vast majority of current clinical pathology is done with brightfield imaging. Taking this a step further the group showed it was possible to achieve image quality similar to that of a $20\times$ microscope lens with a smartphone lens, with the added benefit of increased depth of field achieved by the lower NA lens. The algorithm here was not only improving the spatial resolution, but was able to correct the color distortions from the low-quality lens/camera to that of similar quality from a benchtop microscope [46]. This has even further reaching potential as incredibly low-cost hardware could generate much higher quality diagnostic images allowing for better care in resource-poor nations.

An example of the use of deep learning to increase depth of field is an implementation of a CNN to allow for rapid automated diagnosis of blood films for malaria [47]. Blood films are thick samples, and interpretation of scanned images requires the collection of multiple focal planes merged in a way that can be interpreted by either a human pathologist or an artificial neural network (ANN). Manescu et al. [47] trained a network with a three-plane input that generated an image close to the quality obtained with 14 different focus plane images. It convincingly outperformed traditional extended-depth-of-field algorithms, which could greatly increase the speed at which automated scanning and diagnosis of malaria could be made.

Increasing depth of field, however, is not always beneficial; there are many methods that allow for the reduction of depth of field to allow for axially confined resolution. Such techniques include structured-illumination microscopy (SIM), confocal microscopy, and computational deconvolution. These methods allow for the acquisition of high-resolution images from thick samples without physically sectioning tissue. Zhang et al. [48] implemented a CNN to reduce the optical depth of widefield fluorescence images without having to employ the optical methods just listed. The largest advantage is the reduced complexity of the microscope, as well as the reduction of artifacts. Stripe artifacts that can be seen in structured illumination images are common and can distract from the content of the image; deep learning can help generate similarly optically thinned images while retaining comparable quality. Application of a traditional deconvolution method also eliminated stripe artifacts, but the resulting image appeared is significantly thicker and lacked the sharpness of the AI-generated counterpart. While not currently in clinical use, lightsheet microscopy for pathology has been explored by Ref. [49] and proved especially useful in the evaluation of prostate biopsies. The ability to capture 3D datasets allowed more accurate assessment of Gleason scoring (a prognostic factor for prostate tumors) which could in turn lead to a better quality of care for patients.

Beyond increasing resolution or affecting depth of field, another contribution of AI that can markedly improve image quality is reduction of noise. Images with low signals can be difficult to interpret; this can make in vivo imaging particularly challenging since the data typically must be acquired quickly and with low (safe) light levels. Paired data (low and high noise versions) for developing noise reduction models are relatively easy to acquire or synthesize, meaning that large and representative datasets can be generated quickly. For example, Weigert et al. [50] successfully demonstrated the use of a convolutional neural net trained on multiphoton images using very low laser power and low exposure times as input with the target output being the high-quality images taken with normal exposure times and laser powers (Fig. 7.5C). While not immediately relevant to pathology as it is practiced today, this concept could be applied to all of the previous fluorescent methods to help speed them up. If any of these techniques are to replace the frozen section, they must either offer better-quality histology, or be faster. In addition, these techniques could be used to improve label-free imaging methods, possibly allowing for in vivo microscopic inspection of tumor margins allowing for even better resection margins than obtained via frozen section, as there is no tissue lost due to sectioning or embedding.

This general approach can also be applied to standard super-resolution techniques, such as photoactivated localization microscopy (PALM) or stochastic optical reconstruction microscopy (STORM). Both methods rely on the acquisition of thousands of images to reconstruct structure below the diffraction limit of light microscopy. By training an ANN, Ouyang et al. [51] decreased the number of images required for a PALM reconstruction from 60,000 to a mere 500, representing a difference in acquisition time from 10 min to 9 s. While not currently applicable to pathology, there are some applications of electron microscopy that may be able to be replaced by techniques such as STORM/PALM; and as the field evolves and our understanding of disease processes increases there may be a place for these techniques in clinical pathology.

Increased acquisition time requirements arise not only from a desire to maximize signal-to-noise ratios; many fluorescence image sessions require serial imaging with different sets of filters in order to separate multiple labels. The result is a large increase in imaging times and light exposure to the sample, with attendant potential for phototoxicity or photobleaching. By training a neural net on filter-acquired images, Hershko et al. [52] has shown it is possible to use the chromatic aberration differences related to the use of different wavelengths of light to separate multiple labels from a single image (Fig. 7.5D). The implication of this method is much the same as described previously, namely, the potential for more rapid collection of data, and a reduction in imaging time.

Deep learning for computationally aided diagnosis in histopathology

In the section above, we described the possibility of using AI tools for improving the quality and information salience of images via AI-assisted tools. However, such tools are still regarded with some skepticism on the regulatory side, as they are seen as premature for deployment in high-impact clinical settings. The number of approved AI tools—with or without AI-enhanced images—for pathology is still very small, and for intraoperative guidance even smaller. The notion is that for direct-to-AI-interpretation, the need for an intermediate step of AI-enhancement may be diminished, since extraction of information and reduction of the impact of noise and distortion is implicitly performed by the classifier itself. An example from the neuropathology domain is given below, emphasizing as well the opportunity to combine AI tools with novel rapid histology technology.

A rationale for AI-assisted imaging and interpretation

Serving the US population that grew 8% from 2007 to 2017, the pathology workforce contracted 17% during the same time period [53]. Within certain subspecialties, workforce shortages are even more severe. Approximately 800 neuropathologists cover the 1400 centers performing brain tumor surgery [54]. Worsening deficits in neuropathology are expected with a vacancy rate of approximately 42% in neuropathology fellowships [55]. In neuropathology, the workforce shortage is felt in a number of ways. Although academic centers tend to be well staffed with board-certified neuropathologists, community hospitals rarely have one on staff. Consequently, nonexpert pathologists are compelled to provide services that could better be provided by a more specialized practitioner. Although hard to quantify, lack of neuropathology expertise probably leads to delays in intraoperative diagnosis, unnecessary surgical intervention (where a lymphoma or germinoma is misdiagnosed as a tumor where surgery might be required), and a limitation on how pathology can be used to formulate surgical strategy.

Histologic data have been recognized as central to decision-making in brain tumor surgery since at least 1930 [56]. There are numerous decisions that must be made by surgeons at the time of an operation on a brain lesion. First and foremost, surgeons rely on pathologists to ensure the tissue they have biopsied is indeed lesional and can be used to establish a diagnosis. Beyond that, differentiating neoplastic from nonneoplastic processes in the brain is essential as is differentiating surgical and nonsurgical tumors. With respect to the surgical candidates, differentiating between primary and metastatic tumors, low- and high-grade gliomas, circumscribed and diffuse tumors all have specific implications for decision-making.

While the importance of histologic data in brain tumor surgery is now well established, in modern surgical practice, a chasm remains between the operating room and neuropathology. In most centers, the frozen section lab is off-site or a substantial distance from the operating table, creating a logistic barrier for surgeons interested in viewing slides with the pathologists. Moreover, the process for creating high-quality pathology slides is time- and labor-intensive. Consequently, pathologists will call into an OR with a diagnosis 30−45 min after a specimen is collected. The inefficiency of this process isolates surgeons from histologic data and limits the way it can be used to inform surgical decision-making.

Given the challenges in the modern neuropathology workflow, AI holds great promise in a number of regards: (1) verifying that lesional tissue has been collected, (2) assisting in tissue diagnosis, (3) helping to define surgical endpoints in tumors without gross boundaries, and (4) in the future, predicting actionable and diagnostic molecular markers. In fixed tissue, AI has been applied to classification of epithelial versus stromal regions in breast and colon cancer [57], differentiating necrotic and nonnecrotic regions [58], and differentiating high- and low-grade gliomas [59]. That said, the application of AI for assisting in diagnosis only addresses the challenges associated with establishing diagnosis in neuropathology. With conventional histologic workflows, many of the barriers related to tissue transport and processing remain. To fully leverage the opportunity created by rapid advances in AI-assisted pathologic diagnosis, marriage with a technique for rapid histology is essential.

Approaches to rapid histology interpretations

To this end, several methods for slide-free histology have been proposed and validated to varying degrees. MUSE, stimulated Raman histology (SRH), and light-sheet microscopy are among the most promising tools for imaging unprocessed or minimally processed biological specimens (Fig. 7.6).

While numerous techniques for slide-free histology have been proposed, only SRH has been incorporated into an AI-based diagnostic pipeline validated for brain tumor diagnosis in a clinical setting. Hollon et al. adapted the Inception-V2 CNN to diagnose the 10 most common brain tumors using SRH images and deployed their software on a bedside SRH imager. In a head-to-head clinical trial of 278 patients, Hollon et al. demonstrated that an autonomous diagnostic pathway utilizing SRH and a CNN could predict diagnosis with performance that was noninferior to board-certified neuropathologists interpreting conventional histologic slides in the same patients [61]. The accuracy of both arms was approximately 94% and interestingly the errors in both arms were entirely nonoverlapping (Fig. 7.7). The authors of this study therefore conclude that the SRH + CNN pathway can be used as a stand-alone method for brain tumor diagnosis when pathology resources are unavailable and as a method to improve diagnostic accuracy in neuropathology, even in well-staffed centers. Although the authors limited trial inclusion to common types of brain tumors, they also offered a means of differentiating common and unusual histologic classes in an effort to make their system universal to application in all central nervous system neoplasms. The algorithm was also used to develop a semantic segmentation tool capable of depicting the areas of a histologic image most likely to contain lesional tissue (Fig. 7.8). The authors also conclude that given the features

FIGURE 7.6

Methods for slide-free histology including (A) microscopy with ultraviolet surface excitation, (B) light sheet microscopy, and (C) stimulated Raman histology (SRH), all of which can be performed on minimally processed or unprocessed tissue to generate diagnostic histologic images without the need for the resources of a conventional pathology lab. Each technique relies on optical, rather than physical sectioning of imaged tissue, simplifying the workflow required to generate a diagnostic histologic image. SRH has unique value as a modality for bedside histology as no staining, clearing, or handling of the tissue is required to generate a histological image. In SRH, fresh specimens can be placed into an imager at bedside which rapidly creates a virtual H&E microscopic image through relatively simple spectral band combination and recoloring. To this end, academic-industrial partnership has resulted in the first FDA-registered imager, now employed in several operating rooms across the United States.

Adapted with permission from Orringer DA, Camelo-Piragua S, Fast and slide-free imaging. Nature Biomedical Engineering, *2017;1(12):926–928. https://doi.org/10.1038/s41551-017-0172-z.*

FIGURE 7.7

Prospective clinical trial of SRH plus CNN versus conventional H&E histology. (A) The prediction probabilities for the ground truth classes are plotted in descending order by medical center with indication of correct (green) or incorrect (red) classification. (B) Multiclass confusion matrices for both the control arm and experimental arm. Mistakes in the control arm, traditional H&E histology with pathologist were mostly misclassification of malignant gliomas (10/17). The glial tumors had the highest error rate in the SRH plus CNN arm (9/14). Less common tumors, including ependymoma, medulloblastoma, and pilocytic astrocytomas were also misclassified, likely due to insufficient number of cases for model training, resulting in lower mean class accuracy compared with the control arm. These errors are likely to improve with additional SRH training data. SRH, stimulated Raman histology; CNN, convolutional neural networks (CNN).

Adapted with permission from Hollon TC, et al., Near real-time intraoperative brain tumor diagnosis using stimulated Raman histology and deep neural networks. Nature Medicine, *2020;26(1):52–58. https://doi.org/ 10.1038/s41591-019-0715-9.*

FIGURE 7.8

Semantic segmentation. (A) An SRH mosaic image of a specimen from a glioblastoma patient contains areas of (B) dense tumor infiltration, tumor-brain interface as well as the gliotic peritumoral regions. Tiles from the mosaic are fed into a semantic segmentation algorithm (C) that are classified by a convolutional neural network (CNN) which then assigns a numerical value, depicted by color (red green or blue) corresponding to the likelihood that a given region contains tumor, nondiagnostic tissue, or nonlesional tissue. The classifier provides the likelihood of class membership among 10 categories of the most common brain tumors (D). The entire mosaic can be predicted as a heatmap for each of the 10 categories, 3 of which are shown here (E). SRH, stimulated Raman histology; CNN, convolutional neural networks (CNN).

Adapted with permission from Hollon TC, et al., Near real-time intraoperative brain tumor diagnosis using stimulated Raman histology and deep neural networks. Nature Medicine, *2020;26(1):52—58. https://doi.org/ 10.1038/s41591-019-0715-9.*

that their CNN used to classify brain tumors, similar algorithms could be developed for tumors of other organs in the future.

It is interesting to speculate whether AI-based image enhancement prior to the classification learning step would have improved the performance of the latter.

Future prospects

The entire field of histopathology is experiencing rapid developments across all domains. Opportunities and challenges include:

(a) The wider deployment of conventional whole-slide scanning capabilities that can finally enable the entry of slide-interpretation into the digital realm;

(b) The use of AI to enhance the performance of slide-scanning by interposing color normalization, denoising, sharpening, and depth-of-field enhancements with specialized AI tools prior to classification steps;

(c) The use of AI to dramatically simplify optomechanical requirements for scanners by correcting for lower raw scan performance with computational tools, thus decreasing instrumentation costs, scan times, and inadequate scan performance issues;

(d) Combining novel slide-free imaging hardware and AI to maximize both information content and similarities with conventional H&E-stained slide appearance,

(e) Getting pathologists, surgeons, administrators, the FDA, and payors comfortable with the above.

These are exciting times, as pathology finally seems poised to take advantage of notable advances in microscopy and computation.

References

[1] Russakovsky O, et al. ImageNet large scale visual recognition challenge. International Journal of Computer Vision 2015;115(3):211—52. https://doi.org/10.1007/s11263-015-0816-y.

[2] Cireşan D, Meier U, Masci J, Schmidhuber J. Multi-column deep neural network for traffic sign classification. Neural Networks 2012;32:333—8. https://doi.org/10.1016/j.neunet.2012.02.023.

[3] Krizhevsky A, Sutskever I, Hinton GE. ImageNet classification with deep convolutional neural networks. In: Pereira F, Burges CJC, Bottou L, Weinberger KQ, editors. Advances in neural information processing systems 25. Curran Associates, Inc.; 2012. p. 1097—105.

[4] Simonyan K, Zisserman A. Very deep convolutional networks for large-scale image recognition. ArXiv14091556 Cs. Apr. 2015.

[5] He K, Zhang X, Ren S, Sun J. Deep residual learning for image recognition. In: 2016 IEEE conference on computer vision and pattern recognition (CVPR); 2016. p. 770—8. https://doi.org/10.1109/CVPR.2016.90.

[6] Szegedy C, et al. Going deeper with convolutions. In: 2015 IEEE conference on computer vision and pattern recognition (CVPR); 2015. p. 1—9. https://doi.org/10.1109/CVPR.2015.7298594.

[7] Gurcan MN, Boucheron LE, Can A, Madabhushi A, Rajpoot NM, Yener B. Histopathological image analysis: a review. IEEE Reviews in Biomedical Engineering 2009;2:147—71. https://doi.org/10.1109/RBME.2009.2034865.

[8] Gatys LA, Ecker AS, Bethge M. A neural algorithm of artistic style. ArXiv150806576 Cs Q-Bio. Sep. 2015.

[9] Gatys LA, Ecker AS, Bethge M. Image style transfer using convolutional neural networks. In: 2016 IEEE conference on computer vision and pattern recognition (CVPR), las vegas, NV, USA; 2016. p. 2414−23. https://doi.org/10.1109/CVPR.2016.265.

[10] Izadyyazdanabadi M, et al. Fluorescence image histology pattern transformation using image style transfer. Frontiers in Oncology 2019;9. https://doi.org/10.3389/fonc.2019.00519.

[11] Goodfellow I, Bengio Y, Courville A. Deep learning. The MIT Press; 2016.

[12] LeCun Y, Bengio Y, Hinton G. Deep learning. Nature 2015;521(7553):436−44. https://doi.org/10.1038/nature14539.

[13] Yosinski J, Clune J, Bengio Y, Lipson H. How transferable are features in deep neural networks? In: Ghahramani Z, Welling M, Cortes C, Lawrence ND, Weinberger KQ, editors. Advances in neural information processing systems 27. Curran Associates, Inc.; 2014. p. 3320−8.

[14] Long J, Shelhamer E, Darrell T. Fully convolutional networks for semantic segmentation. In: 2015 IEEE conference on computer vision and pattern recognition (CVPR); 2015. p. 3431−40. https://doi.org/10.1109/CVPR.2015.7298965.

[15] He K, Gkioxari G, Dollár P, Girshick R. Mask R-CNN. In: 2017 IEEE international conference on computer vision (ICCV); 2017. p. 2980−8. https://doi.org/10.1109/ICCV.2017.322.

[16] Ronneberger O, Fischer P, Brox T. U-net: convolutional networks for biomedical image segmentation. In: Medical image computing and computer-assisted intervention − MICCAI 2015, cham; 2015. p. 234−41. https://doi.org/10.1007/978-3-319-24574-4_28.

[17] Fang L, et al. Deep learning-based point-scanning super-resolution imaging. BioRxiv 2019. preprint.

[18] Goodfellow I, et al. Generative adversarial nets. In: Ghahramani Z, Welling M, Cortes C, Lawrence ND, Weinberger KQ, editors. Advances in neural information processing systems 27. Curran Associates, Inc.; 2014. p. 2672−80.

[19] Ledig C, et al. Photo-realistic single image super-resolution using a generative adversarial network. In: 2017 IEEE conference on computer vision and pattern recognition (CVPR); 2017. p. 105−14. https://doi.org/10.1109/CVPR.2017.19.

[20] Radford A, Metz L, Chintala S. Unsupervised representation learning with deep convolutional generative adversarial networks. ArXiv151106434 Cs. Jan. 2016.

[21] Zhu J-Y, Park T, Isola P, Efros AA. Unpaired image-to-image translation using cycle-consistent adversarial networks. In: 2017 IEEE international conference on computer vision (ICCV), Venice; 2017. p. 2242−51. https://doi.org/10.1109/ICCV.2017.244.

[22] Topol EJ. High-performance medicine: the convergence of human and artificial intelligence. Nature Medicine 2019;25(1):44−56. https://doi.org/10.1038/s41591-018-0300-7.

[23] Shaban MT, Baur C, Navab N, Albarqouni S. Staingan: stain style transfer for digital histological images. In: 2019 IEEE 16th international symposium on biomedical imaging (ISBI 2019); 2019. p. 953−6. https://doi.org/10.1109/ISBI.2019.8759152.

[24] de Haan K, Rivenson Y, Wu Y, Ozcan A. Deep-learning-based image reconstruction and enhancement in optical microscopy. Proceedings of the IEEE 2020;108(1):30−50. https://doi.org/10.1109/JPROC.2019.2949575.

[25] Perez L, Wang J. The effectiveness of data augmentation in image classification using deep learning. ArXiv171204621 Cs. Dec. 2017.

[26] Ciompi F, et al. The importance of stain normalization in colorectal tissue classification with convolutional networks. In: 2017 IEEE 14th international symposium on biomedical imaging (ISBI 2017); 2017. p. 160–3. https://doi.org/10.1109/ISBI.2017.7950492.

[27] Janowczyk A, Basavanhally A, Madabhushi A. Stain normalization using sparse AutoEncoders (StaNoSA): application to digital pathology. Computerized Medical Imaging and Graphics 2017;57:50–61. https://doi.org/10.1016/j.compmedimag.2016.05.003.

[28] Ruifrok AC, Johnston DA. Quantification of histochemical staining by color deconvolution. Analytical and Quantitative Cytology and Histology 2001;23(4):291–9.

[29] Azevedo Tosta TA, de Faria PR, Neves LA, do Nascimento MZ. Computational normalization of H&E-stained histological images: progress, challenges and future potential. Artificial Intelligence in Medicine 2019;95:118–32. https://doi.org/10.1016/j.artmed.2018.10.004.

[30] Roy S, kumar Jain A, Lal S, Kini J. A study about color normalization methods for histopathology images. Micron 2018;114:42–61. https://doi.org/10.1016/j.micron.2018.07.005.

[31] Bug D, et al. Context-based normalization of histological stains using deep convolutional features. In: Deep learning in medical image analysis and multimodal learning for clinical decision support, Cham; 2017. p. 135–42. https://doi.org/10.1007/978-3-319-67558-9_16.

[32] F. G. Zanjani, S. Zinger, and B. E. Bejnordi, "Histopathology stain-color normalization using generative neural networks," p. 16.

[33] Chen X, Duan Y, Houthooft R, Schulman J, Sutskever I, Abbeel P. InfoGAN: interpretable representation learning by information maximizing generative adversarial nets. In: Lee DD, Sugiyama M, Luxburg UV, Guyon I, Garnett R, editors. Advances in neural information processing systems 29. Curran Associates, Inc.; 2016. p. 2172–80.

[34] Kingma DP, Welling M. Auto-encoding variational bayes. ArXiv13126114 Cs Stat. May 2014.

[35] Tellez D, et al. Quantifying the effects of data augmentation and stain color normalization in convolutional neural networks for computational pathology. Medical Image Analysis 2019;58:101544. https://doi.org/10.1016/j.media.2019.101544.

[36] Rivenson Y, Liu T, Wei Z, Zhang Y, de Haan K, Ozcan A. PhaseStain: the digital staining of label-free quantitative phase microscopy images using deep learning. Light: Science & Applications 2019;8(1):1–11. https://doi.org/10.1038/s41377-019-0129-y.

[37] Combalia M, Perez-Anker J, García-Herrera A. Digitally stained confocal microscopy through deep learning. In: Proceedings of the 2nd international conference on medical imaging with deep learning (PMLR), 102; 2019. p. 121–9.

[38] Borhani N, Bower AJ, Boppart SA, Psaltis D. Digital staining through the application of deep neural networks to multi-modal multi-photon microscopy. Biomedical Optics Express 2019;10(3):1339–50. https://doi.org/10.1364/BOE.10.001339.

[39] Nygate YN et al. *HoloStain: holographic virtual staining of individual biological cells.* p. 20.

[40] Christiansen EM, et al. In silico labeling: predicting fluorescent labels in unlabeled images. Cell 2018;173(3):792–803. https://doi.org/10.1016/j.cell.2018.03.040. e19.

[41] Rana A, Yauney G, Lowe A, Shah P. Computational histological staining and destaining of prostate core biopsy RGB images with generative adversarial neural networks.

In: 2018 17th IEEE international conference on machine learning and applications (ICMLA), Orlando, FL; 2018. p. 828—34. https://doi.org/10.1109/ICMLA.2018.00133.

[42] Rivenson Y, et al. Virtual histological staining of unlabelled tissue-autofluorescence images via deep learning. Nature Biomedical Engineering 2019;3(6):466—77. https://doi.org/10.1038/s41551-019-0362-y.

[43] Ounkomol C, Seshamani S, Maleckar MM, Collman F, Johnson GR. Label-free prediction of three-dimensional fluorescence images from transmitted-light microscopy. Nature Methods 2018;15(11):917—20. https://doi.org/10.1038/s41592-018-0111-2.

[44] Wang H, et al. Deep learning enables cross-modality super-resolution in fluorescence microscopy. Nature Methods 2019;16(1):103—10. https://doi.org/10.1038/s41592-018-0239-0.

[45] Rivenson Y, Göröcs Z, Günaydin H, Zhang Y, Wang H, Ozcan A. Deep learning microscopy. Optica 2017;4(11):1437—43. https://doi.org/10.1364/OPTICA.4.001437.

[46] Rivenson Y, et al. Deep learning enhanced mobile-phone microscopy. ACS Photonics 2018;5(6):2354—64. https://doi.org/10.1021/acsphotonics.8b00146.

[47] Manescu P, et al. Deep learning enhanced extended depth-of-field for thick blood-film malaria high-throughput microscopy. ArXiv190607496 Cs Eess. Jun. 2019.

[48] Zhang X, et al. Deep learning optical-sectioning method. Optics Express 2018;26(23):30762—72. https://doi.org/10.1364/OE.26.030762.

[49] Reder NP, Glaser AK, McCarty EF, Chen Y, True LD, Liu JTC. Open-top light-sheet microscopy image atlas of prostate core needle biopsies. Archives of Pathology & Laboratory Medicine 2019;143(9):1069—75. https://doi.org/10.5858/arpa.2018-0466-OA.

[50] Weigert M, et al. Content-aware image restoration: pushing the limits of fluorescence microscopy. Nature Methods 2018;15(12):1090—7. https://doi.org/10.1038/s41592-018-0216-7.

[51] Ouyang W, Aristov A, Lelek M, Hao X, Zimmer C. Deep learning massively accelerates super-resolution localization microscopy. Nature Biotechnology 2018;36(5):460—8. https://doi.org/10.1038/nbt.4106.

[52] Hershko E, Weiss LE, Michaeli T, Shechtman Y. Multicolor localization microscopy and point-spread-function engineering by deep learning. Optics Express 2019;27(5):6158—83. https://doi.org/10.1364/OE.27.006158.

[53] Metter DM, Colgan TJ, Leung ST, Timmons CF, Park JY. Trends in the US and Canadian pathologist workforces from 2007 to 2017. JAMA Network Open 2019;2(5):e194337. https://doi.org/10.1001/jamanetworkopen.2019.4337.

[54] Orringer DA, et al. Rapid intraoperative histology of unprocessed surgical specimens via fibre-laser-based stimulated Raman scattering microscopy. Nature Biomedical Engineering 2017;1(2):1—13. https://doi.org/10.1038/s41551-016-0027.

[55] Robboy SJ, et al. Pathologist workforce in the United States: I. Development of a predictive model to examine factors influencing supply. Archives of Pathology & Laboratory Medicine 2013;137(12):1723—32. https://doi.org/10.5858/arpa.2013-0200-OA.

[56] Eisenhardt L, Cushing H. Diagnosis of intracranial tumors by supravital technique. The American Journal of Pathology 1930;6(5):541—552.7.

[57] Xu J, Luo X, Wang G, Gilmore H, Madabhushi A. A Deep convolutional neural network for segmenting and classifying epithelial and stromal regions in histopathological images. Neurocomputing 2016;191:214—23. https://doi.org/10.1016/j.neucom.2016.01.034.

[58] Sharma H, Zerbe N, Klempert I, Hellwich O, Hufnagl P. Deep convolutional neural networks for automatic classification of gastric carcinoma using whole slide images in

digital histopathology. Computerized Medical Imaging and Graphics 2017;61:2—13. https://doi.org/10.1016/j.compmedimag.2017.06.001.

[59] Barker J, Hoogi A, Depeursinge A, Rubin DL. Automated classification of brain tumor type in whole-slide digital pathology images using local representative tiles. Medical Image Analysis 2016;30:60—71. https://doi.org/10.1016/j.media.2015.12.002.

[60] Orringer DA, Camelo-Piragua S. Fast and slide-free imaging. Nature Biomedical Engineering 2017;1(12):926—8. https://doi.org/10.1038/s41551-017-0172-z.

[61] Hollon TC, et al. Near real-time intraoperative brain tumor diagnosis using stimulated Raman histology and deep neural networks. Nature Medicine 2020;26(1):52—8. https://doi.org/10.1038/s41591-019-0715-9.

Precision medicine in digital pathology via image analysis and machine learning

Peter D. Caie, BSc, MRes, PhD [1], **Neofytos Dimitriou, B.Sc** [2],
Ognjen Arandjelović, M.Eng. (Oxon), Ph.D. (Cantab) [2]

[1]*School of Medicine, QUAD Pathology, University of St Andrews, St Andrews, United Kingdom;*
[2]*School of Computer Science, University of St Andrews, St Andrews, United Kingdom*

Introduction
Precision medicine

The field of medicine is currently striving toward more accurate and effective clinical decision-making for individual patients. This can be through many forms of analysis and be put into effect at multiple stages of a patient's disease progression and treatment journey. However, the overarching goal is for higher treatment success rates with lower side effects from potentially ineffectual, but toxic, therapies, and of course better patient well-being and overall survival. For example, understanding if a specific treatment for an individual patient's cancer may help their treatment or in fact be detrimental to their overall survival, as is the case with cetuximab treatment in colorectal cancer. This process of treating the patient as an individual, and not as a member of a broader and heterogeneous population, is commonly termed precision medicine and has traditionally been driven by advances in targeted drug discovery with accompanying translatable companion molecular tests. These tests report on biomarkers measured from patient samples and inform if specific drugs will be effective for patients, normally based on the molecular profile of their diagnostic tissue sample. The tests may derive from our knowledge of biological process, like designing inhibitors against EGFR receptor pathways, or from machine learning—based mining of large multiomic datasets to identify novel drug targets or resistance mechanisms. In the current era of digital medicine, precision medicine is being applied throughout the clinical workflow from diagnosis, prognosis, and prediction. Large flows of data can be tapped from multiple sources and no longer solely through molecular pathology. This is made possible by the digitization, and availability, of patient history and lifestyle records, clinical reports, and through the adoption of digital pathology and image analysis in both the realm of research and the clinic. In fact, prior to the interrogation of digitized histopathological datasets by image analysis, in vitro high-content biology-based drug screens were being developed

Artificial Intelligence and Deep Learning in Pathology. https://doi.org/10.1016/B978-0-323-67538-3.00008-7

by the pharmaceutical industry [1]. These screens also applied image analysis, but to cultured cells exposed to genetic of small molecular manipulation, to segment and classify cellular structures before capturing large multiparametric datasets that inform on novel targets or drug efficacy. Similar methodology taken from high-content biology and image analysis can be applied to digital pathology. This is the case for classical object threshold—based image analysis or for artificial intelligence. The overarching aim being to either quantify and report on specific biomarkers or histological patterns of known importance, or by capturing unbiasedly collected multiparametric data and pattern recognition across segmented objects and whole-slide images (WSI). The aim of distilling and reporting on the extracted data from digital pathology images is to allow for the stratification of patients into distinct groups that may inform the clinician on their optimal and personalized treatment regimen.

Digital pathology

Digital pathology, the high-resolution digitization of glass-mounted histopathological specimens, is becoming more common place in the clinic. This disruptive technology is on track to replace the reporting of glass slides down a microscope, as has been the tradition for centuries. There remain certain obstacles to overcome for wide-scale adoption of digital pathology; such as IT infrastructure, scanning workflow costs, and the willingness of the pathology community. However, as more institutes trend to full digitization, these obstacles diminish. The adoption of digital pathology holds advantages over traditional microscopy in teaching, remote reporting and image sharing, and not least the ability to perform image analysis on the resultant digitized specimens.

In essence, the technology is currently moving from the glass slide and microscope to the digital image and high-resolution screen, although the manual viewing and diagnosis remains the same. Clinical applications using digital pathology and WSIs are currently restricted to the primary diagnosis of H&E stained slides. However, future applications, such as immunofluorescence, can bring advantages to digital pathology. Indeed, scanner vendors are frequently combining both brightfield and multiplexed immunofluorescence visualization into their platforms. Immunofluorescence allows the identification, classification, and quantification of multiple cell types or biomarkers colocalized at the single-cell resolution and on a single tissue section. The importance of this capability is becoming increasingly apparent as we realize that the complex intercellular and molecular interactions within the tumor microenvironment, on top of cellular morphology, play a vital role to a tumor's progression and aggressiveness.

Humans are as adept at reporting from digital pathology samples as they are from glass mounted ones. They do this by identifying diagnostic and prognostic patterns in the tissue, while at the same time disregarding artifact and nonessential histology. However, an inherent human setback in the field of pathology has been the standardization and consistency of inter- and intraobserver reporting. This is specifically true for the identification and semiquantification of more discrete and subtle morphologies as well as, for example, the counting of specific cell types, mitotic figures, or biomarker expression across WSIs [2—4]. The automated analysis of such features by computer algorithms can overcome these flaws and provide objective and standardized quantification. With ongoing research providing much needed evidence of the capability of image analysis and artificial intelligence to accurately quantify and report on molecular and morphological features, it is only a matter of time before these too translate into the clinic.

The use of image analysis and artificial intelligence can be knowledge driven or data driven. The next section of this chapter will discuss how both methodologies can be applied to digital pathology before we expand on the theory and concepts behind the various artificial intelligence models commonly used in the field.

Applications of image analysis and machine learning
Knowledge-driven image analysis

The first applications of image analysis in digital pathology were the quantification of previously identified histopathological features or immunohistochemical results of known pathological significance. This image analysis typically relies on user-defined thresholds of either color or fluorescence intensity coupled with classifications based on object shape, extent, or texture. Examples of histopathological features quantified in such a manner include the quantification of tumor buds, lymphovascular density and invasion, or immune infiltrate [5,6]. Similarly, the quantification of protein expression through immunolabeling, such as pHH3, PDL-1, or EGFR, whether studying predictive or prognostic outcomes, can also be quantified in such a manner [7—9]. This image analysis can be applied to user-defined regions of interest through manual annotations, or across WSIs. A further advantage of the automatic reporting of such features, over and above reproducibility, is that they can be quantified across a continuum instead of traditional semiquantified categorical reporting. The analysis of continuous data is far more amenable to personalized pathology through machine learning than creating distinct categories to group patients.

Machine learning for image segmentation

Pathologists regularly quantify features from specific locations within the tissue section, for example, only within the tumor or stromal cells, or at the cancer's invasive margin. However, to manually annotate images to differentiate these regions of interest prior to performing image analysis is a subjective and tedious task, specifically if needed to be applied to the large patient cohorts required for statistically relevant studies. One can therefore apply machine learning algorithms, such as random forest, directly to the images to overcome the need for manual annotations. This machine learning—based classification relies on the user teaching the algorithm what the specific regions are that they want to segment. They do so by selecting examples across a training subset of images. Once the algorithm has learned the difference between the regions to be differentiated, it can be applied to a larger sample set in order to automatically segment the image of the tissue. An example of this would be using an antibody against cytokeratin to label the tumor and use this marker, on top of the cancer cell morphology, to differentiate the tumor from the stroma (Fig. 8.1A). Once this is performed, one can employ the before-mentioned threshold-based image analysis to quantify, for example, Ki67 expression in only the tumor (Fig. 8.1B), tumor buds only at the invasive margin [10], or CD3 and CD8 positive lymphocytic infiltration within either the tumor core or invasive margin [6] (Fig. 8.2).

Deep learning for image segmentation

There exists great inter- and intrapatient heterogeneity, specifically in the molecular and phenotypic makeup of a patient's tumor. This also equates to great variation within the images, not only morphologically, but also when applying a specific marker

FIGURE 8.1 Automated tumor to stroma segmentation and cellular classification.

(A) A machine learning approach for automatic tissue segmentation using Definiens Tissue Studio software. In this example, segmenting the tumor from the stroma. Ai) A colorectal TMA core labeled by immunofluorescence for tumor (Pan Cytokeratin, green) and nuclei (Hoechst, blue). Aii) The software automatically segments the image based on pixel heterogeneity (blue outline). Aiii) The user tags segmented example objects of the features to be segmented, here turquoise for stroma and purple for tumor. The machine learning algorithm learns these features and automatically segments the rest of the images in the project, as demonstrated in Aiv. (B) The same TMA core was labeled for ki67, which is coregistered in Bi in red. Bii) shows all nuclei automatically segmented (blue outline) by the Definiens software, prior to the exclusion of stroma nuclei (gray) and the retaining of tumor nuclei (blue) in Biii. Biv) shows the tumor nuclei being classified positive for ki67 expression (yellow).

FIGURE 8.2 Quantification of lymphocytic infiltration with the tumor's invasive margin or core.

(A) A whole slide image of a colorectal cancer tissue section labeled for tumor cells (green) and nuclei (blue). The image analysis in this figure is performed using Indica Labs HALO software. The red outline is the automatically detected deepest invasion of tumor cells and the inset shows a zoomed in example of the image segmented into an invasive margin (green) and the tumor core (blue). The purple square denotes where Figure (B and C) originate from in the invasive margin. (B) Multiplexed immunofluorescence visualized CD3 (yellow) and CD8 (red) positive lymphocytes. (C) Automated quantification of these lymphocytes within just the invasive margin of the tumor.

to differentiate regions of interest for image analysis. Furthermore, the tissue specimen is imperfect, and so, therefore, is the digitized WSI. These imperfections can originate from multiple stages of tissue preparation. They can result in folds, tears, or uneven thickness of the tissue to more subtle morphological differences due to the ischemia or fixation times. If performing immunolabeling, nonspecific staining, edge-effect, or autofluorescence can further create confounding issues for automated image analysis. Examples of such artifacts can be seen in Fig. 8.3. All of the above

FIGURE 8.3 Examples of image artifact within digital pathology.

(A–E) Examples of artifact from brightfield image capture. (A) Folded over section of a TMA core. (B) Cutting artifact (dark pink line) and piece of dust (gray) on an H&E-stained image. (C) Out of focus and incorrectly stitched image of an H&E-stained image. (D) Tear and fold in H&E-labeled tissue. (E) Out-of-focus section bordered by a foreign object on the H&E-labeled specimen. (F–J) Examples of artifact from fluorescence image capture. (F) A tear in a tissue section resulting in nonspecific fluorescence. (G) Cutting artifact (bright lines). (H) Out-of-focus nuclei. (I) Illumination artifact resulting in large blue squares. (J) Autofluorescence from hair in a urine cytology sample (blue lines).

may cause inaccurate reporting, such as false positives, when applying image analysis and machine learning to segment tissue across large patient cohorts. However, many of these issues can be overcome by employing deep learning architecture to segment the digital WSI. To do this, trained experts can annotate the regions of interest selected for quantification, while further identifying and training the algorithm to ignore the tissue artifact [11]. The human brain is extraordinary at pattern recognition and the pathologist routinely and automatically ignores imperfect tissue specimens in order to hone in on the area containing the information needed to make their diagnosis or prognosis. The ever developing sophistication of deep learning architectures now allows this level of analysis by automated algorithms.

For accurate tissue segmentation, using either machine learning or deep learning methodology, a strong and standardized signal to noise is required within the feature one is using to differentiate regions of interest. However, the inherently heterogeneous sample is also reflected in the marker used for segmentation, and this may vary in brightness or intensity between patient samples; and even within the same sample. Image color and intensity standardization algorithms can be employed prior to the analysis of the image by artificial intelligence [12]. This can lead to a more accurate fully automated tissue segmentation across diverse and large patient cohorts; however, there is controversy over whether this is the best method to achieve this goal and whether this methodology may reduce real diagnostic information.

   Deep learning is not only being applied to segment tissue prior to biomarker or cellular quantification but also has the ability to recognize histopathological patterns in digitized H&E-stained tissue sections (Fig. 8.4). This has been demonstrated in studies where the expert pathologist has annotated features of significance in order to train the deep learning algorithms to identify these in unseen test and validation sets [13,14]. The clinical application and methodology that allow the computer to visualize and recognize more subtle prognostic associated patterns are covered in

FIGURE 8.4 Tissue segmentation performed by deep learning.

When segmenting tumor from stroma without the aid of a tumor visualization marker, shallow learning—based image segmentation is usually inaccurate. Deep learning can be applied in this instance for accurate tissue segmentation. These examples utilize Indica Labs HALO AI software to segment tumor from stroma. (A) A TMA core stained with only hematoxylin. (B) HALO AI algorithm trained to recognize only tumor cells (red) within the hematoxylin-stained digital image. (C) The software next classifies each tumor nuclei (dark blue). (D) Deep learning algorithm's ability to be trained to recognize tumor (green overlay) from stroma (red overlay) and from H&E-stained digital images.

more detail elsewhere in this book. Algorithms such as these are being developed to aid the pathologist in their diagnosis, and it is only a matter of time until they are applied routinely in the clinical workflow of pathology departments. Currently, these algorithms are not being designed to automatically report on patient samples, without any human verification, rather to act as an aid to the pathologist in order to increase the speed of their reporting, for example, by highlighting the areas of interest, as a method to triage urgent cases or as a second opinion. However, as deep learning becomes more sophisticated, there is a strong possibility that in the future, computer vision algorithms may perform an aspect of autonomous clinical reporting. Later in this chapter, we discuss what regulatory concerns to address when designing an algorithm for translation into the clinic.

Deep learning architectures are now able to predict patient molecular subgroups from H&E-labeled histology. They do this from only the morphology and histological pattern of the tissue sample [15,16]. This may be quite remarkable to imagine; however, the histopathologist would most likely have predicted this to be possible. They have been fully aware of the complex and important variations of morphology present in the tissue and how they affect patient outcome; even if they have not been able to link these to molecular subtypes. This, however, has real implications beyond academic research. Molecular testing is expensive and requires complex instrumentation. If the same information, relevant to personalized pathology, can be gleaned from the routine and cheap H&E-labeled section, this could have significant monetary impact when calculating health economics.

Spatial resolution

We have briefly covered the importance of reporting the tissue architecture in the field of precision medicine when quantifying biomarkers of interest, as opposed to other molecular technology that destroys the tissue and thus the spatial resolution of its cellular components. Histopathologists know that context is key to an accurate diagnosis and prognosis. The tumor microenvironment is complex, with many cellular and molecular interactions that play a role in inhibiting or driving tumor progression and responses to therapy. The quantification of a stand-alone biomarker, even by image analysis, may not be enough to predict accurate prognosis or prediction for an individual patient. This is the case for PDL-1 immunohistochemical testing, where even patients with PDL-1 positive tumors may not respond to anti-PDL-1 therapy [17]. Similarly, there is an advantage to quantifying prognostic histopathological features such as lymphocytic infiltration or tumor budding in distinct regions within the tumor microenvironment. Traditionally, image analysis has quantified a single prognostic feature across a single tissue section and with proven success at patient stratification. However, by applying multiplexed immunofluorescence, it is now possible to visualize multiple biomarkers and histological features within a single tissue section. Image analysis software can furthermore calculate and export the exact x and y spatial coordinates of each feature of interest across the WSI, or recognize specific patterns within the interacting cellular milieu of the tumor microenvironment (Fig. 8.5). This not only brings the advantage of measuring more than one prognostic feature, but also allows new insights into the understanding of disease progression based on quantifying novel interactions at the spatial resolution of the tissue. This was demonstrated by Nearchou et al. who showed that the density of tumor budding and immune infiltrate were significantly associated with stage II colorectal cancer survival, but furthermore that their specific interaction added value to a combined prognostic model [6]. Studies such as this show that complex spatial analysis may be key to the success of accurate prognosis for the individual patient.

Machine learning on extracted data

The image analysis solutions described above allow accurate image segmentation and cellular and molecular classifications of known biomarkers or histopathological features. The quantification of these known features can be utilized and applied to deliver personalized pathology. However, image analysis can further extract a wealth of unbiasedly collected data across multiple classified objects and their spatial interactions. Such data may be the specific density of specific objects surrounding others, or their distance to each other, as well as a wealth of extent, shape, and texture measurements of individual objects. The value of these data is often not known *a priori*

FIGURE 8.5 Quantifying the spatial resolution of cellular subpopulations.

This figure demonstrates how CD3 and CD8 positive lymphocyte densities can be mapped to tumor cells when multiplexed immunofluorescence is quantified using Indica Lab HALO software. Immunofluorescence labeled CD3 (yellow) and CD8 (red) positive lymphocytes (A) segmented and quantified (B). (C) Tumor cells (green) captured from the same image as (A) and segmented and quantified (D). The exported x and y spatial coordinates of the tumor cells (green dots) are plotted alongside the coordinates of the CD3 (yellow dots) and CD8 (red dots) positive lymphocytes(E). This allows for the spatial statistics of the lymphocytes within a 50-μm diameter of a tumor cell being calculated.

and is difficult, if not impossible, to sort and analyze by eye. Machine learning can be applied to large datasets from both molecular and digital pathology in order to understand the optimal features that allow patient stratification, and thus clinical decision-making, in the field of personalized medicine. However, caution must be taken when deciding on which machine learning algorithm to apply to your data. If one model is superior at analyzing one dataset, based on, e.g., the search for the optimal area under the receiver operator, it does not mean that the same algorithm will be as successful at analyzing a second and distinct dataset under similar computational restrictions. This forms part of the "no free lunch theorem" [18] of which we will touch upon again later in the chapter. In plain terms, different machine learning algorithms are superior to others when applied to specific datasets. For example, some algorithms excel at analyzing data with low dimensionality (such as K-Nearest Neighbor) and, however, become intractable or return poor results when the data dimensions increase. On the other hand, random forests excel at analyzing high-dimensional data. Similarly, some models are better than others at separating data in a linear fashion. As we rarely know *a priori* which model, or which settings of their hyperparameters, is optimal at separating a specific dataset, it is prudent to test multiple machine learning methodologies across a single dataset. Automated workflows can be designed that split data into balanced training and test sets, apply feature reduction algorithms (if needed), test multiple machine learning models, and set their hyperparameters before returning the model and features used to best separate ones data and answer the clinical question being asked [19].

An example that demonstrates the usefulness of combining many of the topics that we have discussed in this chapter is that of Schmidt et al., who designed an image analysis and deep learning workflow to better predict a patient's response to ipilimumab [20]. They combined basic image analysis thresholding to classify lymphocytic infiltrating cells and applied deep learning to negate artifact and necrosis in the images. Furthermore, they used pathologist annotations to train for specific regions of interest, where they compartmentalized the tumor and stroma prior to quantification of the lymphocytic contexture. Finally, they applied multiple methods of analyzing their resultant data before reporting the final optimal model that predicts response to treatment.

Beyond augmentation

To make deep learning an effective method for patient diagnosis in the clinic, there must be a sufficient amount of labeled annotations and a wide variety of samples to be representative of the larger population. In the case of deep learning, this requires training and validation on 1000s of patient samples, obtained from multiple international institutes and prepared by multiple individuals. This is not an easy or fast task to perform. A major drawback to the field is a lack of such large well-annotated and curated datasets that are available to data scientists. However, there is a wealth of data held in each hospital located in their glass microscope slide archives and that go back decades. These data can be traced back to each patient treated in that institute along with their clinical reports. A sample tissue section from each patient in the archive will be stained with H&E, and as each prospective patient's samples are also stained with H&E, it makes sense to concentrate deep learning efforts on digital pathology samples prepared with this stain. The bottleneck is therefore not access to patient samples but the expert's digitized annotations of regions of interest that pertain to diagnosis. To overcome this bottleneck, researchers are forgoing image level annotations and developing weakly supervised deep learning architectures that rely only on slide level annotations, namely the diagnosis of the patient. Simply put, the computer is not told where in the image the cancer is, rather that somewhere in the image there are cancer cells. This methodology has been shown to be effective and relies on the data-driven analysis of patients, where the computer vision algorithm identifies subtle and complex morphologies that relate to diagnosis or prognosis. Thus, the machine can now inform the human on what is of pathological significance within the patient's individual tissue specimen. These patterns may have gone unnoticed to date, or have been too complex to allow for a standardized reporting protocol to be produced by human effort. This type of methodology has been tested in colorectal cancer [21], prostate cancer, and lymph nodal metastasis of breast cancer [22]. Further information on these methodologies can be found in the following chapter.

Practical concepts and theory of machine learning
Machine learning and digital pathology

The existing work in the realm of digital pathology, which analyzes various types of clinical data, could be conceptually organized in a variety of ways, that is, according to different criteria. Considering the diversity of pathologies of possible interest, one approach would be to consider solutions developed with specific diseases in mind, or indeed tissues or populations; another criterion would be based on the type of annotations that is training feedback, available for learning; yet another could distinguish between different types of input data and the modalities used to acquire them.

For reasons which will become apparent as we develop our narrative, herein we found it useful to start with a broad categorization of work in the area into two categories in terms of their technical approach to the problem. The first of these could be roughly described as involving "conventional" (or "traditional") computer vision, and the second one as deep learning based. This distinction is somewhat loose but in that it reflects the current trends in the field, namely the shift in focus from the former to the latter, it will be useful for illustrating the driving challenges and opportunities in the field, as well as for highlighting potential pitfalls and limitations of the current thinking, and for explaining our thoughts and recommendations for future work.

Considering the variety of challenges that a pathologist has to deal with in the analysis of real-world cases, it should come as no great surprise to the reader that algorithmic solutions addressing a wide range of possibly useful tasks have been explored and proposed. Much, indeed probably most, of research has focused on diagnostic tasks or prognostic stratification (e.g., high vs. low risk). Others provide a more assistive role to a human expert by providing automatic or semiautomatic segmentation of images, classification of cells, detection of structures of interest (cells, tissues types, tumors, etc.) from images, and so on. Although future work may lead to the fully automatic diagnosis of patients, currently the drive is for clinically transferable tools to aid the pathologist in their diagnosis.

Common techniques

The common clinical questions highlighted in the previous section can all be broadly seen as to have the same form as the two most frequently encountered machine learning paradigms: namely those of classification (e.g., "is a disease present or not?" and "is the patient in the high risk category or not"?) and regression (e.g., "what is the severity of disease?" and "what is the patient's life expectancy?"). Therefore it can hardly come as much of a surprise to observe that most of the work in the area to date involves the adoption and adaptation of well-known and well-understood existing techniques, and their application on pathology data. Here we give the reader a flavor of the context, and pros and cons, of some of these that have been applied to analyzing the multiparametric data extracted from the image analysis of digital pathology specimens.

Supervised learning

Even the mere emergence of digitization to clinical pathology, that is the use of computerized systems for storing, logging, and linking information, has led to the availability of vast amounts of labeled data as well as the associated meta-data. The reduced cost of computing power and storage, increased connectivity, and widespread adoption of technology have all contributed greatly to this trend which has escalated yet further with the rising recognition of the potential of artificial intelligence. Consequently, supervised machine learning in its various forms has attracted a great amount of research attention and continues to be one of the key focal points of ongoing research efforts.

Both shallow and deep learning algorithms have been successfully applied to clinical problems. Deep learning strategies based on layer depth and architecture of neural network—based models have been discussed in detail in Chapters 2—4. This section will therefore focus on the mathematical underpinnings of shallow learning algorithms such as Naïve Bayes, logistic regression, support vector machines, and random forests. In contrast, the mathematics of deep learning models are highly complex, as they encompass multilayer perceptron models, probabilistic graphical models, residual and recurrent networks, reinforcement and evolutionary learning, and so on. Detailed overview of these is presented in Chapters 2—4, but the mathematics involved are beyond the scope of the book. For a rigorous mathematical treatment of deep learning, see *Deep Learning* by Goodfellow, Bengio, and Courville, or any of the other modern texts in the field.

Naïve Bayes assumption—based methods

Naïve Bayes classification applies the Bayes theorem by making the "naïve" assumption of feature independence. Formally, given a set of n features $x_1,..., x_n$, the associated pattern is deemed as belonging to the class y which satisfies the following condition:

$$y = \arg \max_j P(C_j) \prod_{i=1}^{n} p(x_i|C_j) \qquad 8.1$$

where P (C_j) is the prior probability of the class C_j and $p(x_i|C_j)$ is the conditional probability of the feature x_i given class C_j (readily estimated from data using a supervised learning framework) [23].

The key potential weakness of naïve Bayes—based algorithms, be they regression or classification oriented, is easily spotted, and it lies in the unrealistic assumption of feature independence. Yet, somewhat surprisingly at the first sight, these simple approaches often work remarkably well in practice and often outperform more complex and, as regards the fundamental assumptions of feature relatedness, more expressive and more flexible models [19].

There are a few reasons why this might be the case. One of these includes the structure of errors—if the conceptual structure of data relatedness under a given representation is in a sense symmetrical, errors in the direction of overestimating conditional probabilities and those in the direction of underestimating them can cancel out in the aggregate, leading to more accurate overall estimates [24]. Another equally important factor contributing to often surprisingly good performance of methods which make the naïve Bayes assumption emerges as a consequence of the relationship between the amount of available training data (given a problem of a specific complexity) and the number of free parameters of the adopted model. It is often the case, especially considering that in digital pathology class imbalance poses major practical issues, that more complex models cannot be sufficiently well trained; thus, even if in principle able to learn a more complex functional behavior, this theoretical superiority cannot be exploited.

While a good starting point and a sensible baseline, naïve Bayes—based methods are in the right circumstances outperformed by more elaborate models, some of which we summarize next.

Logistic regression—based methods

Logistic regression is another widely used, well-understood, and often well-performing supervised learning technique. In logistic regression, the conditional probability of the dependent variable (class) y is modeled as a logit-transformed multiple linear regression of the explanatory variables (input features) $x_1, ..., x_n$:

$$P_{LR}(y = \pm 1|\mathbf{x}, \mathbf{w}) = \frac{1}{1 + e^{-y\mathbf{w}^T\mathbf{x}}}. \qquad 8.2$$

The model is trained (i.e., the weight parameter w learned) by maximizing the likelihood of the model on the training dataset, given by:

$$\prod_{i=1}^{2} Pr(y_i|\mathbf{x}_i, \mathbf{w}) = \prod_{i=1}^{2} \frac{1}{1 + e^{-y_i \mathbf{w}^T \mathbf{x}_i}}, \qquad 8.3$$

penalized by the complexity of the model:

$$\frac{1}{\sigma\sqrt{2\pi}} \, e^{-\frac{1}{2\sigma^2}\mathbf{w}^T\mathbf{w}}, \qquad 8.4$$

which can be restated as the minimization of the following regularized negative log-likelihood:

$$\mathfrak{L} = C \sum_{i=1}^{2} \log\left(1 + e^{-y_i \mathbf{w}^T \mathbf{x}_i}\right) + \mathbf{w}^T \mathbf{w}. \qquad 8.5$$

A coordinate descent approach, such as the one described by Yu et al. [25], can be used to minimize L.

Support vector–based methods

Support vector machines perform classification by constructing a series of class separating hyperplanes in a high-dimensional (potentially infinitely dimensional) space into which the original input data are mapped [26]. For comprehensive detail of this regression technique, the reader is referred to the original work by Vapnik [27]; herein we present a summary of the key ideas.

In the context of support vector machines, the seemingly intractable task of mapping data into a very high-dimensional space is achieved efficiently by performing the aforesaid mapping implicitly, rather than explicitly. This is done by employing the so-called *kernel trick* which ensures that dot products in the high-dimensional space are readily computed using the variables in the original space. Given labeled training data (input vectors and the associated labels) in the form $\{(x_1, y_1), \ldots, (x_n, y_n)\}$, a support vector machine aims to find a mapping which minimizes the number of misclassified training instances, in a regularized fashion. As mentioned earlier, an implicit mapping of input data $x \rightarrow \Phi(x)$ is performed by employing a Mercer-admissible kernel [28] $k(x_i, x_j)$ which allows for the dot products between mapped data to be computed in the input space: $\Phi(x_i) \cdot \Phi(x_j) = k(x_i, x_j)$. The classification vector in the transformed, high-dimensional space of the form

$$w = \sum_{i=1}^{n} c_i y_i \Phi(x_i) \qquad 8.6$$

is sought by minimizing

$$\sum_{i=1}^{n} c_i - \frac{1}{2} \sum_{i=1}^{n} \sum_{j=1}^{n} y_i c_i k(x_i, x_j) y_j c_j \qquad 8.7$$

subject to the constraints $\sum_{i=1}^{n} c_i y_i = 0$ and $0 \leq c_i \leq 1/(2n\lambda)$. The regularizing parameter λ penalizes prediction errors. Support vector—based approaches usually perform well even with relatively small training datasets and have the advantage of well-understood mathematical behavior (which is an important consideration in the context of regularly compliance, among others).

Stepping back for a moment from the technical detail, intuitively what is happening here is that the algorithm is learning which class exemplars are the "most problematic" ones, i.e., which exemplars are nearest to the class boundaries and thus most likely to be misclassified. These are the support vectors that give the approach its name. Inspection of these is insightful. Firstly, a large number of support vectors (relative to the total amount of training data) should immediately raise eyebrows as it suggests overfitting. Secondly, by examining which exemplars end up as support vectors, an understanding of the nature of learning that took place can be gain as well as of the structure of the problem and data representation, which can lead to useful and novel clinical insight.

Nonparametric, k-nearest neighbor—based methods

The k-nearest neighbor classifier classifies a novel pattern comprising features x1, ..., xn to the class dominant in the set of k-nearest neighbors to the input pattern (in the feature space) among the training patterns with known class memberships [29]. The usually employed similarity metric used is the Euclidean distance.

Random forests

Random forest classifiers fall under the broad umbrella of ensemble-based learning methods [30]. They are simple to implement, fast in operation, and have proven to be extremely successful in a variety of domains [31,32]. The key principle underlying the random forest approach comprises the construction of many "simple" decision trees in the training stage and the majority vote (mode) across them in the classification stage. Among other benefits, this voting strategy has the effect of correcting for the undesirable property of decision trees to overfit training data [33]. In the training stage, random forests apply the general technique known as bagging to individual trees in the ensemble. Bagging repeatedly selects a random sample with replacement from the training set and fits trees to these samples. Each tree is grown without any pruning. The number of trees in the ensemble is a free parameter which is readily learned automatically using the so-called out-of-bag error [29].

Much like in the case of naïve Bayes— and k-nearest neighbor—based algorithms, random forests are popular in part due to their simplicity on the one hand, and generally good performance on the other. However, unlike the former two approaches, random forests exhibit a degree of unpredictability as regards the structure of the final trained model. This is an inherent consequence of the stochastic nature of tree building. As we will explore in more detail shortly, one of the key reasons why this characteristic of random forests can be a problem in regulatory reasons— clinical adoption often demands a high degree of repeatability not only in terms of the ultimate performance of an algorithm but also in terms of the mechanics as to how a specific decision is made.

Unsupervised learning

We have already mentioned the task of patient stratification. Indeed, the need for stratification emerges frequently in digital pathology, for example, due to the hetero-geneity of many diseases or differential response of different populations to treat-ment or the disease itself [19].

Given that the relevant strata are often unknown a priori, often because the lim-itations imposed by previously exclusively manual interpretation of data and the scale at which the data would need to be examined to draw reliable conclusions, it is frequently desirable to stratify automatically. A common way of doing this is by means of unsupervised learning, by applying a clustering algorithm such as a Gaussian mixture model or more frequently due to its simplicity and fewer free pa-rameters, the k-means algorithm [21]. Then any subsequent learning can be per-formed in a more targeted fashion by learning separate models for each of the clusters individually.

Let $X = \{x_1, x_2, ..., x_n\}$ be a set of d-dimensional feature vectors. The k-means algorithm partitions the points into K clusters, $X_1, ..., X_K$, so that each datum be-longs to one and only one cluster. In addition, an attempt is made to minimize the sum of squared distances between each data point and the empirical mean of the cor-responding cluster. In other words, the k-means algorithm attempts to minimize the following objective function:

$$J(X_1, ..., X_k) = \sum_{i=1}^{k} \sum_{x \in X_i} \|c_i - x\|^2,$$

8.8

where the empirical cluster means are calculated as:

$$c_i = \sum_{x \in X_i} x / |X_i|.$$

8.9

The exact minimization of the objective function in Ref. [1] is an NP-hard prob-lem [34]. Instead, the k-means algorithm only guarantees convergence to a local minimum. Starting from an initial guess, the algorithm iteratively updates cluster centers and data-cluster assignments until (1) a local minimum is attained, or (2) an alternative stopping criterion is met (e.g., the maximal desired number of itera-tions or a sufficiently small sum of squared distances). The k-means algorithm starts from an initial guess of cluster centers.

Often, this is achieved simply by choosing k data points at random as the centers of the initial clusters, although more sophisticated initialization methods have been proposed [35,36]. Then, at each iteration $t = 0, ...$ the new datum-cluster assignment is computed:

$$X_i^{(t)} = \left\{ x : x \in X \wedge \arg \min_j \left\| x - c_j^{(t)} \right\|^2 = i \right\}. \qquad 8.10$$

In other words, each datum is assigned to the cluster with the nearest (in the Euclidean sense) empirical mean. Lastly, the locations of cluster centers are recomputed from the new assignments by finding the mean of the data assigned to each cluster:

$$c_j^{(t+1)} = \sum_{x \in X_i^{(t)}} x / \left| X_i^{(t)} \right| \qquad 8.11$$

The algorithm is guaranteed to converge because neither of the updates in Ref. [3] nor [4] can ever increase the objective function of Ref. [1]. Various extensions of the original k-means algorithm include fuzzy c-means [37], k-medoid [38], kernel k-means [39], as well as discriminative k-means when partial labeling is available [40]. The interested reader is referred to the cited publications for further information.

Image-based digital pathology

Probably one of the most interesting areas of research in digital pathology, both in terms of practical potential and the nature of intellectual challenges, concerns the use of images.

Due to the inherent complexity of images of interest in pathology, the aforementioned distinction between what we termed "conventional" machine learning— and deep learning—based methods is particularly pronounced in this realm of digital pathology. In an outline, the former usually take on a modular, pipeline form whereby explicitly engineered features (sometimes referred to as "handcrafted" features) are extracted from input images first, and then fed into a machine learning algorithm of the sort described in the previous section. In contrast, in deep learning—based approaches, the process is not atomized [41] in this manner—good features, as complex functions of directly sensed data (e.g., pixel intensities), are learned automatically from labeled training data. This distinction has often led to deep learning—based methods being characterized as "data agnostic" [42]; colloquially put, the idea is that no matter what the input is, the algorithm will learn what good features are. However, to describe deep learning in this manner would be a misnomer and highly misleading. For any learning to take place, the model has to be constrained and by virtue of these constraints contain implicit information about the problem at hand; succinctly put, a tabular rasa cannot learn. Indeed, one of the theorems popularly known as "no free lunch theorem" implicitly says the very same:

> *Any two optimization algorithms are equivalent when their performance is averaged across all possible problems.*

Ref. [18]

Thus, deep learning algorithms too are not endowed with a quasi-magical ability to overcome this fundamental limitation but are also constrained by some prior knowledge (and are hence not agnostic). In particular, a deep neural network contains constraints, which emerge from the type of its layers, their order, and the number of neurons in each layer, the connectedness of layers, and other architectural aspects. This is important to keep in mind and not see deep learning as necessarily superior to "conventional" approaches or see them as the universal solution to any problem.

Conventional approaches to image analysis

As mentioned already, the first broad category of algorithms that have been proposed a means of analyzing images used in clinical pathology is one which uses what we term conventional, or traditional, computer vision. By this, we primarily refer to the first stage in the processing, which concerns the extraction of a priori, explicitly defined features. The key premise is appealing and intuitively sensible to use human expertize to identify what elementary, low level elements of an image are salient in that they capture important discriminative information on the one hand, and are yet compact enough to facilitate computational efficiency and reliable learning from available data.

Having demonstrated success on a wide variety of images of so-called natural scenes (to say the least, they have rather revolutionarized the field) [43], local appearance descriptors originally proposed for more day-to-day applications of computer vision (e.g., location recognition, synthetic panoramic image generation, object localization, etc.) have been adopted first and applied on a diverse range of pathology image types [44,45]. Popular and widely used examples include local binary pattern (LBP) [46], scale invariant feature transform (SIFT) [47], and histogram of oriented gradients (HOG) [48] based descriptors.

While also "handcrafted" in contrast to the above general purpose descriptor—based features are features which directly and explicitly exploit domain-specific information, that is, human expert knowledge of pathology. Thus, body of interest counts (e.g., tumor and immune cells, etc.), their morphology quantifiers (e.g., size, eccentricity), or spatial statistics are some of the widely used ones. The appeal of these is twofold. First, by their very nature they can be reasonably expected to exhibit saliency in the context of pathology slide analysis. Moreover, they are usually rather effortlessly measured (extracted) from images: different staining and imaging modalities or biomarkers can be used to highlight the targets of interest, and simple image processing or computer vision algorithms (such as flood fill algorithms [49], morphological operators [50], blob detectors [45], etc.) usually suffice as regard to the computational side.

Deep learning on images

One of the reasons why deep learning has become such a popular area of research lies in its success when applied to many computer vision problems, including a number of those which have been prohibitively challenging using more traditional approaches [51]. Its application to image analysis in digital pathology has not disappointed either, with deep learning quickly establishing the state-of-the-art performance in the context of a number of diverse tasks. Considering that the technical detail specifically of deep learning is addressed by several other chapters in the present volume, herein we focus our attention on the bigger picture with the aim of highlighting the key trends in the field, the main challenges, and inherent advantages and disadvantages of deep learning.

Rather than joining the choir singing praises to deep learning, a more useful, insightful, and instructive question to ask concerns the outstanding limitations. If the key obstacle were merely the availability of sufficient data (undoubtedly a difficulty encountered by virtually any single research group, perhaps save for the few tech giants), the solution would be merely a matter of time and concerted effort. Unfortunately from the practical point of view, or fortunately from the point of view of intellectual challenge, the answer is more nuanced. In particular, the major problem to current methods is posed by the sheer size of individual images which are often in excess of 10 GB each. Training deep neural network images of this size (and bear in mind that deep learning methods are very training data hungry) is computationally impractical.

A survey of existing work in the field shows two main ways of dealing with the problem posed by the size of WSIs. The first of these involves severe downsampling—a multiple gigapixel image is scaled down to an image with mere tens of thousands of pixels. The second approach consists of dividing a WSI into small patches (usually nonoverlapping), performing learning on these as individual images, and then aggregating patch level decisions to arrive at a slide level decision. Both approaches can be seen to lead to information loss, albeit in different ways. As formally demonstrated by Nyquist in the 1930s, but equally easy understood intuitively, the type of information loss incurred by the downsampling approach comes in the form of loss of fine detail (i.e., high spatial frequencies). Even to a human expert, this information is important in the interpretation of a tissue slide, and can be expected to be even more so to computer-based methods which do not suffer from many of the imperfections of the human visual system. The type of information loss that takes place in patch-based algorithms is rather different and more nuanced so it is useful to highlight a few influential works before continuing the discussion.

In the simplest form, patches are treated entirely separately from one another. This approach has yielded promising results in patch level distinction between tumorous and normal tissues [52] and the segmentation of precursor lesions [53], but on prognostic tasks the success has been much more limited [54]. Moving away from patch level decision as the ultimate aim, Hou et al. [55] proposed a method whereby a deep neural network is trained on individual patches, and patch level decisions aggregated by virtue of voting to make slide level predictions. Recently, a few methods which address the challenges of intraslide heterogeneity have been introduced, broadly comprising adaptive selection of patches, phenotype-based patch clustering, automatic clustering selection, and learned aggregation of cluster level predictions. Initial attempts were disappointing [56], but more subsequent refinements of the methodology have led to much more promising results [21].

What the above fly-through the field brings out to the fore are some of the key limitations of patch-based methods, which dominate the existing literature. First, by decomposing a WSI into patches, it is virtually unavoidable but to resort to a form of ad hoc labeling of patches, usually attaching the whole slide label to all of the patches extracted from it. This is clearly a rather unattractive proposition as not every region in a slide containing a pathology is equally informative; indeed some may contain perfectly healthy tissue. Hence the learning algorithm is effectively fed incorrect data. Moreover, problems arise in the aggregation stage too. Lastly, there is a loss of spatial information effected by the separation of patches and the arbitrariness of the loci of patch boundaries with respect to the imaged physical tissue.

Regulatory concerns and considerations

Thus far our focus was on the fundamental challenges associated with the use of images for tasks in digital pathology, the manner in which these have shaped the field to date, and the trends most likely to yield advances in future. Related to these, equally important in practice though somewhat different in nature, are requirements and demands associated with the adoption of artificial intelligence in everyday clinical processes. Oftentimes these are imposed by various regulatory bodies, such as the Food and Drug Administration (FDA) in the United States or more loosely the end users themselves. While a comprehensive examination of this topic is beyond the scope of this chapter, it is important to draw the reader's attention to some of the key issues within this area. In particular, we highlight three issues:

- Explainability,
- Repeatability, and
- Generalizability.

Explainability in the context of relevance here concerns the ability for a decision made by an algorithmic, artificial intelligence—based solution to be communicated to a human on a semantically appropriate level. In other words, the question being asked is not just what the decision is but rather how or why the algorithm made that decision. As alluded to before, for many of the algorithms covered under the umbrella of conventional approaches to image understanding, this is reasonably straightforward. For example, in k-nearest neighbor—based solutions, the nearest neighbors, that is, previously seen and human labeled examples which exhibit the greatest similarity to a new example under consideration can be brought up. With support vector–based methods, the closest examples (in a kernel sense) or the support vectors which define class boundaries can be similarly used to gain insight into what was learned and how a decision was made. With random forests, a well-known method of substituting features with dummy features can be used to quantify which features are the most important ones in decision-making and "sanity checked" by an expert. This process can be not only confirmatory but can also lead to novel clinical insight. While explainability has for a long time been seen as a potential disadvantage (cf. with human memory and brain: can one localize where the concept of "cake" is stored?) of deep learning–based approaches, which used to be seen as proverbial "black boxes," recent years have seen huge strides of progress in this area [57]. For example, looking at which neurons in a network fire together (cf. the mantra of biological reinforcement learning "what fires together wires together") can be insightful. A higher (semantic) level of insight can be gained by looking at different layers and visualizing features learned—typically layers closer to input tend to learn simple, low-level appearance elements, which are then combined to compose more complex visual patterns downstream [58]. Another ingenious technique involves so-called "occlusion" whereby parts of an input image are occluded by a uniform pattern (thus effecting localized information loss) and quantifying the impact such occlusion has on the decision—the greater the impact, the greater the importance of a particular image locus [59].

The issues of repeatability and reproducibility have gained much prominence in academic circles, and wider, in recent years. The difference between the two concepts has been convincingly highlighted and discussed by Drummond [60], but this nuance does not appear to have penetrated regulatory processes as of yet. In particular, the practical impossibility of perfect reproducibility of experimental outcomes for some machine learning algorithms poses a major obstacle in their adoption in clinical practice due to the stochastic nature of their operation. We have already alluded to this in the previous section in our overview of random forests. In particular, even if the same training data are used and the same manner of training employed, the parameters of a trained random forest or neural network will differ from instance to instance. This is an inherent consequence of the stochastic elements of their training processes and is something that does not sit comfortably with some. While this sentiment is not difficult to relate to, it does illustrate what can be argued to be an inconsistency in how human and machine expertize are treated. In particular, the former has been shown to exhibit major interpersonal variability (two different, competent, and experienced pathologists arriving at different conclusions from the same data), as well as intrapersonal one (e.g., depending on the degree of fatigue, time of day, whether the decision is made in the anteprandial or postprandial period, etc.). This kind of double standard is consistent with a broad range of studies involving human-human and human-machine interaction and is neurologically well understood, with the two types of engagement differently engaging important brain circuitry such as the ventromedial prefrontal cortex and the amygdala [61]. Generalizability is a concept that pervades machine learning. It refers to the ability of an algorithm to learn from training data some information contained within it which would allow it to make good decisions on previously unseen input, often seemingly rather different from anything seen in the training stage. The issue of generalizability underlies the tasks of data representation, problem abstraction, mathematical modeling of learning, etc. Herein we are referring to generalizability in a very specific context. Namely, a major challenge in the practice of pathology concerns different protocols and conditions in which data are acquired. Put simply, the question being asked is what performance can I expect to see from an algorithm evaluated using data a technician acquired using particular equipment on one cohort of patients in a specific lab, when it is applied on data acquired by a different technician in a different lab from a different cohort. It can be readily seen that slight changes in the data acquisition (such as the duration of exposure to a dye), different physical characteristics of lab instruments, or indeed different demographics of patients all pose reasonable grounds for concern. Indeed, at present, most of the work in digital pathology is rather limited in this regard, in no small part due to the variety of obstacles in data sharing: there are issues of ethics and privacy, as well as financial interests at stake.

Acknowledgments

The authors would like to acknowledge Inés Nearchou for kindly providing images for the figures within this chapter.

References

[1] Caie PD, Walls RE, Ingleston-Orme A, Daya S, Houslay T, Eagle R, et al. High-content phenotypic profiling of drug response signatures across distinct cancer cells. Molecular Cancer Therapeutics 2010;9(6):1913–26.

[2] Deans GT, Heatley M, Anderson N, Patterson CC, Rowlands BJ, Parks TG, et al. Jass' classification revisited. Journal of the American College of Surgeons 1994;179(1):11–7.

[3] Lim D, Alvarez T, Nucci MR, Gilks B, Longacre T, Soslow RA, et al. Interobserver variability in the interpretation of tumor cell necrosis in uterine leiomyosarcoma. The American Journal of Surgical Pathology 2013;37(5):650–8.

[4] Chandler I, Houlston RS. Interobserver agreement in grading of colorectal cancers—findings from a nationwide web-based survey of histopathologists. Histopathology 2008;52(4):494–9.

[5] Caie PD, Zhou Y, Turnbull AK, Oniscu A, Harrison DJ. Novel histopathologic feature identified through image analysis augments stage II colorectal cancer clinical reporting. Oncotarget 2016;7(28):44381–94.

[6] Nearchou IP, Lillard K, Gavriel CG, Ueno H, Harrison DJ, Caie PD. Automated analysis of lymphocytic infiltration, tumor budding, and their spatial relationship improves prognostic accuracy in colorectal cancer. Cancer Immunology Research 2019;7(4):609–20.

[7] Khameneh FD, Razavi S, Kamasak M. Automated segmentation of cell membranes to evaluate HER2 status in whole slide images using a modified deep learning network. Computers in Biology and Medicine 2019;110:164–74.

[8] Widmaier M, Wiestler T, Walker J, Barker C, Scott ML, Sekhavati F, et al. Comparison of continuous measures across diagnostic PD-L1 assays in non-small cell lung cancer using automated image analysis. Modern Pathology 2019;33.

[9] Puri M, Hoover SB, Hewitt SM, Wei BR, Adissu HA, Halsey CHC, et al. Automated computational detection, quantitation, and mapping of mitosis in whole-slide images for clinically actionable surgical pathology decision support. Journal of Pathology Informatics 2019;10:4.

[10] Brieu N, Gavriel CG, Nearchou IP, Harrison DJ, Schmidt G, Caie PD. Automated tumour budding quantification by machine learning augments TNM staging in muscle-invasive bladder cancer prognosis. Scientific Reports 2019;9(1):5174.

[11] Brieu N, Gavriel CG, Harrison DJ, Caie PD, Schmidt G. Context-based interpolation of coarse deep learning prediction maps for the segmentation of fine structures in immunofluorescence images. SPIE; 2018.

[12] Roy S, kumar Jain A, Lal S, Kini J. A study about color normalization methods for histopathology images. Micron 2018;114:42−61.

[13] Cruz-Roa A, Gilmore H, Basavanhally A, Feldman M, Ganesan S, Shih NNC, et al. Accurate and reproducible invasive breast cancer detection in whole-slide images: a deep learning approach for quantifying tumor extent. Scientific Reports 2017;7:46450.

[14] Litjens G, Bandi P, Ehteshami Bejnordi B, Geessink O, Balkenhol M, Bult P, et al. 1399 H&E-stained sentinel lymph node sections of breast cancer patients: the CAMELYON dataset. GigaScience 2018;7(6).

[15] Coudray N, Ocampo PS, Sakellaropoulos T, Narula N, Snuderl M, Fenyö D, et al. Classification and mutation prediction from non−small cell lung cancer histopathology images using deep learning. Nature Medicine 2018;24(10):1559−67.

[16] Sirinukunwattana K, Domingo E, Richman S, Redmond KL, Blake A, Verrill C, et al. Image-based consensus molecular subtype classification (imCMS) of colorectal cancer using deep learning. bioRxiv 2019:645143.

[17] Havel JJ, Chowell D, Chan TA. The evolving landscape of biomarkers for checkpoint inhibitor immunotherapy. Nature Reviews Cancer 2019;19(3):133−50.

[18] Wolpert DH, Macready WG. No free lunch theorems for optimization. Transactions on Evolutionary Computation 1997;1(1):67−82.

[19] Dimitriou N, Arandjelović O, Harrison DJ, Caie PD. A principled machine learning framework improves accuracy of stage II colorectal cancer prognosis. NPJ Digital Medicine 2018;1(1):52.

[20] Harder N, Schonmeyer R, Nekolla K, Meier A, Brieu N, Vanegas C, et al. Automatic discovery of image-based signatures for ipilimumab response prediction in malignant melanoma. Scientific Reports 2019;9(1):7449.

[21] Yue X, Dimitriou N, Arandjelovic O. Colorectal cancer outcome prediction from H&E whole slide images using machine learning and automatically inferred phenotype profiles. February 01, 2019. Available from: https://ui.adsabs.harvard.edu/abs/2019arXiv190203582Y.

[22] Campanella G, Hanna MG, Geneslaw L, Miraflor A, Werneck Krauss Silva V, Busam KJ, et al. Clinical-grade computational pathology using weakly supervised deep learning on whole slide images. Nature Medicine 2019;25(8):1301−9.

[23] Bishop CM. Pattern recognition and machine learning. New York, USA: Springer- Verlag; 2007.

[24] Vente D, Arandjelović O, Baron V, Dombay E, Gillespie S. Using machine learning for automatic counting of lipid-rich tuberculosis cells influorescence microscopy images.

In: Proc. AAAI conference on artificial intelligence workshop on health intelligence; 2019.

[25] Yu H-F, Huang F-L, Lin C-J. Dual coordinate descent methods for logistic regression and maximum entropy models. Machine Learning 2011;85(1−2):41−75.

[26] Schölkopf B, Smola A, Müller K. Advances in Kernel methods − SV learning, chapter Kernel principal component analysis. Cambridge, MA: MIT Press; 1999. p. 327−52.

[27] Vapnik V. The nature of statistical learning theory. Springer-Verlag; 1995.

[28] Mercer J. Functions of positive and negative type and their connection with the theory of integral equations. Philosophical Transactions of the Royal Society A 1909;209: 415−46.

[29] Cunningham P, Delany SJ. k-nearest neighbour classifiers. Multiple Classifier Systems 2007:1−17.

[30] Breiman L. Random forests. Machine Learning 2001;45(1):5−32.

[31] Cutler DR, Edwards TC, Beard KH, Cutler A, Hess KT, Gibson J, Lawler JJ. Random forests for classification in ecology. Ecology 2007;88(11):2783−92.

[32] Ghosh P, Manjunath B. Robust simultaneous registration and segmentation with sparse error reconstruction. IEEE Transactions on Pattern Analysis and Machine Intelligence 2013;35(2):425−36.

[33] Zadrozny B, Elkan C. Obtaining calibrated probability estimates from decision trees and naive Bayesian classifiers. Proceedings IMLS International Conference on Machine Learning 2001;1:609−16.

[34] Dasgupta S. The hardness of k-means clustering. Technical Report CS2007-0890. San Diego: University of California; 2007.

[35] Khan SS, Ahmadb A. Cluster center initialization algorithm for k- means clustering. Pattern Recognition Letters 2004;25(11):1293−302.

[36] Peña JM, Lozano JA, Larrañaga P. An empirical comparison of four initialization methods for the k-means algorithm. Pattern Recognition Letters 1999;20(10):1027−40.

[37] Dunn JC. A fuzzy relative of the ISODATA process and its use in detecting compact well-separated clusters. Journal of Cybernetics 1973;3(32−57).

[38] Kaufman L, Rousseeuw PJ. Finding groups in data: an introduction to cluster analysis. Wiley; 2005.

[39] Schölkopf B, Smola A, Müller K-R. Nonlinear component analysis as a kernel eigenvalue problem. Neural Computation 1998;10(5):1299−319.

[40] Arandjelović O. Discriminative k-means clustering. In: Proc. IEEE international joint conference on neural networks; 2013. p. 2374−80.

[41] Arandjelović O. A more principled use of the p-value? Not so fast: a critique of Colquhoun's argument. Royal Society Open Science; 2019.

[42] Kooi T, Litjens G, Van Ginneken B, Gubern-Mérida A, I Sánchez C, Mann R, den Heeten A, Karssemeijer N. Large-scale deep learning for computer aided detection of mammographic lesions. Medical Image Analysis 2017;35:303−12.

[43] Niemeyer M, Arandjelović O. Automatic semantic labelling of images by their content using non-parametric Bayesian machine learning and image search using synthetically generated image collages. In: Proc. IEEE international conference on data science and advanced analytics; 2018. p. 160−8.

[44] Alhindi TJ, Kalra S, Ng KH, Afrin A, Tizhoosh HR. Comparing lbp, hog and deep features for classification of histopathology images. In: 2018 International joint conference on neural networks (IJCNN). IEEE; 2018. p. 1−7.

[45] Xing F, Yang L. Robust nucleus/cell detection and segmentation in digital pathology and microscopy images: a comprehensive review. IEEE Reviews in Biomedical Engineering 2016;9:234−63.

[46] Fan J, Arandjelović O. Employing domain specific discriminative information to address inherent limitations of the LBP descriptor in face recognition. In: Proc. IEEE international joint conference on neural networks; 2018. p. 3766−72.

[47] Lowe DG. Distinctive image features from scale-invariant keypoints. International Journal of Computer Vision 2003;60(2):91−110.

[48] Arandjelović O. Object matching using boundary descriptors. In: Proc. British machine vision conference; 2012. https://doi.org/10.5244/C.26.85.

[49] Mehta N, Raja'S A, Chaudhary V. Content based sub-image retrieval system for high-resolution pathology images using salient interest points. In: 2009 Annual international conference of the IEEE engineering in medicine and biology society. IEEE; 2009. p. 3719−22.

[50] Karunakar Y, Kuwadekar A. An unparagoned application for red blood cell counting using marker controlled watershed algorithm for android mobile. In: 2011 Fifth international conference on next generation mobile applications, services and technologies. IEEE; 2011. p. 100−4.

[51] Zhu J-Y, Park T, Isola P, Efros AA. Unpaired image-to-image translation using cycle-consistent adversarial networks. In: Proceedings of the IEEE international conference on computer vision; 2017. p. 2223−32.

[52] Jamaluddin MF, Fauzi MFA, Abas FS. Tumor detection and whole slide classification of h&e lymph node images using convolutional neural network. In: Proc. IEEE International conference on signal and image processing applications; 2017. p. 90−5.

[53] Albayrak A, Ünlü A, Çalık N, Bilgin G, Türkmen İ, Çakır A, Ça- par A, Töreyin BU, Ata LD. Segmentation of precursor lesions in cervical cancer using convolutional neural networks. In: Proc. Signal processing and communications applications conference; 2017. p. 1−4.

[54] Mackillop WJ. The importance of prognosis in cancer medicine. TNM Online; 2003.

[55] Hou L, Samaras D, Kurc TM, Gao Y, Davis JE, Saltz JH. Patch-based convolutional neural network for whole slide tissue image classification. In: Proc. IEEE conference on computer vision and pattern recognition; 2016. p. 2424−33.

[56] Zhu X, Yao J, Zhu F, Huang J. Wsisa: making survival prediction from whole slide histopathological images. In: IEEE conference on computer vision and pattern recognition; 2017. p. 7234−42.

[57] Erhan D, Bengio Y, Courville A, Vincent P. Visualizing higher-layer features of a deep network. University of Montreal 2009;1341(3):1.

[58] Cooper J, Arandjelović O. Visually understanding rather than merely matching ancient coin images. In: Proc. INNS conference on big data and deep learning; 2019.

[59] Schlag I, Arandjelović O. Ancient Roman coin recognition in the wild using deep learning based recognition of artistically depicted face profiles. In: Proc. IEEE international conference on computer vision; 2017. p. 2898−906.

[60] Drummond C. Replicability is not reproducibility: nor is it good science. 2009.

[61] Kätsyri J, Hari R, Ravaja N, Nummenmaa L. The opponent matters: elevated fmri reward responses to winning against a human versus a computer opponent during interactive video game playing. Cerebral Cortex 2013;23(12):2829−39.

Artificial intelligence methods for predictive image-based grading of human cancers

Gerardo Fernandez, Abishek Sainath Madduri, Bahram Marami, Marcel Prastawa, Richard Scott, Jack Zeineh, Michael Donovan

Department of Pathology, Icahn School of Medicine at Mount Sinai, New York, NY, United States

Introduction

Surgical pathology and the practice of general medicine are often described as having legitimate components of art as well as science. That perception is perhaps less relevant in the current information age and with the adoption of genomic medicine, in large part due to the growth in disease-specific causal knowledge. As a surgical pathologist, gestalt and intuition are words you may not use to describe how you arrive at a specific patient's diagnosis, but it is certainly understood that with experience, in particular with a deep immersion in a subspecialty, comes an understanding of histopathology that cannot easily be transmitted or formalized. This is not in any way to delegitimize pathology or relegate it to the unscientific, rather to illustrate a strength of the human brain. For well over 100 years using a microscope, pathologists have been applying this strength to group and separate disease entities into diagnoses and their subtypes. The brain seems to be good at pattern recognition, filtering noise, and dealing with variability, and from a histopathology perspective, this has complemented the medical need quite well for over a century. Although the concept of tumor differentiation and its relationship to clinical outcome dates back to the early days of histopathology until fairly recently, limited treatment options diminished the necessity for more precise and standardized grading.

Over the past several decades, however, treating physicians and patients have seen increasingly sophisticated therapeutic options, directed at narrower oncologic disease states and have therefore become more and more reliant on accurate tumor classification to make informed decisions on the overall best treatment choice. The relevant information in this current era of personalized medicine ranges from robust prognostic information about specific diagnoses to the presence or absence of biomarkers that may dictate a targeted therapy. Although accurate classification clearly starts with tumor diagnosis, relevant subtypes, and even target biomarkers, it is not complete without robust and reproducible grading schemes providing reliable prognostic information. Although grade is emphasized in this review, it is important to

Artificial Intelligence and Deep Learning in Pathology. https://doi.org/10.1016/B978-0-323-67538-3.00009-9

understand that clinically relevant prognostic clinical models rely on both the AJCC cancer staging system and histologic grade to guide treatment decisions and project outcomes. In addition, these clinical models have further evolved with the advent of molecular phenotyping and the interplay with these same clinical features.

If we restrict ourselves to one organ system or further to one cell of origin, there are many examples where tumor type and subtype provide the prognostic information required to guide treatment and therefore grading schemes are either less important or not applicable, as is the case, for example, with prognostically favorable tubular or medullary carcinomas of the breast and prognostically unfavorable small cell lung cancer. For many cancers, however, it is the degree of differentiation that determines the aggressiveness of the tumor and therefore the grade. This makes intuitive sense as the degree of differentiation is a measure of a tumor's morphologic departure from the normal histologic pattern of the organ. The greater the tumor's departure from normal histology, the more malignant, unchecked, and aggressive it is.

Grading schemes over the years represent attempts to create a histopathology-based prognostic model, capturing the degree of differentiation and providing treating clinicians with the most reliable insight into the potential aggressive behavior of a cancer and therefore risk to the patient. These models incorporate a range of histologic features that are quantitatively or semiquantitatively determined microscopically by the pathologist. Some grading schemes incorporate very few features or focus on a narrow group of features as is the case in the Fuhrman grading system for renal clear-cell carcinoma which only uses nuclear features (size, shape, chromatin pattern, and nucleolar prominence) [1]. Other grading schemes incorporate a combination of features such as architectural or proliferative activities. Architectural features in carcinomas generally reflect the degree to which the tumor's epithelial component differs from the organ's normal epithelial component. Grading schemes for adenocarcinoma of the colon, adenoid cystic carcinoma of salivary gland, and adenocarcinoma of prostate all primarily rely on architectural features [2–4]. Proliferative activity, namely mitotic figure counts or proliferative (Ki67) indices, is occasionally primarily relied on, such as in gastrointestinal stromal tumors and some neuroendocrine tumors of the gastrointestinal tract, whereas it is frequently a part of multiple-feature grading schemes including breast's Nottingham modification of the Bloom-Richardson grade which additionally incorporates nuclear morphology and glandular architecture [5–8].

The battleground in histopathologic grading has been between complexity and reproducibility where many schemes capture nuance at the expense of reproducibility. Numerous studies in different subspecialties have documented less than optimal reproducibility of grading systems, be it intra- or interobserver or whether the comparison is against a consensus of experts or general pathologists [9–12]. Recent efforts by international organizations representing subspecialties have tried consensus to guide grading recommendations in the direction of increased reproducibility and clinical utility, perhaps none more than in the case of prostate cancer. The Gleason grading scheme has undergone a number of modifications to simplify ambiguity in the pattern categories. Most recently the International Society of Urological Pathology (ISUP) focusing on clinical utility modified how the score is reported to match pathologically defined subgroups to clinically relevant risk and treatment groups [13].

Prognostic models to establish risk for patients with cancer have evolved beyond grade and stage. In their simplest form, they have combined or incorporated the two to better assess prognosis. The Nottingham Prognostic Index, for example, combined grade with tumor size and lymph node status to arrive at clinically relevant prognostic groupings [14]. There are also numerous nomogram variations that combine grade with stage and clinical variables such as the Kattan preoperative and postoperative nomograms for prostate cancer [15,16].

Despite strategies for improving the reproducibility of grade by simplifying schemes or combining it with other predictive features such as stage or clinical variables for improved prognostic value, the central issue has not been addressed until recently. As long as humans are visually quantifying grading scheme features, there will always be a significant reproducibility problem. Not all feature quantitation suffers equally; in breast cancer, for example, we are significantly better at reproducibly assessing tubule formation than nuclear pleomorphism or mitotic counts [11,12]. In all cases, however, a tool for quantitative assessment has been missing. Although image analysis with traditional machine vision (MV) approaches has been slowly inching its way into this role, the recent feasibility of artificial intelligence (AI) approaches such as deep learning promises to change the field in the next half-decade.

To date, there are no clinically validated let alone clinically accepted AI-based grading schemes, although there have been a few traditional MV-based models that combine morphometric assessment and biomarker quantitation to risk stratify patients [17−20]. Much more common in the literature are MV- and AI-based algorithms that focus on quantitating histologic features, and some have created models that correlate features to grade [21−23]. Although the latter, probably best described as computer-aided diagnosis (CAD), is a useful first step, the ultimate goal is to generate models that use these features to create a better prognostic tool, in terms of patient clinical outcome, than current grading schemes. The sections below will roughly follow a pipeline (Fig. 9.1) for developing an image analysis−based multivariate system, with attention drawn in each subsection to inherent obstacles and published state of the art, as well as to our own experience with solutions.

Tissue preparation and staining

A few basic principles and common factors related to tissue preparation and staining are worth mentioning that impact the design of an algorithm development cohort and the feature engineering strategy. Preanalytical factors known to affect the antigenicity of tissue [24,25], such as length of fixation, tissue processing, and age of cut slides, can introduce significant variability into the set of biomarker-stained images used for algorithm development. This variability/noise

> ⟶ Tissue preparation and staining (H&E, IF, IHC)
> ⟶ Image acquisition
> ⟶ Stain normalization or unmixing of IF spectral images
> ⟶ Automated region detection in whole-slide images
> ⟶ Image segmentation
>   ⟶ Nuclear and epithelial segmentation in IF and H&E images
>   ⟶ Mitotic Figures
>   ⟶ Ring segmentation
> ⟶ Protein Biomarker features
> ⟶ Morphological features
> ⟶ Modeling with patient outcome
> ⟶ Ground truth data for AI-based features

FIGURE 9.1

Pathology image analysis pipeline.

particularly affects absolute biomarker intensity features that look for a correlation between raw intensity values and a clinical endpoint. H&E or IHC stain reagents, protocol variations, as well as cut tissue thickness can further affect color intensities and distribution. This variability is not only important when evaluating and optimizing feature performance, but also when scaling any algorithm for broader use outside of the training environment where preanalytics and staining protocols are less controlled. Creating tissue microarrays when blocks are available can be an effective way to mitigate some of this variability in training, by combining many patient samples on a single slide, although it does significantly limit the area of tumor analyzed and does not address preanalytical issues with fixation or the scaling for a broader population [26]. Some other strategies to mitigate the effect of these variables will be discussed below.

Image acquisition

There are many different instruments available for digital image capture. It is perhaps the relative abundance and accessibility of digital image data that, along with advances in computing technology, account for the recent interest and progress made in the field of computational pathology. Regulatory approval for the use of these systems as primary diagnostics tools will additionally increase the accessibility of digital images for development purposes [27]. A detailed discussion of each image capture technology is beyond the scope of this chapter, but we should mention some general categories. Whole slide digital scanners have been around for over a decade; improved color fidelity, focal plane algorithms, and scanning speed have made these high-throughput devices the cornerstone of generating large digital image databases. Multispectral fluorescent scopes including confocal image capture have been around for even longer but until recently have been limited to static image capture. Whole slide fluorescent scanners are available; however, true multispectral whole slide scanning is variably limited by speed.

Stain normalization

Color and intensity variations in histology images can not only cause inconsistencies in interpretation between pathologists but can also significantly impact the performance of CAD systems. These variations are in part due to variability in preparation, staining, and digitization of histological samples. These include preanalytic factors such as fixation and tissue preservation, paraffin embedding, deparaffinization, slide thickness, stain reagents, stain protocols, and mounting medium, as well as color fidelity algorithms of the digitization device. In order to compensate for this type of input variability, stain normalization strategies are often employed, in which the color and intensity range of an image is transformed to match those of another image. A review of the major techniques for stain normalization of digitized histologic images is discussed here.

An early method, originally developed for nonmedical images [28] and later applied to stain normalization of histology images [29], transforms the typical RGB image into an alternate color space ($l\alpha\beta$) which allows a statistical color distribution in each channel to match the reference image. This method, however, does not take into account the independent contribution of stain dyes to the final color and can result in improper color mapping [30]. Macenko et al. [31] proposed to convert the image to an optical density space and find the optimal stain vectors by means of singular value decomposition. This method does not preserve all information from the source image in the processed image and performs poorly in the presence of strong staining variations. The algorithm proposed by Vahadane et al. [32] preserves all the structure of the source image by using a sparse nonnegative matrix factorization method. Although this method outperforms all previous supervised stain separation methods, it is computationally costly and the algorithm might reach a nonrepresentative local optimal solution [33]. A whole slide color standardization algorithm was proposed in Ref. [34] in which two chromatic distributions and one density distribution are computed for hematoxylin, eosin, and background in the image after applying an RGB-to-HSD model. The source image is then transformed to the space of the reference image by a weighted sum of three nonlinear transformations between the distributions. This algorithm has a high processing time and does not preserve all the source image information such as background and red blood cells color.

More recently, deep generative models have been used as style transfer and generative learning for stain normalization of histopathology images. BenTaieb et al. [35] used a generative adversarial network (GAN) for learning stain normalization across different datasets and integrated it with a task-specific discriminative model for supervised classification. Moreover, Shaban et al. [30] proposed StainGAN, using cycle-consistent adversarial networks (CycleGAN) for image-to-image unpaired translation between two datasets. This method does not require picking a reference image for stain normalization, and the processed image has a good visual similarity to the reference domain. We have compared the performance of five different methods in Fig. 9.2.

FIGURE 9.2

Comparison of stain normalization methods: the source and the reference images are extracted from TCGA [36] and Mount Sinai Hospital whole slide images, respectively. (A) Reference; (B) Shaban-StainGAN; (C) Bejnordi; (D) Vahadane; (E) Macenko; (F) Reinhard; (G) Source.

Unmixing of immunofluorescence spectral images

The multispectral immunofluorescent microscope (e.g., Vectra imaging system [37]) acquires a spectral stack, a set of grayscale images taken at a series of wavelengths separated by 10 or 20 nm intervals. These images show proteins of interest tagged by fluorescent biomarkers, mixed with autofluorescence and other unwanted signals.

The unmixing process extracts the desired signals from the spectral stack, either for structural biomarkers, designed to respond to anatomical compartments, e.g., nuclei (DAPI) and glands (CK18/pan-Cytokeratin), or for functional biomarkers such as cancer-related proteins, e.g., androgen receptor (AR) in the prostate or estrogen receptor (ER) and progesterone receptor (PR) in the breast (Fig. 9.3). The unmixing algorithm for functional biomarkers is designed to produce a linear response proportional to the protein present in the tissue, typically using a deconvolution-type algorithm [38]. Careful calibration of staining and microscope is required to ensure that biomarker spectral profiles are stable over different images and tissues. For structural biomarkers, where the goal is to obtain an image which can be correctly segmented, the unmixing algorithm has more leeway to compensate for weak staining or other variations in spectral profiles. For prostate samples, we use a semisupervised approach based on nonnegative matrix factorization [39]. Fig. 9.3 Panel A shows a typical unmixed image output for CK18.

FIGURE 9.3

Structural (A and B) and functional (D and E) immunofluorescent biomarkers in high-grade prostate cancer (20× objective lens), Gleason pattern 4, after unmixing. Panel F combines four biomarkers by showing the maximum value biomarker at each pixel, with AR (purple), Ki67 (yellow), DAPI (blue), and CK18 (gold). Compare with H&E stain of the same tissue in panel (C). (A), CK18; (B), DAPI; (C), H&E; (D), AR; (E), Ki67; (F), Max biomarker.

Automated detection of tumor regions in whole-slide images
Localization of diagnostically relevant regions of interest in whole-slide images

A digital whole-slide image (WSI) obtained from scanning glass slides often has more than a billion pixels in the highest resolution (40×). However, only small regions within the slide contain diagnostic information. The relevant region in the image is usually less than 50% of the digitized area. Additionally, artifacts such as ink, mounting medium air bubbles, tissue folds, crushed nuclei, and out-of-focus regions could potentially mislead feature extraction, segmentation, and detection algorithms.

A multiscale framework using high- and low-resolution imaging features was proposed in Ref. [40] to rapidly identify the high-power fields of interest in the WSIs. Bahlmann et al. [41] developed a classification method for discriminating between statistics of relevant versus irrelevant regions. They used visual descriptors that captured the distribution of color intensities observed for nuclei and cytoplasm. Moreover, Mercan et al. in Ref. [42] extracted regions of interest (ROIs) by tracking records of pathologists' actions, such as zooming, panning and fixating. They developed a visual bag-of-words model based on color and texture features of the extracted regions to predict diagnostically relevant ROI in the WSIs. We developed an automatic technique for detecting diagnostically important ROIs within the WSIs using convolutional neural networks (CNN). We trained the CNN to identify multiple tissue types in the images excluding abovementioned regions from analysis. Using this tool, only diagnostically relevant regions are localized (orange color in Fig. 9.4B) and used for further processing and analysis. Localization of these ROIs not only significantly reduces the computational load for other processes but also improves the accuracy of these downstream processes by focusing on relevant areas and decreasing the possibility of artifact interference.

Tumor detection

Automated tumor detection in digital histopathology images is by itself quite a broad subject, with numerous techniques, from traditional features—based MV to deep learning approaches, with many different intended uses. Automated deep learning approaches to tumor detection have flourished over the past several years over traditional MV approaches as deep learning methods aim to automatically learn relevant characteristics and complex relationships directly from the data, and therefore require less supervision and actually perform better [43,44]. Although there is certainly overlap, the intended use and functional requirements tend to drive the technical design of the algorithm. These fall into a few categories which include screening applications, tumor classification or diagnosis, and tumor volume assessment.

Screening tools tend to be less supervised as the classification problem can be done at the ROI level and does not require manual annotations or object segmentation. For instance, Campanella et al. [45] employed a deep learning approach under the multiple instance learning assumption for prostate cancer diagnosis using over 12,000 needle biopsy slides, where only the overall slide diagnosis was available. Tumor classification and volume assessment can similarly require little input supervision if the requirement does not demand, for example, to differentiate distinct architectural patterns as would be required to separate in situ carcinoma or scattered normal structures mixed in with invasive carcinoma of breast. Cruz-Roa et al. [46] developed a CNN-based classifier for automatic detection of tumor (including both

(A)   **(B)**

FIGURE 9.4

Localization of region of interest in the H&E whole-slide image. Colors in the region of interest (ROI) detector represent the different regions of the slide. (A) H&E whole-slide image; (B) ROI detector output.

invasive and in situ carcinoma) on breast WSIs. Annotated tumor on the WSIs were used for patch-based training of the CNN classifier. They further developed their work in Ref. [43] by creating a fast high-throughput CNN-based method for automatic detection of invasive breast tumor on WSIs. For this, they used an efficient adaptive and iterative sampling method based on probability gradients to efficiently identify the precise extent of the invasive breast cancer, obtaining comparative results to those using dense sampling. Bejnordi et al. in Ref. [47] assessed and compared the performance of deep learning algorithms submitted to a public challenge to detect metastases in H&E tissue sections of lymph nodes in women with breast cancer. Seven out of 32 deep learning algorithms submitted to this competition showed greater discriminating performance than a panel of 11 pathologists in a simulated time-constrained diagnostic setting.

The task becomes more complicated when attempting to both detect tumor and classify architectural heterogeneity on WSIs. This can be as simple as separating benign from malignant to distinguishing invasive disease, in situ carcinoma, proliferative entities, reactive patterns, and normal structures. Machine learning and more specifically deep learning techniques have provided state-of-the-art results in automated detection and morphologic classification in histopathology images. Bardou et al. [44] developed and compared two approaches for the classification of breast cancer histology images into benign and malignant classes, as well as their subclasses. In the first method, they extracted a set of handcrafted features encoded by bag-of-words and locality-constrained linear coding descriptors, and used support vector machines for the classification of features. In the second approach, they trained a CNN for the classification of a large labeled image dataset. Although the deep learning approach has many advantages including outperforming the handcrafted approach as well as automated feature generation, it is worth mentioning that one of the drawbacks of this approach is that the features are not transparent as they are embedded in the neural network architecture. Using a context-aware stacked CNN approach, Bejnordi et al. [48] classified whole slide breast images into normal/benign, in situ, and invasive classes. They first trained a deep CNN with high pixel resolution, but small image size, to classify the tissue into different classes. Then, they fed much larger images to the model and used the extracted feature responses generated by the initial model as input to a second CNN. This architecture allowed them to use a larger input image to learn the global interdependence of various structures or context in different lesion categories.

We have developed a robust ensemble CNN-based technique for classification of clinically significant architectural and morphologic patterns into four types: normal tissue, benign (proliferative) entities, in situ carcinoma, and invasive cancer. We incorporated image perturbation models specifically designed for digital pathology images for training the classifiers, which increased robustness and generalizability of the classifier to real-world image data variability [49]. A review of the state-of-the-art methods with their performance and collective results on a public challenge is given in Ref. [50]. Fig. 9.5 shows the results of our developed technique applied specifically to the histologically relevant areas of the WSI given in Fig. 9.4.

FIGURE 9.5

Representation of colors in the tumor detector: invasive: red, DCIS: orange, benign: green, normal: blue, nontissue: gray. Tumor detection is only applied on the tissue region of Fig. 9.4. (A) Tumor detector output; (B) Zoomed region.

Image segmentation

Deep learning as described above is capable of learning complex relationships in histopathology images and has successfully been applied to learning differences in large sets of images to separate or classify them as either containing or not containing tumor. This black box or top-down approach certainly has its merits particularly as a screening tool when the requirement is to detect areas of interest for a pathologist to pay special attention to. This approach, although arguably less clinically useful, has also been used to classify tumors into distinct patterns or grades [22]. Using deep learning approaches to classify images according to outcome though is a whole different endeavor, which will be discussed in more detail below, but at the highest level, is difficult because large enough development cohorts with outcome are not generally available at the necessary scale.

This is where traditional machine vision handcrafted features and deep learning have converged with machine learning modeling to create the real possibility of automated histopathology image—based grading. We have shown that a bottom-up approach—segmenting and characterizing histologic compartments morphologically combined with protein expression on multiplexed immunofluorescent images—yields handcrafted feature—based models that provide a significant advantage over conventional grading for risk stratifying patients [17]. This has never been done with H&E image—based models in large part due to the difficulties handcrafted features have in handling color variability and the lack of contrast between compartments. Leveraging deep learning's ability to distinguish subtlety in large datasets, the next step in automated grading of H&E images is to apply a bottom-up approach, segmenting histologic compartments for direct characterization and feature engineering.

Nuclear and epithelial segmentation in IF images

The goal of nuclear and epithelial segmentation is to delineate their borders in un-mixed images (Fig. 9.6), accurately separating touching or overlapping objects and

FIGURE 9.6

Structural IF biomarkers (A-gland, C-nuclei) and their segmentations (B and D respectively) in low-grade prostate cancer, Gleason pattern 3 (20× objective lens). See Fig. 9.8 for segmentation of H&E images of the same tissue by deep NN. (A), CK18; (B), CK18 segmentation; (C), DAPI; (D), DAPI segmentation.

identifying each gland or nucleus with a unique label. A classic algorithm for IF nuclear segmentation is Ref. [51], which operates according to a popular nuclear detection pattern, by first finding seed points, one per nucleus, and then growing the seeds according to proximity, size, and shape constraints to find the nuclear boundaries. Many variations of this algorithm have been proposed for H&E and IHC images also, *e.g.*, Ref. [52], but they all share a common problem which is that the irregular texture and holes, the result of chromatin clumping and margination in high-grade nuclei, lead to the detection of multiple seed points per nucleus, producing fragmented segmentations. A second (inverse) problem is that closely packed nuclei may be merged together when too few seed points are detected or the nuclear borders are missed. A comprehensive review of nuclei segmentation algorithms [53] shows the successful application of deep neural networks to these problems.

A distinct problem, common in epithelium segmentation of IF images, is the inconsistency of cytokeratin intensity throughout the cytoplasm, often magnified by the negative impression where the nucleus sits, or the DAPI holes. This problem has been addressed by combining epithelial with nuclear segmentation, as in Ref. [54], by filling in nuclear holes in the cytokeratin (the inverse of the DAPI image) along the gland border where the nuclei are clustered and the staining is often weaker. In order to compensate for unmixing errors, which may result in strong background signal or in weak response along gland borders, we have developed a combined unmixing/segmentation algorithm which is robust against typical under- and over-segmentation errors.

Nuclei detection and segmentation in H&E images

Although not part of the Gleason grading system, manually characterizing nuclei is a common thread throughout most grading schemes and often one of the least reproducible [11,12]. As described above in IF images, H&E segmentation of nuclei

FIGURE 9.7

Annotation for nuclei detection compared with segmentation. From left to right: H&E image, image overlaid with boxes indicating detected nuclei, and image overlaid with nuclei boundary segmentation. In a detection task, the objective is to determine presence of nuclei without exact boundaries. In a segmentation task, the objective is to determine nuclei membership for each pixel accounting for overlaps and touching boundaries. The required annotation for a segmentation task is more demanding than detection.

suffers from similar challenges including variability of size, shape, and chromatin textures, as well as touching and overlapping. Accounting for this variability is particularly challenging in H&E with a handcrafted approach. By leveraging large datasets, deep learning has the potential to generate robust and reproducible algorithms for both detecting the presence of and determining the boundaries of nuclei. These two tasks have somewhat different complexities and requirements for annotated data. Nuclei detection specifically is a task where an algorithm counts nuclei, often identifying them with bounding boxes. Segmentation algorithms, on the other hand, determine the precise pixels that form each nucleus with boundaries defined explicitly. Detecting and counting nuclei is comparatively simpler than segmenting nuclei, where the exact boundary is defined, distinguishing overlapping and touching nuclei. Fig. 9.7 shows the difference between these two tasks.

Nuclei detection with deep learning is typically performed by generating probability maps derived from training a CNN that is applied to image patches in a sliding window fashion or a fully convolutional neural network (FCN), and then finding local maximas within the nuclei probability map [55]. Naylor et al. proposed the use of an FCN for nuclei segmentation [56], combined with a watershed algorithm for splitting touching nuclei. Nuclei segmentation provides more details and more flexibility in developing a cancer grading feature. Bounding boxes from a nuclei detector can only generate an approximation of sizes, while boundaries from a nuclei segmenter can provide measures such as elongation, orientation angle, and smoothness of chromatin boundaries.

Epithelial segmentation in H&E images

The task of epithelial segmentation in H&E images is considerably harder, due to color variations and low contrast between cytoplasm and stroma, particularly in activated tumor-associated stroma. A good solution to these problems is to use deep neural networks, as seen in Fig. 9.8.

(A)   **(B)**   **(C)**

FIGURE 9.8

H&E with deep NN segmentation on the same tissue as Fig. 9.6 (40× objective lens). Note the low contrast of glands, and nonuniform nuclei in panel A, well segmented in panels B and C. (A), H&E; (B), H&E epithelial segmentation; (C), H&E nuclei segmentation.

In colon cancer, the GlaS (gland segmentation) challenge [57] has inspired an impressive series of improvements to this gland-instance segmentation problem [58–60], using deep neural networks trained to define boundaries and separate distinct epithelial regions. Chen et al. [58] used a modified version of the FCN with an explicit representation of gland contours. Ronnenberger et al. proposed a method called U-Net [61], which is also fully convolutional, with a penalty function for misclassifying pixels in the gaps between glands. Al-Milaji et al. [62] proposed a method that combines a CNN with an unsupervised classifier, where deep learning provides image features and unsupervised region segmentation refines the boundary of the epithelial segmentation. Bulten et al. [63] developed a segmentation approach for epithelium in prostate cancer using U-Net where they leveraged immunohisto-chemistry markers (P63 and CK8/18) to create initial ground truth that is corrected manually and then mapped to H&E images.

Mitotic figure detection

Establishing proliferative activity is central in determining the aggressive potential of many if not most tumors. Grading schemes call for manual mitotic counts or occasion-ally incorporate the use of immunohistochemical stains such as Ki67. The importance of proliferation in the prognostic evaluation of tumors is reinforced by a number of prognostic gene panels that include or are dominated by proliferation-associated genes [64]. As with the evaluation of nuclear features, mitotic counts are generally among the less reproducible components of grading schemes [11,12].

The same issues that make mitotic figures difficult to reproducibly count manually are the same that make them challenging to detect automatically, namely that they are relatively rare events, heterogeneously distributed, morphologically diverse, and with a number of nonmitotic objects that share similar properties. Cells undergoing cell division can be visually recognized at a number of morphologically different stages some, in the middle and later stages of the cycle, easier to identify than the earlier stages. Even in the later stages the morphologic variability is quite pronounced and the difference between mitotic objects and nonmitotic mimics can be as subtle as boundary fuzziness. Deep learning with large datasets is well suited for these types of subtle morphologic distinctions. One aspect of mitotic figure detection that is challenging for deep learning is that of class imbalance between mitotic figures, nonmitotic background objects such as regular nuclei and lymphocytes, and mimics such as apoptotic cells. This is generally handled by oversampling the mitotic figure class or by adjusting the loss function for training to account for the lower sample count. Ciresan et al. [65] developed a CNN approach for mitotic figure detection that is trained on image patches. Training of the neural network included enrichment of the limited mitotic training data by generating rotated and flipped versions of the images. These additional training examples helped alleviate the class imbalance issue and resulted in a robust network that had the best performance in the Assessment of Mitosis Detection Algorithms 2013 (AMIDA13) challenge [66]. Chen et al. [67] proposed the use of a cascade of two CNNs. The first network generating a coarse classification of objects that are likely to be mitosis and may include other similar structures, and a second network performing finer discrimination and verification to determine the final mitotic figure classification. Their approach utilized a specialized network that analyzed subtle patterns in images to reduce false-positive identifications. Albarqouni et al. [68] utilized data obtained from untrained annotators (crowds) in a CNN that contains an aggregation layer. Crowdsourcing provides enrichment of training data for mitosis, with noise handled using an explicit data aggregation step in training.

Ring segmentation

Gland structures, in general, are three-dimensional objects composed of tubules of varying width and length, with rounded ends, connected in a branching structure at lower grades, or forming an interconnected network at higher grades. Confocal microscopy of prostate samples in Ref. [69] and stacked histology slices in Ref. [70] show how the 3D geometry of glands relates to patterns in 2D histology. In the fragmented pattern of prostate cancer, illustrated with increasing grade on the right descending side of the Gleason diagram [71], tubules wrapped in stroma shrink down to small clusters and single cells, and central lumens disappear. In the cribriform and solid patterns, on the left descending side of the diagram, tubules are fused together without intervening stroma, as lumen size and frequency decreases. The morphogenesis from low grade to high grade, suggested by the Gleason diagram, is confirmed by 3D studies of gland structure to be a process of continuous growth along these two axes of variation.

There are a number of patterns that lumen, epithelium, and stroma can take in relation to one another. These patterns can be seen in many different kinds of cancer, with the frequency of occurrence and prognostic significance varying by organ. The cribriform pattern in breast, prostate, colon, lung, and other organs is discussed in Ref. [72]. From an engineering point of view, it is useful to identify organ-specific gland morphologic tendencies and their prognostic implications, to design segmentation strategies and features that correlate with the underlying biological processes, and so lead to accurate characterization of tumor differentiation.

This motivates the segmentation of gland rings, which we define as complete or fragmented tubules, appearing either as a ring of epithelial nuclei surrounding a gland lumen, or as a gland fragment with a few epithelial nuclei surrounded by stroma [73]. By looking at the adjacency between rings, stromal, and lumen regions, an algorithm can detect and evaluate these patterns across all grades of cancer.

Our ring segmentation algorithm works by forming a compact triangulation of epithelial nuclei centers, known as the Delaunay triangulation (characterized by the property that the interior of each triangle's circumcircle contains no other vertices). The algorithm then clusters the triangles across epithelial and lumen regions, to form broad areas separated by relatively short edges between ring nuclei, as shown in Fig. 9.9. This algorithm was originally developed based on IF epithelial and nuclear segmentation and has been validated as part of a clinical test [17] for risk stratification of prostate cancer patients. With the advent of accurate deep learning segmentations, rings and ring features can be applied to H&E images also with similar results, Fig. 9.14.

Few existing algorithms make the distinction between epithelial and gland ring segmentation, focusing instead on lower grade presentations with one ring of closely spaced nuclei per epithelial unit, surrounding a clear lumen, *e.g.*, Ref. [74]. These algorithms use nuclei as a guide for region-growing, starting from the lumen, an approach which can work well for the colon, less for prostate and breast glands which tend to have a greater frequency of fragmentation and fusion. A notable exception is Ref. [75], which searches for polygonal gland rings using a randomized Markov Chain Monte Carlo approach, based upon approximate gland and nuclei maps. But this algorithm too does not generalize to handle the continuum of presentations between low- and high-grade cancers.

Protein biomarker features

Protein biomarkers provide valuable diagnostic and prognostic information not available in standard H&E-stained tissue. This section provides an overview of a few of the many ways of quantifying biomarkers in an image.

Immunohistochemistry (IHC), in its most popular form, uses a brown chromogenic detection system (3,3-diaminobenzidine or DAB) to tag a protein of interest against a nuclear hematoxylin counterstain, viewed on a brightfield microscope and manually quantified on a scale of 0–3. Multiplexing and automation extend

FIGURE 9.9

Ring segmentation by watershed graph algorithm. (A) Rings and triangulation overlaid on nuclei (prostate, inverted DAPI, 20× objective lens) in fused gland. (B) Illustration of watershed graph segmentation algorithm applied to top of image (A) showing nuclei centers as hilltops, joined by red rings which surround regions where simulated rainfall would flow down to the same valley. The algorithm effectively clusters triangular areas (dark lines, Delaunay triangulation, see text) to form broad regions separated by relatively short (red) edges [73]. (C) Geometry of two fused glands (or one U-tube shaped tubule, or a branching tubule—the 2D histology image can be derived from several different 3D geometries). Tubule size in 3D = gland width in image = the longest triangle edge crossing the ring.

this process to multiple, overlapping biomarkers. One technique stains serial sections with different markers, then coregisters the images with correlation software, for example, putting Ki67 on one slide and a cytokeratin epithelial marker on the next, to count epithelial Ki67 positive nuclei. This method was used in Ref. [76] with Visiopharm software [77] to analyze Ki67, ER, PR, and HER2 in breast cancer.

Alternatively, multiplex immunofluorescence puts a set of up to eight biomarkers on one slide [78,79], for example, analyzing tumor infiltrating lymphocytes (TILs) in melanoma [80], or comparing TIL profiles in multiple tissues [81]. In prostate cancer, the androgen receptor (AR) signaling pathway drives progression of the disease, lowering AR levels in the stroma, while increasing AR in the epithelium [82], and thus the ratio of the two is a powerful prognostic feature [17].

Beyond simple counting and ratio features, distance between different cell types can be used as a filter. In Refs. [83], for instance, the HALO package [84] analyzes colon cancer TIL immunoscore within 50 microns of invasive tumor buds only. Instead of averaging over the image, biomarker features may be calculated for clusters of cells, or for gland rings as in Fig. 9.10, or over other kinds of structural or morphological graphs. For example, in Ref. [85], breast cancer extra cellular matrix (ECM) biomarkers integrin-α 3 and 6 are used to define the connectivity of cell graphs (covered in the next section) from which a set of features are derived.

Morphological features for cancer grading and prognosis

In the process of evaluating a slide, the pathologist takes into consideration features from several levels of image resolution. Although all resolutions are used to evaluate a slide, generally speaking, starting at the lowest resolution, composition (*e.g.*, mucin, necrosis, stroma) and architectural patterns are noticed. At an intermediate resolution, size, shape, and the relationship (*e.g.*, density and streaming) of nuclei to one another are prominent. And finally, nuclear texture, including chromatin pattern, margination, and nucleoli, depend on fine details seen at the highest resolution. Capturing and characterizing these relationships within and between scales is one of the creative sides of developing automated grading systems as many of these potentially prognostic relationships are based on well-accepted histopathological principals, but in and of themselves are difficult to quantitate without computation. This is feature engineering.

Semiautomated attempts to quantify the relative importance of these feature, for example, grading of invasive breast cancer in Ref. [86], or nuclear radius variance for prostate prognosis [87], show good results and encourage the search for fully automated methods.

FIGURE 9.10

Biomarker Features Combined with Morphology. Left: Biomarker intensity image (20× objective lens). Right: Combination of morphology, AR and Ki67 features. Outer rings represents the SL-touch value (see next section), inner rings represent AR epistromal ratio (shown in green for high values, red for low values, i.e., worse outcome/grade). Nuclear AR strength is shown on a blue (low) to purple (high) scale, with Ki67 (yellow) on CK18 (gold) background.

As will be discussed throughout this section, layering is a common theme of feature engineering. Starting with the segmentation outputs discussed above, a variety of different techniques can be layered to quantitate or characterize relationships as well as to normalize features for robustness. Nuclei segmentation, for example, followed by ellipsoid fitting can provide a high-level view of the shape and organization of nuclei within a region of interest, Fig. 9.11. Additionally derived features from the ellipsoidal representations, could include density, shape, orientation, and regularity, among others Fig. 9.12. Nuclear shape, texture, and orientation have recently been shown to be predictive of outcome in estrogen positive, lymph node negative breast cancer [21]. At the highest resolution, color and texture of nuclei successfully distinguish benign and malignant regions in colon cancer, as shown by Jørgensen et al. [88].

Although raw mitotic count may be predictive in TMA cohorts, normalizing to account for variability in the sample volume will stabilize the feature when developing in larger samples and when scaling outside of the test environment. Manual grading schemes generally require counting mitotic figures within a specified area or per a specified number of tumor cells to account for volume variability from patient to patient [89]. This provides a standard mechanism for comparing mitotic activity in different subjects. Applying that concept to an automated scheme, an algorithm applies the same specified area to each slide either randomly or looking for the area of highest proliferation, analogous to the mitotic count requirement of the modified Bloom-Richardson grading scheme for breast cancer. Another similar relative measure could be achieved by combining mitotic count and nuclear count providing a density index that reflects a tumor's proliferative activity.

Characterizing the spatial distribution of epithelial cells and stromal cells in cancer is an evaluation primarily in the domain of computational pathology. Although glandular differentiation or the degree to which tumor glands deviate from normal is

FIGURE 9.11

Example nuclear segmentation and ellipse fitting (left: input H&E image, right: segmentation results with fitted ellipsoids).

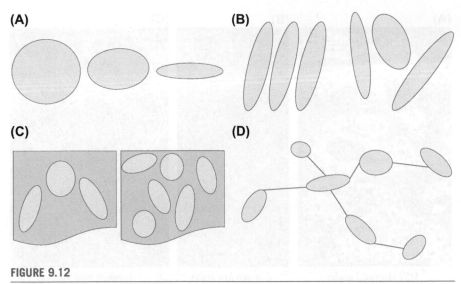

FIGURE 9.12

Example nuclear features. Elongation of an individual nucleus can be computed from the ratio of major and minor axes of the ellipsoid. The variability of the orientation of the major axis provides a measure of the level of organization in a tissue. Density of nuclei within a given compartment is measured as count of nuclei (or area of nuclei) divided by the area of the compartment. Graphs can be used to provide a summary of the morphological relationships and structure of nuclei clusters.

part of a number of grading schemes, computational pathology and graphs specifically offer a more bottom-up approach which can support gland segmentation as noted above, but can also provide a framework for more free-form characterizations. We can construct graphs describing the adjacency and spatial relationships of nuclear and epithelial regions, providing a way to summarize the complexity of the tissue. Higher grade cancer typically yields more irregular, complex graphs. We then search for graph features or statistics that predict grade and patient outcome.

The simplest predictive graph is perhaps the minimum spanning tree (MST) based on epithelial nuclei as vertices (Fig. 9.13). The MST is the minimum connected subset of the Delaunay triangulation (see Fig. 9.9). From this tree, we can extract measures such as the average edge length and the degree of vertices (number of edges connected to a vertex). In low-grade cancer where the epithelial nuclei are arranged in tightly spaced rings, MST edge length is short and vertex degree is mostly equal to two, corresponding to the two neighbors in the ring, whereas in high-grade cancer edge length is longer and a greater proportion of vertices has three or more neighbors.

Graphs based on clustering or segmentation of nuclei are better able to represent the higher level structure of glands and different cell types. The cell cluster graph (CCG) [90], a popular hierarchical graph which contains clusters of nuclei, which in turn are probabilistically connected to nearby clusters, has been used to define

(A) MST degree 3 nodes   **(B)** L-touch low (red)   **(C)** L-touch high (green)

FIGURE 9.13

Graph Features for Prostate Cancer. (A) Minimum spanning tree (MST) showing three-way vertices with red halos. The proportion of degree three vertices is a strong feature for grade and prognosis. (B) Gland rings in fragmented pattern, adjacent to stroma without lumens, having low value of L-touch (shown in red). (C) Gland rings in fused (cribriform) pattern not touching stroma, with luminal clearings, having high value of L-touch (shown in green).

numerous features such as gland angularity co-occurrence in the prostate [91] and infiltrating lymphocytes in the lung [92]. A challenge in setting up the CCG is that clusters may not correspond to biologically relevant structures and may not adapt to the dynamically changing scales present in the tissue. Good reviews covering pathology graphs and other texture and nuclear features are provided in Refs. [93,94].

The gland ring or fragment, introduced in section Ring segmentation, is a natural clustering of nuclei that we have found to produce good features in prostate cancer across all grades, especially when combined with protein biomarker measurements. Since the growth and functioning of the prostate is mediated by signaling across the epithelial-stromal and epithelial-lumen boundaries, we have developed a set of simple ring-stroma-lumen adjacency features which account for the proportion of the ring boundary that is adjacent to stroma, S-touch, and the proportion adjacent to lumen, L-touch, Fig. 9.13. The product of these two, the SL-touch feature, covering gland fusion and fragmentation patterns, is highly prognostic in prostate cancer (Fig. 9.14).

Given features characterizing nuclei clusters or rings, the features are aggregated over the graph representing the image or whole slide by taking the mean, the median

(A)   (B)

IF   *H&E*

FIGURE 9.14

SL-touch Product Feature. The product of stromal adjacency (S-touch) and lumen adjacency (L-touch) scores, with low value in red, high value in green (better prognosis) (compare segmentations in Figs. 9.6 and 9.8), showing similar results for IF and H&E images of the same tissue. Gray lines show the Voronoi diagram, the zone of influence around each epithelial nucleus.

or some other aggregation function. More sophisticated aggregation can use support vector machines (SVMs) learning (see Modeling section) with graph kernels [95], or deep graph neural networks [96].

Modeling

Modeling as the final computational step in creating improved grading schemes combines the output of image-derived features as well as clinically derived features to predict the probability of survival or the expected time until significant progression of the disease in a cohort of patients with known clinical outcome. Standard clinical features that go into models include age, race, sex, etc. as well as pathologic stage, laboratory values, features from radiology and genetic testing [97]. Machine learning algorithms learn the most relevant feature combinations (imaging and clinically derived) and quantify the relative importance of each feature in a model that can then be applied to new patients outside of the training and test environment. Development cohorts for survival analysis are generally split into a set for training the model and a separate set for testing or validating the model. There are a number of disease- and cohort-specific considerations to be taken into account when creating these two groups, but in general they should look very similar in terms of disease types, subtypes, grades, and outcome. This is to create a balanced testing environment.

Survival analysis involves methods which analyze and predict the time to a medical event such as death, disease recurrence, or disease progression [98]. The survival function, denoted by $S(t)$, is the probability that the patient has not experienced the event at time t and survives past this time. As time goes by, the probability of survival decreases, as shown in the Kaplan-Meier plot in Fig. 9.15 [99].

Concordance index (C-Index), a widely used measure of algorithm performance, is a form of rank correlation between the model predictions and the actual survival times, which takes into account missing or censored data (see below) [100]. The C-index has some elegant properties: it is the probability that the model correctly predicts which of a random pair of patients has the longer survival time, which in the binary outcome case is the area under the ROC curve—the curve that plots model true positive rate (sensitivity) against false-positive rate (1-specificity). The C-Index lies in the range 0—1, with a value of 0.5 meaning that the model results

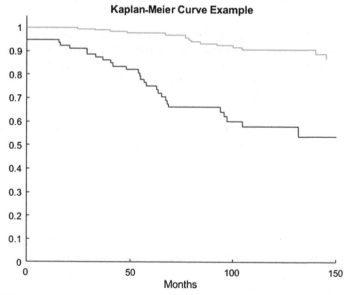

FIGURE 9.15

An example, Kaplan-Meier (K-M) curve, plotting survival probability decreasing with time, in the range 0—1 on the y-axis against survival months on the x-axis, for two treatments. Top treatment (green) has better survival rates than bottom treatment (red).

are no better than chance. Although a useful measure, some caveats are important to remember. C-Index indicates the discrimination power of an algorithm but not the predictive power. Since the index only looks at the proportion of correctly ordered pairs, it is agnostic to the actual predicted times.

Survival analysis can be treated as a regression problem of predicting survival times of which there are many methods [98], most of which, however, do not handle the problem of missing data caused by patients dropping out of the study over time. Missing information from these patients is known as censored data [101]. Patients who have experienced the event of interest (*e.g.*, PSA recurrence, death, or metastasis) are considered events. Right-censored patients are ones being followed at the end of the study who have not experienced the event or have dropped out of the study, and left-censored patients are patients who had an event but the timing is not clear.

Traditional ways of dealing with censored data in statistics include removing the sample points, treating them as nonevents, or more elaborate ways such as repeating the data points once as an event and once as a nonevent. There are also imputing methods which estimate the missing values before training on a survival model. Inevitably, however, all these methods introduce a bias to the resulting model. To rectify this, there are a variety of methods that can handle censored information, these are outlined in the paragraphs below.

Cox proportional hazards model

One of the first and most popular methods of handling censored information is the Cox proportional hazards model [102]. In this model, the hazard function or risk (the slope of the survival function, $h_i(t)$) is proportional for any two individuals. The proportionality is set up by taking the product of a baseline hazard function ($h_0(t)$) with baseline features, and an exponential function of weighted feature values, with the weights indicating the importance of each feature. The biggest caveat when using this model, is to detect and account for time-varying effects where the proportionality assumption may break down [103], as is the case in many biological applications. The reliability of the Cox model (and other models) is not sound if the number of features is greater than the number of events.

Neural networks

In their earliest and simplest form, neural networks for survival analysis [104] learned the relationship between features and the hazard functions. Unfortunately, this method performed about the same as a linear Cox model. DeepSurv, a relatively new method which is rooted in the Cox model, uses deep learning to predict the risk of a patient experiencing an event [105]. It is a simple application of a multilayer neural network with one output node that predicts patient risk. The main advantage of DeepSurv is that, while the Cox model evaluates efficacy as a whole for the group of patients, DeepSurv produces a risk score tailored to each patient. DeepHit, a higher performing improvement that does not make assumptions about the structure of the relationship between features and risk [106], learns the distribution of survival times directly. The structure of the network is more complicated than DeepSurv, with fully connected layers and a single softmax layer as the output layer. A disadvantage of using deep neural networks for survival analysis is that, in order to build robust models with reliable predictions, these algorithms tend to require large quantities of clinically annotated patient data (i.e., outcome), which is often not available at the necessary scale.

Decision trees and random forests

Tree-based methods can be used to solve problems in classification and regression by growing conceptual trees [107]. A simple traversal algorithm walks from the root to one of the leaves of the tree, choosing each branch limb depending on the value of a feature relative to a threshold the algorithm selects for that branching point. A regression value is therefore computed at each branch and leaf, creating a regression tree. Creating too many branching points overfits the data, and conversely, not creating a deep-enough tree risks not learning the appropriate structure of the data. Decision trees are unfortunately sensitive to noise, and small perturbation in the data can result in vastly different models due to the recursive identification of branch points.

Random forest [108] is a conceptual modification of the decision tree approach that introduces two main random components to generate multiple trees whose outputs are then aggregated. Random modifications include bootstrap aggregation of the data and random selection of features for each node. Using this modification to the decision-tree learning algorithm, multiple trees are generated are combined by averaging and arriving at a solution which reduces the bias and variance in the decision-tree models.

Random survival forest (RSF) is an extension of the random forest method [109], which includes the computation of an ensemble cumulative hazards function (EHF). The central idea of RSF is that the survival difference between low- and high-risk patients is maximized in the tree. For a given set of features, for every tree, a path is followed to a unique terminal node and EHF value. This is averaged over all survival trees to compute the survival estimate for the patient.

SVM-based methods: Survival-SVM, SVCR, and SVRc

Support vector machine, introduced in the early 1990s [110], is a classification algorithm that learns to distinguish between binary labels of given data. SVM is a linear method, extended to encapsulate nonlinear problems through projecting the data to a higher dimensional space. This method has enjoyed particular success in its ease of handling high-dimensional data and the interpretability of its linear models. This method was also extended to solving regression problems, known as support vector regression. Essentially, the SVM algorithm is an optimization algorithm that works by maximizing the margin of a data set and finding the separating hyperplane that neatly divides the data. The margin is the smallest distance between a data point and the separating hyperplane. Implicitly, we have assumed that the data we are trying to classify and learn are perfectly separable by a hyperplane, but if this is not the case, we can still find an approximation by optimizing the distance to the separating hyperplane (pink box), Fig. 9.16, with error variables (blue box), subject to constraints (red box).

$$\min_{W,b} \quad \frac{1}{2}\|W\|^2 + C\sum_{n}^{i=1}(\xi_i + \xi_i^*)$$

given the constraints

$$y_i - (W \cdot \phi(x_i) + b) \leq \epsilon + \xi_i$$

$$(W \cdot \phi(x_i) + b) - y_i \leq \epsilon + \xi_i^*$$

$$\xi_i, \xi_i^* \geq 0 \quad i = 1, ..., n$$

FIGURE 9.16

Support vector machine (SVM) equations. SVM is an optimization algorithm to find the optimal hyperplane that separates two classes of data in a given higher dimensional feature space. The operation of the algorithm is explained in three boxes. Pink box: minimize the weight of all features. The distance between a point of one class and the optimal hyperplane can be represented as 1. We want to maximize this distance or equivalently, minimize the denominator W, $\|W\|$. Blue box: penalize imperfectly separated data using error (slack) variables, with penalty factor C. Red box: constrain the slack variables to separate the data. Larger slack variables, with greater penalty, are needed for points whose projection to higher dimensional feature space by $\phi(x_i)$ is further than ε from the target value [111]. The two constraint lines deal with points on either side of the hyperplane, or when extended to survival regression, to early predictions in the first line, and late predictions in the second line. The kernel trick is a way of speeding up the computation by calculating the matrix multiplication $W.\phi$ once, and reusing the result for every data point. In SVCR (censored regression), the two hyper-parameter penalty values, C and ε, are used for early and late predictions and for censored data and events—an overly restrictive model. SVRc effectively extends the model by using separate penalty parameters for early/late and censored/event data. These eight hyper-parameters were optimized in advance over a set of cohorts by particle swarm optimization (see text).

SVCR, a simple extension of SVMs for survival analysis that accounts for censoring [112], ignores constraints where the prediction time is later than the censor time (right censoring, second line in red box). In this model, errors in events and nonevents and in early and late predictions are penalized identically, which creates a problem in that late prediction of an event is generally a far more serious error than early prediction, having consequences for patient treatment decisions.

SVRc, an effective and efficient solution to this problem, improves the handling of censored data by applying separate penalty factors [113]. The algorithm applies the most severe penalty to late prediction of events, followed by a lesser penalty to early prediction of nonevents, then early prediction of events, and finally a negligible penalty is applied to late prediction of nonevents (censored data). Optimal values for these parameters may be found using a hyper-parameter tuning algorithm to learn the values over multiple data sets. We have successfully used particle swarm optimization [114] to set up these parameters.

Feature selection tools

The feature development sections above can generate many features often anywhere between several hundreds to multiple thousands per application. Considering that for modeling purposes there must be a limit and an optimal balance between features and events, methods for reducing the number of features must be a part of any modeling strategy. There are four possible classes of features—strongly relevant, weakly relevant, redundant, and irrelevant [115]. As the names suggest, relevant features are important for achieving good results [116]. Irrelevant features do not affect the result but may affect algorithm efficiency. Redundant features are those that contain the same information as another or a subset of features. Removing irrelevant and redundant features is the function of feature selection algorithms, with the goal of improving results and reducing computation time. Let us assume there are m features associated with a problem. To find the best subset of features, one needs to evaluate all $2^m - 1$ subsets, a computationally infeasible task. Hence, there is a need for approximation algorithms that can perform feature selection. Broadly there are three classes of feature selection methods: Filter, Wrapper and Embedded methods [117].

Filter methods filter out irrelevant features by some mechanism that computes a score of importance. For example, Pearson's correlation measures the linear dependency of two random variables. This could be used to compute the correlation coefficients of features with respect to the target variable and then select the top features as input to the algorithm. Another coefficient, mutual information (MI) better captures nonlinear relationships between features and target variables.

Wrapper methods for feature selection are those methods that use the classification algorithm itself as a black box predictor and use the performance of the resulting model as an indicator of how good the feature subset is. Obviously, as explained above, not all subsets can be evaluated and thus, wrapper methods use clever algorithms to prune and search the space of feature subsets to arrive at an optimal subset.

Broadly these methods can be classified as sequential search algorithms and heuristic search algorithms. Forward selection and backward elimination are examples of the sequential search methods. In forward selection, we start with an empty set and add the feature that results in the best performance. Sequentially, we keep adding features and stop when there is no further improvement. Backward elimination works in a similar fashion where we start with the entire set of features and progressively remove features. These are both examples of greedy methods, where one hopes that sequentially taking the best step will result in a globally optimal solution. But this is not usually the case when there are complicated interactions between features. Alternatively, heuristic-based wrapper algorithms, like particle swarm optimization and genetic algorithms tend to find better locally optimal solutions. Given that feature selection is a problem for which no efficient algorithms exist, these solutions are the best we can do in a reasonable time.

Embedded methods perform feature selection as an intrinsic part of the classification algorithm, for example, decision trees only consider splits that result in best performance. The features that do not contribute to the model are not considered. Regularization is an important, optional addendum to linear feature selection models that falls under the class of embedded methods. When learning a linear model (linear regression, linear SVMs), lasso (least absolute shrinkage and selection operator) regularization is invoked by adding a term to the cost function. Linear models operate by learning the coefficients of the model that best fit the data, often including many small weights which do not meaningfully improve the model, and which do not generalize well to unseen data. To get over this limitation, we need to force some of the coefficients to zero and adjust other coefficients. This is done by adding an extra term to the cost function which penalizes the nonzero weights. In practice, this extra term limits the sum of the absolute value of the coefficients.

Ground truth data for AI-based features

Deep learning algorithms are heavily data dependent, and to ensure scalability outside of the development environment, these large datasets must conform to clinical reality both in terms of absolute numbers and in variety of representation. It is critical to not only represent different grades and morphologic subtypes but also different staining conditions and tissue quality. In addition to large datasets in a supervised or semisupervised setting, deep learning also demands ground truth annotations. This can be as simple as assigning a grade or binary label of tumor or nontumor to an input image, all the way to digitally drawing outlines around target objects for detection or segmentation. The choice of annotation strategy is dependent on the algorithms functional output. For example, if the output is boundary segmentation of an object, then precise boundaries must be part of the ground truth. If, on the other hand, the task is detection then the annotation may involve putting a bounding box around or a seed in the target object. Clearly segmentation provides much greater flexibility downstream in creating features, but it comes at a much higher upfront cost in terms of annotation.

Rapid outlining using semiautomatic methods can reduce the work demand for expert annotators, using minimal gestures and mouse clicks to initialize algorithms that create complete boundaries for structures of interest. Example algorithms include segmentation based on active contour evolution [118,119] where users provide an initial boundary and the algorithm evolves it to match an image boundary. This type of algorithm has been applied successfully for a variety of outlining tasks in medicine [120]. Random walker [121] is another algorithm that automatically generates contours, where the user provides a rough initial labeling of the different objects. This approach has less burden compared with active contour approaches as it does not require a complete definition of an outline. An alternative approach to contour initialization uses the watershed algorithm [122], which simulates the flooding of water in image valleys (low-intensity values surrounded by high values) to detect objects separated by boundaries. Annotators can interactively specify thresholds for the watershed algorithm and select pixel clusters that form the object of interest.

Due to the dependence of deep learning on large datasets, virtually all deep learning—based approaches conduct training of the neural network using data augmentation where training data are transformed to expand the existing datasets. Transformations are performed geometrically via rotations or flips, and they can also be performed based on color (e.g., stain transformation, contrast adjustment, etc.). Crowdsourcing also has great potential for generating larger datasets. Consistency and detection of low-quality annotations is a critical issue for such an approach, necessitating a data aggregation step such as the one proposed by Albarqouni et al. [68].

Conclusion

The importance of accurate histopathologic diagnosis in patient care is often underestimated. This perception is changing among treating clinicians as our molecular understanding of disease has exploded and targeted therapies and new specific treatment protocols continue to emerge. Having precise and reproducibly characterized disease remains an important component in developing these specific treatment protocols. To this end the use of deep learning methods for interrogating images and artificial intelligence to analyze complex interrelated datasets are changing this landscape. The promise of this technological and knowledge revolution ultimately is to improve patient outcomes by creating a more robust basis for linking patients with the most effective treatments.

References

[1] Fuhrman SA, Lasky LC, Limas C. Prognostic significance of morphologic parameters in renal cell carcinoma. The American Journal of Surgical Pathology 1982;6(7): 655−63.

[2] Bosman FT, Carneiro F, Hruban RH, Theise ND, et al. WHO classification of tumours of the digestive system, vol. 4. World Health Organization; 2010.

[3] Seethala RR. Histologic grading and prognostic biomarkers in salivary gland carcinomas. Advances in Anatomic Pathology 2011;18(1):29−45.

[4] Gleason DF, Mellinger GT. Prediction of prognosis for prostatic adenocarcinoma by combined histological grading and clinical staging. The Journal of Urology 1974; 111(1):58−64.

[5] Mutch DG. The new figo staging system for cancers of the vulva, cervix, endometrium and sarcomas. Gynecologic Oncology 2009;115(3):325−8.

[6] Miettinen M, Lasota J. Gastrointestinal stromal tumors: pathology and prognosis at different sites. In: Seminars in diagnostic pathology, vol. 23. Elsevier; 2006. p. 70−83.

[7] Klimstra DS, Modlin IR, Coppola D, Lloyd RV, Suster S. The pathologic classification of neuroendocrine tumors: a review of nomenclature, grading, and staging systems. Pancreas 2010;39(6):707−12.

[8] Elston C, Ellis I. Assessment of histological grade. The Breast 1998;13:356−84.

[9] Gleason DF. Histologic grading of prostate cancer: a perspective. Human Pathology 1992;23(3):273−9.

[10] Allsbrook Jr WC, Mangold KA, Johnson MH, Lane RB, Lane CG, Epstein JI. Interobserver reproducibility of gleason grading of prostatic carcinoma: general pathologist. Human Pathology 2001;32(1):81−8.

[11] Boiesen P, Bendahl P-O, Anagnostaki L, Domanski H, Holm E, Idvall I, Johansson S, Ljung- berg O, Ringberg A. Histologic grading in breast cancer: reproducibility between seven pathologic departments. Acta Oncologica 2000;39(1):41−5.

[12] Meyer JS, Alvarez C, Milikowski C, Olson N, Russo I, Russo J, Glass A, Zehnbauer BA, Lister K, Parwaresch R. Breast carcinoma malignancy grading by bloom−richardson system vs pro- liferation index: reproducibility of grade and advantages of proliferation index. Modern Pathology 2005;18(8):1067.

[13] Epstein JI, Egevad L, Amin MB, Delahunt B, Srigley JR, Humphrey PA. The 2014 inter- national society of urological pathology (isup) consensus conference on gleason grading of prostatic carcinoma. The American Journal of Surgical Pathology 2016; 40(2):244−52.

[14] Galea MH, Blamey RW, Elston CE, Ellis IO. The nottingham prognostic index in primary breast cancer. Breast Cancer Research and Treatment 1992;22(3):207−19.

[15] Greene KL, Meng MV, Elkin EP, Cooperberg MR, Pasta DJ, Kattan MW, Wallace K, Carroll PR. Validation of the kattan preoperative nomogram for prostate cancer recurrence using a community based cohort: results from cancer of the prostate strategic urological research endeavor (capsure). The Journal of Urology 2004;171(6 Part 1):2255−9.

[16] Stephenson AJ, Scardino PT, Eastham JA, Bianco Jr FJ, Dotan ZA, DiBlasio CJ, Reuther A, Klein EA, Kattan MW. Postoperative nomogram predicting the 10-year probability of prostate cancer recurrence after radical prostatectomy. Journal of Clinical Oncology: Official Journal of the American Society of Clinical Oncology 2005; 23(28):7005.

[17] Donovan MJ, Fernandez G, Scott R, Khan FM, Zeineh J, Koll G, Gladoun N, Charytonowicz E, Tewari A, Cordon-Cardo C. Development and validation of a novel automated gleason grade and molecular profile that define a highly predictive prostate cancer progression algorithm-based test. Prostate Cancer and Prostatic Diseases 2018; 21(4):594.

[18] Beck AH, Sangoi AR, Leung S, Marinelli RJ, Nielsen TO, Van De Vijver MJ, West RB, Van De Rijn M, Koller D. Systematic analysis of breast cancer morphology uncovers stromal features associated with survival. Science Translational Medicine 2011;3(108):108ra113.

[19] Donovan MJ, Khan FM, Fernandez G, Mesa-Tejada R, Sapir M, Zubek VB, Powell D, Fogarasi S, Vengrenyuk Y, Teverovskiy M, et al. Personalized prediction of tumor response and cancer progression on prostate needle biopsy. The Journal of Urology 2009;182(1):125–32.

[20] Blume-Jensen P, Berman DM, Rimm DL, Shipitsin M, Putzi M, Nifong TP, Small C, Choudhury S, Capela T, Coupal L, et al. Development and clinical validation of an in situ biopsy- based multimarker assay for risk stratification in prostate cancer. Clinical Cancer Research 2015;21(11):2591–600.

[21] Lu C, Romo-Bucheli D, Wang X, Janowczyk A, Ganesan S, Gilmore H, Rimm D, Madab- hushi A. Nuclear shape and orientation features from H&E images predict survival in early-stage estrogen receptor-positive breast cancers. Laboratory Investigation 2018;98(11):1438.

[22] Arvaniti E, Fricker KS, Moret M, Rupp N, Hermanns T, Fankhauser C, Wey N, Wild PJ, Rueschoff JH, Claassen M. Automated gleason grading of prostate cancer tissue microarrays via deep learning. Scientific Reports 2018;8.

[23] Couture HD, Williams LA, Geradts J, Nyante SJ, Butler EN, Marron J, Perou CM, Troester MA, Niethammer M. Image analysis with deep learning to predict breast cancer grade, er status, histologic subtype, and intrinsic subtype. NPJ Breast Cancer 2018; 4(1):30.

[24] Mirlacher M, Kasper M, Storz M, Knecht Y, Dürmüller U, Simon R, Mihatsch MJ, Sauter G. Influence of slide aging on results of translational research studies using immunohistochemistry. Modern Pathology 2004;17(11):1414.

[25] Grillo F, Pigozzi S, Ceriolo P, Calamaro P, Fiocca R, Mastracci L. Factors affecting immunoreactivity in long-term storage of formalin-fixed paraffin-embedded tissue sections. Histochemistry and Cell Biology 2015;144(1):93–9.

[26] Rimm DL, Camp RL, Charette LA, Costa J, Olsen DA, Reiss M. Tissue microarray: a new technology for amplification of tissue resources. Cancer Journal (Sudbury, Mass.) 2001;7(1):24–31.

[27] Mukhopadhyay S, Feldman MD, Abels E, Ashfaq R, Beltaifa S, Cacciabeve NG, Cathro HP, Cheng L, Cooper K, Dickey GE, et al. Whole slide imaging versus microscopy for primary diagnosis in surgical pathology: a multicenter blinded randomized noninferiority study of 1992 cases (Pivotal study). The American Journal of Surgical Pathology 2018;42(1):39.

[28] Reinhard E, Adhikhmin M, Gooch B, Shirley P. Color transfer between images. IEEE Computer Graphics and Applications 2001;21(5):34–41.

[29] Magee D, Treanor D, Crellin D, Shires M, Smith K, Mohee K, Quirke P. Colour normalisation in digital histopathology images. In: Proc. optical tissue image analysis in microscopy, histopathology and endoscopy (MICCAI workshop), vol. 100. Daniel Elson; 2009.

[30] Shaban MT, Baur C, Navab N, Albarqouni S. Staingan: stain style transfer for digital histological images. 2018. arXiv preprint arXiv:1804.01601.

[31] Macenko M, Niethammer M, Marron JS, Borland D, Woosley JT, Guan X, Schmitt C, Thomas NE. A method for normalizing histology slides for quantitative analysis. In: 2009 IEEE international symposium on biomedical imaging: from nano to macro. IEEE; 2009. p. 1107–10.

[32] Vahadane A, Peng T, Sethi A, Albarqouni S, Wang L, Baust M, Steiger K, Schlitter AM, Es- posito I, Navab N. Structure-preserving color normalization and sparse stain separation for histological images. IEEE Transactions on Medical Imaging 2016;35(8):1962–71.

[33] Roy S, kumar Jain A, Lal S, Kini J. A study about color normalization methods for histopathology images. Micron 2018;114.

[34] Bejnordi BE, Litjens G, Timofeeva N, Otte-Höller I, Homeyer A, Karssemeijer N, van der Laak JA. Stain specific standardization of whole-slide histopathological images. IEEE Transactions on Medical Imaging 2016;35(2):404–15.

[35] BenTaieb A, Hamarneh G. Adversarial stain transfer for histopathology image analysis. IEEE Transactions on Medical Imaging 2018;37(3):792–802.

[36] Network CGA, et al. Comprehensive molecular portraits of human breast tumours. Nature 2012;490(7418):61.

[37] Akoya biosciences, vectra imaging system. Available from: https://www.akoyabio.com/phenopticstm/instruments.

[38] Zimmermann T. Spectral imaging and linear unmixing in light microscopy. In: Microscopy techniques. Springer; 2005. p. 245–65.

[39] Gillis N, Vavasis SA. Fast and robust recursive algorithms for separable nonnegative matrix factorization. IEEE Transactions on Pattern Analysis and Machine Intelligence 2014;36(4):698–714.

[40] Huang C-H, Veillard A, Roux L, Loménie N, Racoceanu D. Time-efficient sparse analysis of histopathological whole slide images. Computerized Medical Imaging and Graphics 2011;35(7–8):579–91.

[41] Bahlmann C, Patel A, Johnson J, Ni J, Chekkoury A, Khurd P, Kamen A, Grady L, Krupinski E, Graham A, et al. Automated detection of diagnostically relevant regions in h&e stained digital pathology slides. In: Medical imaging 2012: computer-aided diagnosis, vol. 8315. International Society for Optics and Photonics; 2012. p. 831504.

[42] Mercan E, Aksoy S, Shapiro LG, Weaver DL, Brunyé TT, Elmore JG. Localization of diagnostically relevant regions of interest in whole slide images: a comparative study. Journal of Digital Imaging 2016;29(4):496–506.

[43] Cruz-Roa A, Gilmore H, Basavanhally A, Feldman M, Ganesan S, Shih N, Tomaszewski J, Madabhushi A, González F. High-throughput adaptive sampling for whole-slide histopathology im- age analysis (hashi) via convolutional neural networks: application to invasive breast cancer detection. PloS One 2018;13(5):e0196828.

[44] Bardou D, Zhang K, Ahmad SM. Classification of breast cancer based on histology images using convolutional neural networks. IEEE Access 2018;6:24680–93.

[45] Campanella G, Silva VWK, Fuchs TJ. Terabyte-scale deep multiple instance learning for classification and localization in pathology. 2018. arXiv preprint arXiv:1805.06983.

[46] Cruz-Roa A, Gilmore H, Basavanhally A, Feldman M, Ganesan S, Shih NN, Tomaszewski J, González FA, Madabhushi A. Accurate and reproducible invasive breast cancer detection in whole-slide images: a deep learning approach for quantifying tumor extent. Scientific Reports 2017;7:46450.

[47] Bejnordi BE, Veta M, Van Diest PJ, Van Ginneken B, Karssemeijer N, Litjens G, Van Der Laak JA, Hermsen M, Manson QF, Balkenhol M, et al. Diagnostic assessment of deep learning algorithms for detection of lymph node metastases in women with breast cancer. JAMA 2017;318(22):2199—210.

[48] Bejnordi BE, Zuidhof G, Balkenhol M, Hermsen M, Bult P, van Ginneken B, Karssemeijer N, Litjens G, van der Laak J. Context-aware stacked convolutional neural networks for classification of breast carcinomas in whole-slide histopathology images. Journal of Medical Imaging 2017;4(4):044504.

[49] Marami B, Prastawa M, Chan M, Donovan M, Fernandez G, Zeineh J. Ensemble network for region identification in breast histopathology slides. In: International conference image analysis and recognition. Springer; 2018. p. 861—8.

[50] Aresta G, Araújo T, Kwok S, Chennamsetty SS, Safwan M, Alex V, Marami B, Prastawa M, Chan M, Donovan M, et al. Bach: grand challenge on breast cancer histology images. 2018. arXiv preprint arXiv:1808.04277.

[51] Al-Kofahi Y, Lassoued W, Lee W, Roysam B. Improved automatic detection and segmentation of cell nuclei in histopathology images. IEEE Transactions on Biomedical Engineering 2010;57(4):841—52.

[52] Veta M, Van Diest PJ, Kornegoor R, Huisman A, Viergever MA, Pluim JP. Automatic nuclei segmentation in H&E stained breast cancer histopathology images. PloS One 2013;8(7):e70221.

[53] Xing F, Yang L. Robust nucleus/cell detection and segmentation in digital pathology and microscopy images: a comprehensive review. IEEE Reviews in Biomedical Engineering 2016;9:234—63.

[54] Ajemba P, Al-Kofahi Y, Scott R, Donovan M, Fernandez G. Integrated segmentation of cellular structures. In: Medical imaging 2011: image processing, vol. 7962. International Society for Optics and Photonics; 2011. 79620I.

[55] Hofener H, Homeyer A, Weiss N, Molin J, Lundstrom CF, Hahn HK. Deep learning nuclei detection: a simple approach can deliver state-of-the-art results. Computerized Medical Imaging and Graphics 2018;70:43—52. https://doi.org/10.1016/j.compmedimag.2018.08.010.

[56] Naylor P, La M, Reyal F, Walter T. Nuclei segmentation in histopathology images using deep neural networks. In: 2017 IEEE 14th international symposium on biomedical imaging. ISBI 2017; 2017. p. 933—6. https://doi.org/10.1109/ISBI.2017.7950669.

[57] Sirinukunwattana K, Pluim JP, Chen H, Qi X, Heng P-A, Guo YB, Wang LY, Matuszewski BJ, Bruni E, Sanchez U, et al. Gland segmentation in colon histology images: the glas challenge contest. Medical Image Analysis 2017;35:489—502.

[58] Chen H, Qi X, Yu L, Heng P-A. Dcan: Deep contour-aware networks for accurate gland segmentation. In: 2016 IEEE conference on computer vision and pattern recognition (CVPR); 2016. p. 2487—96.

[59] Xu Y, Li Y, Wang Y, Liu M, Fan Y, Lai M, Eric I, Chang C. Gland instance segmentation using deep multichannel neural networks. IEEE Transactions on Biomedical Engineering 2017;64(12):2901—12.

[60] Manivannan S, Li W, Zhang J, Trucco E, McKenna SJ. Structure prediction for gland segmentation with hand-crafted and deep convolutional features. IEEE Transactions on Medical Imaging 2018;37(1):210—21.

[61] Ronneberger O, Fischer P, Brox T, U-net. Convolutional networks for biomedical image segmentation. In: Medical image computing and computer-assisted intervention MICCAI 2015. Springer International Publishing; 2015. p. 234241.

[62] Al-Milaji Z, Ersoy I, Hafiane A, Palaniappan K, Bunyak F. Integrating segmentation with deep learning for enhanced classification of epithelial and stromal tissues in H&E images. Pattern Recognition Letters 2019;119:214−21. https://doi.org/10.1016/j.patrec.2017.09.015. Deep Learning for Pattern Recognition.

[63] Bulten W, Bándi P, Hoven J, Loo Rv d, Lotz J, Weiss N, Laak Jv d, Ginneken Bv, Hulsbergen-van de Kaa C, Litjens G. Epithelium segmentation using deep learning in H&E-stained prostate specimens with immunohistochemistry as reference standard. Scientific Reports 2019;9(1):864. https://doi.org/10.1038/s41598-018-37257-4.

[64] Sotiriou C, Pusztai L. Gene-expression signatures in breast cancer. New England Journal of Medicine 2009;360(8):790−800.

[65] Cireşan DC, Giusti A, Gambardella LM, Schmidhuber J. Mitosis detection in breast cancer histology images with deep neural networks. In: Mori K, Sakuma I, Sato Y, Barillot C, Navab N, editors. Medical image computing and computer-assisted intervention − MICCAI 2013. Berlin, Heidelberg: Springer Berlin Heidelberg; 2013. p. 411−8.

[66] Veta M, van Diest PJ, Willems SM, Wang H, Madabhushi A, Cruz-Roa A, Gonzalez F, Larsen AB, Vestergaard JS, Dahl AB, Cirean DC, Schmidhuber J, Giusti A, Gambardella LM, Tek FB, Walter T, Wang C-W, Kondo S, Matuszewski BJ, Precioso F, Snell V, Kittler J, de Campos TE, Khan AM, Rajpoot NM, Arkoumani E, Lacle MM, Viergever MA, Pluim JP. Assessment of algorithms for mitosis detection in breast cancer histopathology images. Medical Image Analysis 2015;20(1):237−48. https://doi.org/10.1016/j.media.2014.11.010.

[67] Chen H, Dou Q, Wang X, Qin J, Heng P. Mitosis detection in breast cancer histology images via deep cascaded networks. 2016.

[68] Albarqouni S, Baur C, Achilles F, Belagiannis V, Demirci S, Navab N. Aggnet: deep learning from crowds for mitosis detection in breast cancer histology images. IEEE Transactions on Medical Imaging 2016;35(5):1313−21. https://doi.org/10.1109/TMI.2016.2528120.

[69] Verhoef EI, van Cappellen WA, Slotman JA, Kremers G-J, Ewing-Graham PC, Houtsmuller AB, van Royen ME, van Leenders GJ. Three-dimensional analysis reveals two major architectural subgroups of prostate cancer growth patterns. Modern Pathology 2019:1.

[70] Tolkach Y, Thomann S, Kristiansen G. Three-dimensional reconstruction of prostate cancer architecture with serial immunohistochemical sections: hallmarks of tumour growth, tumour compartmentalisation, and implications for grading and heterogeneity. Histopathology 2018;72(6):1051−9.

[71] Epstein JI. Prostate cancer grading: a decade after the 2005 modified system. Modern Pathology 2018;31(S1):S47.

[72] Branca G, Ieni A, Barresi V, Tuccari G, Caruso RA. An updated review of cribriform carcinomas with emphasis on histopathological diagnosis and prognostic significance. Oncology Reviews 2017;11(1).

[73] Scott R, Khan FM, Zeineh J, Donovan M, Fernandez G. Gland ring morphometry for prostate cancer prognosis in multispectral immunofluorescence images. In: International conference on medical image computing and computer-assisted intervention. Springer; 2014. p. 585−92.

[74] Nguyen K, Sabata B, Jain AK. Prostate cancer grading: gland segmentation and structural features. Pattern Recognition Letters 2012;33(7):951−61.

[75] Sirinukunwattana K, Snead DR, Rajpoot NM. A stochastic polygons model for glandular structures in colon histology images. IEEE Transactions on Medical Imaging 2015;34(11):2366−78.

[76] Stålhammar G, Martinez NF, Lippert M, Tobin NP, Mølholm I, Kis L, Rosin G, Rantalainen M, Pedersen L, Bergh J, et al. Digital image analysis outperforms manual biomarker assessment in breast cancer. Modern Pathology 2016;29(4):318.

[77] Visiopharm a/s, hoersholm, Denmark. Available from: https://www.visiopharm.com.

[78] Carvajal-Hausdorf DE, Schalper KA, Neumeister VM, Rimm DL. Quantitative measurement of cancer tissue biomarkers in the lab and in the clinic. Laboratory Investigation 2015;95(4):385.

[79] Stack EC, Wang C, Roman KA, Hoyt CC. Multiplexed immunohistochemistry, imaging, and quantitation: a review, with an assessment of tyramide signal amplification, multispectral imaging and multiplex analysis. Methods 2014;70(1):46−58.

[80] Wong PF, Wei W, Smithy JW, Acs B, Toki MI, Blenman KR, Zelterman D, Kluger HM, Rimm DL. Multiplex quantitative analysis of tumor-infiltrating lymphocytes and immunotherapy outcome in metastatic melanoma. Clinical Cancer Research 2019;25.

[81] Gorris MA, Halilovic A, Rabold K, van Duffelen A, Wickramasinghe IN, Verweij D, Wortel IM, Textor JC, de Vries IJM, Figdor CG. Eight-color multiplex immunohistochemistry for simultaneous detection of multiple immune checkpoint molecules within the tumor microenvironment. The Journal of Immunology 2018;200(1):347−54.

[82] Leach D, Buchanan G. Stromal androgen receptor in prostate cancer development and progression. Cancers 2017;9(1):10.

[83] Nearchou IP, Lillard K, Gavriel CG, Ueno H, Harrison DJ, Caie PD. Automated analysis of lymphocytic infiltration, tumor budding, and their spatial relationship improves prognostic accuracy in colorectal cancer. Cancer Immunology Research 2019;7(4):609−20.

[84] Indica labs, albuquerque, nm. Available from: https://www.indicalab.com.

[85] Oztan B, Shubert KR, Bjornsson CS, Plopper GE, Yener B. Biologically-driven cellgraphs for breast tissue grading. In: 2013 IEEE 10th international symposium on biomedical imaging. IEEE; 2013. p. 137−40.

[86] Khan N, Afroz N, Rana F, Khan M. Role of cytologic grading in prognostication of invasive breast carcinoma. Journal of Cytology/Indian Academy of Cytologists 2009;26(2):65.

[87] Veltri RW, Isharwal S, Miller MC, Epstein JI, Partin AW. Nuclear roundness variance predicts prostate cancer progression, metastasis, and death: a prospective evaluation with up to 25 years of follow-up after radical prostatectomy. The Prostate 2010; 70(12):1333−9.

[88] Jørgensen AS, Rasmussen AM, Andersen NKM, Andersen SK, Emborg J, Rge R, Østergaard LR. Using cell nuclei features to detect colon cancer tissue in hematoxylin and eosin stained slides. Cytometry, Part A 2017;91(8):785−93.

[89] Dowsett M, Nielsen TO, Ahern R, Bartlett J, Coombes RC, Cuzick J, Ellis M, Henry NL, Hugh JC, Lively T, et al. Assessment of ki67 in breast cancer: recommendations from the international ki67 in breast cancer working group. Journal of the National Cancer Institute 2011;103(22):1656−64.

[90] Ali S, Veltri R, Epstein JA, Christudass C, Madabhushi A. Cell cluster graph for prediction of biochemical recurrence in prostate cancer patients from tissue microarrays. In: Medical imaging 2013: digital pathology, vol. 8676. International Society for Optics and Photonics; 2013. 86760H.

[91] Lee G, Sparks R, Ali S, Shih NN, Feldman MD, Spangler E, Rebbeck T, Tomaszewski JE, Madabhushi A. Co-occurring gland angularity in localized subgraphs: predicting biochemical recurrence in intermediate-risk prostate cancer patients. PloS One 2014;9(5):e97954.

[92] Lu C, Wang X, Prasanna P, Corredor G, Sedor G, Bera K, Velcheti V, Madabhushi A. Feature driven local cell graph (fedeg): predicting overall survival in early stage lung cancer. In: International conference on medical image computing and computer-assisted intervention. Springer; 2018. p. 407–16.

[93] Sharma H, Zerbe N, Lohmann S, Kayser K, Hellwich O, Hufnagl P. A review of graph-based methods for image analysis in digital histopathology. Diagnostic Pathology 2015:1–61.

[94] Gurcan MN, Boucheron L, Can A, Madabhushi A, Rajpoot N, Yener B. Histopathological image analysis: a review. IEEE Reviews in Biomedical Engineering 2009;2:147.

[95] Ghosh S, Das N, Gonçalves T, Quaresma P, Kundu M. The journey of graph kernels through two decades. Computer Science Review 2018;27:88–111.

[96] Wu Z, Pan S, Chen F, Long G, Zhang C, Yu PS. A comprehensive survey on graph neural networks. 2019. arXiv preprint arXiv:1901.00596.

[97] Ackerman DA, Barry JM, Wicklund RA, Olson N, Lowe BA. Analysis of risk factors associated with prostate cancer extension to the surgical margin and pelvic node metastasis at radical prostatectomy. The Journal of Urology 1993;150(6):1845–50.

[98] Cox DR. Analysis of survival data. Routledge; 2018.

[99] Kaplan EL, Meier P. Nonparametric estimation from incomplete observations. Journal of the American Statistical Association 1958;53(282):457–81.

[100] Caetano S, Sonpavde G, Pond G. C-statistic: a brief explanation of its construction, interpretation and limitations. European Journal of Cancer 2018;90:130–2.

[101] Klein JP, Moeschberger ML. Survival analysis: techniques for censored and truncated data. Springer Science & Business Media; 2006.

[102] Cox DR. Regression models and life-tables. Journal of the Royal Statistical Society: Series B (Methodological) 1972;34(2):187–202.

[103] Bellera CA, MacGrogan G, Debled M, de Lara CT, Brouste V, Mathoulin-Pélissier S. Variables with time-varying effects and the cox model: some statistical concepts illustrated with a prognostic factor study in breast cancer. BMC Medical Research Methodology 2010;10(1):20.

[104] Faraggi D, Simon R. A neural network model for survival data. Statistics in Medicine 1995;14(1):73–82.

[105] Katzman JL, Shaham U, Cloninger A, Bates J, Jiang T, Kluger Y. Deepsurv: personalized treatment recommender system using a cox proportional hazards deep neural network. BMC Medical Research Methodology 2018;18(1):24.

[106] Lee C, Zame WR, Yoon J, van der Schaar M. Deephit: a deep learning approach to survival analysis with competing risks. In: Thirty-second AAAI conference on artificial intelligence; 2018.

[107] Friedman J, Hastie T, Tibshirani R. The elements of statistical learning. Springer Series in Statistics, vol. 1; 2001. New York.

[108] Breiman L. Random forests. Machine Learning 2001;45(1):5–32.

[109] Ishwaran H, Lu M. Random survival forests. Wiley StatsRef: Statistics Reference Online. 2008. p. 1–13.

[110] Boser BE, Guyon IM, Vapnik VN. A training algorithm for optimal margin classifiers. In: Proceedings of the fifth annual workshop on Computational learning theory. ACM; 1992. p. 144—52.

[111] Fouodo CJ, König IR, Weihs C, Ziegler A, Wright MN. Support vector machines for survival analysis with R. R Journal 2018;10(1).

[112] Shivaswamy PK, Chu W, Jansche M. A support vector approach to censored targets. In: Seventh IEEE international conference on data mining (ICDM 2007). IEEE; 2007. p. 655—60.

[113] Khan FM, Zubek VB. Support vector regression for censored data (svrc): a novel tool for survival analysis. In: 2008 Eighth IEEE international conference on data mining. IEEE; 2008. p. 863—8.

[114] Eberhart R, Kennedy J. Particle swarm optimization. In: Proceedings of the IEEE international conference on neural networks, vol. 4. Citeseer; 1995. p. 1942—8.

[115] Chandrashekar G, Sahin F. A survey on feature selection methods. Computers and Electrical Engineering 2014;40(1):16—28.

[116] Saeys Y, Inza I, Larrañaga P. A review of feature selection techniques in bioinformatics. Bioinformatics 2007;23(19):2507—17.

[117] Guyon I, Elisseeff A. An introduction to variable and feature selection. Journal of Machine Learning Research 2003;3(Mar):1157—82.

[118] Zhu SC, Yuille A. Region competition: unifying snakes, region growing, and bayes/mdl for multi- band image segmentation. IEEE Transactions on Pattern Analysis and Machine Intelligence 1996;(9):884—900.

[119] Sethian JA. Level set methods and fast marching methods: evolving interfaces in computational geometry, fluid mechanics, computer vision, and materials science, vol. 3. Cambridge university press; 1999.

[120] Yushkevich PA, Piven J, Hazlett HC, Smith RG, Ho S, Gee JC, Gerig G. User-guided 3d active contour segmentation of anatomical structures: significantly improved efficiency and reliability. NeuroImage 2006;31(3):1116—28. https://doi.org/10.1016/j.neuroimage.2006.01.015.

[121] Grady L. Random walks for image segmentation. IEEE Transactions on Pattern Analysis and Machine Intelligence 2006;11:1768—83.

[122] Vincent L, Soille P. Watersheds in digital spaces: an efficient algorithm based on immersion simulations. IEEE Transactions on Pattern Analysis and Machine Intelligence 1991;13(6):583—98. https://doi.org/10.1109/34.87344.

Artificial intelligence and the interplay between tumor and immunity

Joel Haskin Saltz, MD, PhD [1], **Rajarsi Gupta, MD, PhD** [2]

[1]*Professor, Chair, Biomedical Informatics, Stony Brook University, Stony Brook, NY, United States;*
[2]*Assistant Professor, Biomedical Informatics, Stony Brook Medicine, Stony Brook, NY, United States*

Introduction

Over the last 20 years, digital pathology has rapidly grown and evolved alongside advances in immunology, cancer therapeutics, computer science, and artificial intelligence. During this time, there has been increased adoption of digital slide scanners in clinical settings and greater availability of digital whole-slide images (WSIs) of glass slides for a wide spectrum of clinical and research applications. Digital pathology, deep learning, and computational pathology have emerged as powerful and valuable tools in the era of precision medicine and immunotherapy. These technologies and computational methods can revolutionize the clinical subspecialty of pathology, which serves as the central hub of medicine and oncology by providing definitive tissue-based diagnoses that guide patient management and treatment selection in cancer.

Computational image analysis of digital pathology images generates data that are referred to as Pathomics, which refers to the automated quantification of the wide spectrum of phenotypic features of tissues and cells in WSIs. Basic clinically relevant and interpretable Pathomics features include (1) characterization of phenotypically distinct architectural regions such as cancer, benign, and stromal connective tissue, (2) shapes and textures of nuclei, (3) classifications of cell type, and (4) characterization of lymphocytic infiltration. Recently, digital pathology tools have been developed that can quantify and characterize nuanced interactions between cancer and the immune system in digital WSIs of hematoxylin and eosin (H&E)-stained tissue samples from patients, motivated by the guidelines of the International Immuno-Oncology Biomarkers Working Group [1–4].

Image analysis has been employed to study digital pathology images for many years, as described in excellent review articles of algorithmic methods [5–9]. Recently, deep learning and artificial intelligence in Pathomics has led to the development of computational methods that augment and empower qualitative traditional diagnostic histopathologic evaluation, which can substantially accelerate cancer research. Emerging digital pathology and deep learning applications can (1) stratify

Artificial Intelligence and Deep Learning in Pathology. https://doi.org/10.1016/B978-0-323-67538-3.00010-5

patient management through data-driven insights into cancer, (2) identify relevant biomarkers to predict clinical outcomes and treatment response, and (3) enhance our collective understanding of cancer biology to motivate the utilization of novel therapeutic approaches [5—8,10—41]. This chapter introduces and describes a selected set of novel Pathomics-based deep learning methods that have been developed to classify and reproducibly quantify the interplay between tumor cells and the immune response in the tumor microenvironment.

Immune surveillance and immunotherapy

The human immune system is typically described as the sum of the innate and adaptive immune systems, which function together to maintain a state of continuous surveillance through several different types and subtypes of immune cells. These diverse cells are responsible for eliminating the vast majority of infectious agents, aberrant cells with acquired genetic and epigenetic changes, and cancer cells through the recognition and processing of foreign antigens. The cells of the innate immune system have pattern recognition receptors that recognize non-self antigens which generate immediate, short-lived, and nonspecific inflammatory responses, whereas the cells of the adaptive immune response generate highly specific inflammatory responses through antibody-mediated and cell-dependent responses to provide long-lasting defense with the capacity for memory [17,23,25,27].

The innate and adaptive immune systems are hierarchical regulatory mechanisms that are coordinated through many different types of immune cells. These cells are typically divided into broader classes and cell lineages that commonly include B-cells, T-cells (TH_1, TH_2, TH_{17}, T_{REG}, $\gamma\delta$ T-cells, cytotoxic T-cells, and NK/T-cells), neutrophils, macrophages, dendritic cells, mast cells, and NK cells [34,35,42—44]. The major categories of cell types that exist in the tumor microenvironment (TME) include cytotoxic CD8+ T-cells that kill non-self and cancer cells; CD4+ helper T-cells that suppress or regulate immune responses through cytokine signaling; CD4+ regulatory T-cells (CD25+/FOXP3+ Treg) that play an important role in tolerance; natural killer cells (NK cells) that kill cells that are missing self MHC-I markers without requiring cytokine stimulation; and macrophages and dendritic cells that have phagocytic and antigen presenting functions [45,46]. To put the diversity and heterogeneity of the immune landscape into perspective, there are over 100 different populations of immune cell types in the peripheral blood of humans that are characterized by the variable expression of cell surface and intracellular markers across the continuum of various activation and differentiation states [47—50].

The dynamic complexity of the immune system and its ability to respond to diverse stimuli and fight cancer cells is highly unpredictable due to intrinsic differences in the pro-inflammatory and anti-inflammatory cell populations that vary widely across individuals [17,28,29,51—53]. Moreover, immune infiltrates can include all kinds of immune cell types in any given tumor, leading to heterogeneity of the immune landscape across the wide spectrum of different types of cancer, which results in the high variability and diversity of immune cell populations in patients [17,31,33—35,44,54]. Cancer cells evade immune-mediated recognition and elimination through immunosuppressive strategies that disrupt T-cell signaling and induce tolerance in the TME through the production of inhibitory cytokines that prevent the expansion and activation of CD4+ helper and cytotoxic CD8+ T-cells [30,37—39].

The suppression and inactivation of immune detection and immune-mediated cytotoxicity is also accompanied by the ability of cancer cells to actively reprogram immune cells in order to stimulate angiogenesis and accompanying stromal responses that promote the progression of disease through the continued survival of cancer cells. The subversion of normal immunoregulatory mechanisms also leads to the emergence of subsets of tumor cells that are less immunogenic and resistant to apoptosis within the immunosuppressed milieu of the tumor microenvironment. This selection pressure enables cancer cells to adapt and further evade the immune system through the loss of tumor antigens that would normally stimulate complement-mediated and antibody-dependent cell-mediated cytotoxicity from T-cells and natural killer (NK) cells [17,28—39]. The combination of the uncontrolled proliferation and adaptation of cancer cells in the immunosuppressed tumor micro-environment ultimately results in the invasion of neighboring tissues and distant sites beyond the primary site of origin.

The importance of the role of immunity in controlling cancer was observed a century ago by Dr. William Coley in a case of complete remission in advanced inoperable sarcoma secondary to severe *Streptococcus pyogenes* bacterial skin infections [55]. Thus, the concept of stimulating and inhibiting hierarchical immunoregulatory mechanisms of the immune surveillance system as a feasible treatment strategy for cancer was born decades ago [56—58]. Since then, many studies have focused on specific types of immune cell populations and their various functional properties in order to determine the clinical significance of pro-inflammatory and anti-inflammatory temporospatial relationships in numerous types of human disease, including cancer [17,28—30,32,44,52,53,59—65]. During the process of uncontrolled growth in cancer, nuanced differences in protein structure of foreign antigens in infected, aberrant, or tumor cells are detected at the molecular level during antigen processing and processed by the innate and adaptive immune system to coordinate and targeted immune-mediated response. However, the immune system is highly complex and consists of many types and subtypes of immune cells to fight infections and remove aberrant cells, which results in a dynamic interplay between pro-inflammatory and anti-inflammatory functional states that are regulated through cytokine cell signaling and direct interactions between immune cells to generate systemic immune responses to fight cancer.

Despite the intrinsic functional complexities and widely variable composition of the immune system, we are fortunate as a society to have access to first-generation immunotherapeutic options in our current day and age that have been utilized to successfully treat cancer and provide tangible clinical benefits. Currently, available treatment options stimulate immune cells or block immune checkpoint pathways. The best examples of recent success in immunotherapy include monoclonal antibody-based treatment strategies that block cytotoxic T-lymphocyte associated protein 4 (CTLA-4) and programmed cell death protein-1 (PD-1), which have generated substantial interest in identifying other novel clinically actionable targets that can further improve treatment response and clinical outcomes through combinations with existing chemotherapy and other novel pharmacologic options. Other types of treatments that are being explored include chimeric-antigen receptor T-cells (CAR-T) that are produced by genetically modifying T-cells harvested from individual patients; recombinant proteins to stimulate and enhance cytotoxic T-cell activity; cancer vaccines to augment antigen presentation; and oncolytic viruses to initiate systemic anti-tumor immunity in order to target and destroy cancer cells [30,37,38].

Examples of immune checkpoint therapy with CTLA-4 or PD-1/PD-L1 to overcome the immunosuppression mediated by tumor cells [37,38,64,66] include melanoma, renal cancer, and lung cancer [67−71]. Ipilimumab, the monoclonal antibody that blocks CTLA-4, was approved by the Food and Drug Administration (FDA) to treat melanoma in 2011, which was followed by FDA approval for nivolumab to block PD-1 in melanoma and non−small cell lung cancer (NSCLC) in 2014 [50,72]. These success were followed by the introduction of Pembrolizumab, which is considered to be a breakthrough therapy for the treatment of NSCLC because treatment response is significantly improved in tumors that also express high levels of the PD-L1. Nivolumab has also been recently approved to treat patients with advanced metastatic squamous NSCLC with disease progression in combination with or after standard platinum-based chemotherapy [39,71,72]. In order to further improve the therapeutic efficacy of these immune checkpoint inhibitors, combinations of immunotherapy with existing forms of chemotherapy and other forms of targeted therapies are currently being tested and evaluated in patients with locally advanced or metastatic cancer [37,73−76].

Despite this success, the identification and stratification of patients who will likely benefit from immunotherapy is not so straightforward, even though the PD-1 signaling blockade has become an established form of treatment for many types of cancer. Commercially available standardized assays to evaluate the bioactivity of PD-1/PD-L1 lack antigen specificity, even though the overexpression of surface or soluble PD-L1 in multiple tumor types is mostly associated with poor prognosis [67,70,72,76−81]. The histologic assessment of PD-L1 is also challenging due to heterogeneous expression in cancer and benign normal tissues, which is further complicated with unintuitive thresholds and cutoffs for scoring PD-L1 positivity that can vary and lead to known problematic interobserver variability in PD-L1 assessment by pathologists [42,82−84].

As immunotherapy expands, there is a high demand for reliable and standardized bioassays and scoring methods that can characterize antibodies and evaluate expression to select the appropriate patients for PD-1/PD-L blockade therapy. Since checkpoint inhibitors and other forms of emerging immunotherapy rely on the host immune system and tumor infiltrating lymphocytes (TILs) to fight cancer, the utility and pharmacologic effects of these treatments may be limited in current treatment strategies if the host immune system is depleted or not present in the tumor microenvironment. Furthermore, inaccurate patient stratification and the impact of misinterpretation of PD-L1 expression can lead to radically different therapeutic stratification, clinical outcomes, and serious adverse effects that can occur due to subjective scoring around variable thresholds and cutoffs [42,82−84]. In order to meet this unmet clinical need, digital pathology algorithms that can detect and characterize lymphocytes in WSIs of diagnostic surgical pathology specimens may play useful roles to identify and stratify patients for immunotherapy, especially with the recent success of manual assessment of TILs by pathologists in histopathologic specimens in many solid tumor types to provide important prognostic information and established the potential of the role of TILs as a biomarker to predict treatment response [3,4,28,85,86].

Identifying TILs with deep learning

The biological behavior of various types and subtypes of cancer is intrinsically coupled to the characteristics of the tumor microenvironment, which consists of stroma, immune infiltrate, nerves, and lymphovascular vessels [17,31−35,50]. Since these distinct tissue components cohabit the TME with cancer cells, it is widely believed that tumor antigenicity−driven immune responses are likely quite influenced, if not directly dependent, on the type, quantity, and spatial localization of immune cells that are present in the immediate landscape of the TME [17,31,87]. In order to further examine the relationship of immune cells in the TME with cancer cells, the assessment of TILs is gaining importance as a candidate prognostic and predictive biomarker that may be useful to identify and stratify patients with the highest likelihood of responding to immunotherapy treatment options in a variety of cancer types [32−35,88].

Thus, the routine of evaluation of TILs is gaining popularity as a readily available and widely applicable biomarker that needs to be incorporated into diagnostic surgical pathology reports. Even though the implementation of TILs as a routine clinical biomarker has not been achieved yet, the immediate need to incorporate the evaluation of TILs to improve current protocols for immune checkpoint therapy and other forms of immunotherapy is very clear. The evaluation and appropriate characterization of TILs in the TME is also warranted in terms of addressing immunotherapy-related safety issues since serious adverse effects and the lack of long-lasting responses in many patients suggests that the activation of previously tumor-immunosuppressed TILs needs to be carefully controlled [63].

High densities of TILs correlate with favorable clinical outcomes [89], including longer disease-free survival (DFS) or improved overall survival (OS) in multiple cancer types [90]. Moreover, the spatial localization and distribution of TILs in terms of the immune infiltrate in the tumor center and invasive margin have also become important in cancer prognosis [89]. Similarly, the quantification of spatial

TIL density and distribution in different tumor regions has high prognostic value [33,91,92] with respect to cellular heterogeneity within the TME. In terms of the clinical utility of TILs as potentially useful biomarker, the presence of high levels of TILs is consistently associated with a more favorable prognosis in patients with early-stage triple-negative and HER2-positive breast cancer [1,93].

Pathologists routinely utilize H&E-stained tissue sections for diagnostic histo-pathologic examination of biopsy, excision, and surgical resection tissue samples for almost every case of cancer for patients who are undergoing treatment. Currently, large collections of WSIs have been generated by commercially available slide scanners that contain digitized H&E-stained tissue sections for clinical research studies. The increasing availability of collections of WSIs has provided the oppor-tunity to utilize quantitative digital pathology—based methods to assess TILs in H&E WSIs, which have emerged as potential applications that can complement the manual histopathologic examination of TILs in H&E glass slides. Even though the assessment of TILs in H&E glass slides and WSIs do not explicitly shed light on the molecular aspects of tumor immune interactions in the TME, a great deal of clinically useful information can be obtained.

Advances in high-performance computing, deep learning, and artificial intelli-gence have resulted in the capability and capacity to perform image analysis on highly complex images of human tissues, which can be used to identify, delineate, and label specific tissue regions, architectural elements, cell types, and nuclei [41,94—105]. These technological innovations have led to substantially increased focus on deep learning—based techniques to extract and analyze image-based fea-tures from highly complex images in biomedical research and other domains in the past few years [41,94—110]. Therefore, it has not been surprising that deep learning methods are proving to be excellent tools that can identify and characterize TILs in H&E WSIs.

In terms of the approaches to this task in digital pathology from the point of view of computer science and computer vision, one approach to identifying infiltrating lymphocytes segments tissue regions that contain lymphocytes, whereas another complementary approach detects individual lymphocytes. Even though lymphocytes typically have a reasonably uniform appearance in H&E WSIs, deep learning algo-rithms that distinguish lymphocytes from other microanatomic entities have to necessarily contend with tissue-specific, cancer-specific, and disease site—specific confounders. Thus, analyses of TILs typically encompass analysis of spatial interre-lationships between cancer, tumor-associated stroma, and lymphocytes, which can involve the classification of tissue regions and/or the detection and classification of individual cells. Due to the importance of the spatial patterns of distribution of TILs, significant efforts are being dedicated to characterizing the spatial clustering of lymphocytes, as well as the interrelationships between cancer, tumor-associated stroma, and lymphocytes.

Early research efforts to characterize TILs focused on the detection of individual lymphocytes and cancer cells [28,111—113] in solid tumors with a special interest in developing methods to capture the features of the lymphocytic infiltrate in breast cancer. This work leveraged rapidly expanding machine learning methodology in nuclear segmentation, feature extraction, and classification [5,6,9]. Segmentation of nuclei in tissue images proved to be challenging due to (1) variations in nuclear size and morphology, (2) nuclear overlap, (3) complex and irregular visual aspects of histologic structures, and (4) variations and irregularity of H&E staining and image acquisition. Irshad et al. [6] and Gurcan et al. [5] provide excellent surveys of the state of the art as it existed approximately 5–10 years ago in nuclear segmentation and detection. Image processing algorithms of various levels of sophistication were also employed, but the utilization of supervised algorithms was rare. Irshad et al. [6] specifically stated in their review article in 2014 that, "To the best of our knowledge, only few supervised machine learning techniques like Bayesian … SVM (Support Vector Machine) … and AdaBoost are used for nuclei segmentation."

In the past few years since then, deep learning methods have played a rapidly increasing role in both nuclear segmentation and detection (for early examples, see Refs. [114–116]). Janowczyk et al. [21] articulated the advantages of deep learning approaches in an excellent manner by stating, "in order to develop a nuclear segmentation algorithm, one must first understand all of the possible variances in morphology, texture, and color appearances. Subsequently, an algorithmic scheme needs to be developed which can account for as many of these variances as possible while not being too general as to result in false positive results or too narrow as to result in false negative errors. This process can become quite unwieldy as it is often infeasible to view all of the outlier cases a priori, and thus an extensive iterative trial and error approach needs to be undertaken." Winners of the recent MICCAI nuclear segmentation challenges have also utilized deep learning methods [117]. Since the success of deep learning algorithms tends to hinge on training data adequacy, generation of comprehensive training datasets remains crucial and challenging. This is especially challenging due to the wide variability in the appearance of nuclei that can differ between tissue types and can sometimes be difficult to morphologically distinguish and classify in cancer, which is further complicated by the variations in appearance that are due to tissue preparation. A promising approach to reduce the requirements for generating training datasets employs generative adversarial networks (GANs) [118] to generate realistic synthetic nuclei that can be used to enlarge and generalize training sets [119,120].

Early work in lymphocyte detection and characterization efforts also explored the development of a clinical decision support (CDS) system to discriminate among three types of lymphoproliferative disorders and normal blood cells [121], along with lymphocyte detection and centroblast quantification in follicular lymphoma [122]. Currently, algorithms have been developed that can detect and classify lymphocytes as well as other types of cells, which allows for the detailed characterization of the interrelationships between tumor, tumor-associated stroma, and lymphocytes [123]. Corredor et al. recently presented a set of metrics that captures density and spatial co-localization of TILs and tumor cells that were linked to likelihood of early-state NSCLC recurrence [123]. Similarly, Heindl et al. captured metrics of immune cell abundance and spatial heterogeneity that were computed for patients with ER + breast cancer [124] based on a pipeline that segmented and classified nuclei as lymphocytes, cancer, or other types of nuclei to perform analyses in postmenopausal patients with ER + breast cancer treated with tamoxifen or anastrozole over 5 years. The prognostic significance of immune scores was then compared with Oncotype DX 21-gene recurrence score (RS), PAM50 risk of recurrence (ROR) score, IHC4 score, and clinical treatment scores.

The development of methods that classify tissue regions has been facilitated by the rapid development of convolutional neural network (CNN) methods and publicly available software. Recently, a deep learning—based patch classification workflow was utilized to characterize patterns of lymphocytes in WSIs by using a CNN to classify image patches as lymphocyte-positive (i.e., containing lymphocytes) or lymphocyte-negative in combination with a CNN to segment necrotic regions in order to reduce false lymphocyte-positive classifications [41]. This method leveraged a convolutional autoencoder (CAE) that was designed to encode nuclei in image patches into sparse feature maps that encode both the location and appearance of nuclei [105]. A supervised CNN took unsupervised encoded features from the unsupervised CAE for classification. An iterative training effort was carried out with 100×100 pixel image patches (equivalent to a resolution of $50 \times 50\mu m$ patches at $200\times$ magnification) for 5200 images from 13 tumor types using TCGA data.

The approach taken was to progress through tumor types and (1) annotate lymphocyte infiltrated image regions and regions not infiltrated by lymphocytes, (2) train by using all available annotations to generate predictions, and (3) visually assess the predictions while extracting samples of images from regions where the predictions were inaccurate until adequate accuracy was obtained for the given tumor type. After the end of this process, a separate testing dataset was generated across tumor types to evaluate results. Recently, Abousamra et al. utilized all of the publicly available set of annotations generated in this method to train two standard CNN networks, VGG 16 and Inception v4 to generate predictions in the same 5200 TCGA specimens [125]. The accuracy that was obtained by using the standard models on the *aggregated* training set is modestly better than that reported by using the CAE model on the *incrementally* generated training set [41,125].

A variety of other efforts have targeted characterization of region types in specific tumor types. In breast cancer, a fully convolutional network was utilized to carry out pixel level semantic segmentation to identify tumor, stroma, necrosis, and TILs [10]. These training data were gathered through a structured annotation gathering, where the annotation curation process was called "structured crowdsourcing" through participants with varying degrees of expertise who contributed training data. Amgad et al. [11] have also described pixel-level semantic segmentation of tumor, stroma, and necrosis regions linked with the detection of tumor, stroma, and lymphocytic nuclei. This approach also employs a fully convolutional network approach that combines region and nucleus segmentation masks to classify pixels into 12 classes, where each class encodes a combination of region and nucleus membership information. The framework enforces biological constraints, e.g., it does not allow cell classifications within necrotic regions or stromal cells within non-stromal regions.

Other current work that parallels these types of efforts include the combination of automated tumor detection to facilitate the interpretation of the spatial patterns of distribution of TILs within a relevant histologic landscape in order to identify intratumoral and peritumoral TILs. Le et al. have recently developed methods to classify 350×350 pixel image patches (equivalent to a resolution of $85 \times 85\mu m$ patches at $400\times$ magnification) of invasive breast cancer in WSIs that are combined with existing lymphocyte detection method [41,126]. Figs. 10.1 and 10.2 are examples of tumor-TIL maps that can be generated from H&E WSIs with a combination of deep learning methods to provide immediate insight into the spatial distribution of intratumoral and peritumoral TILs in breast cancer and identify whether a specific tumor is "hot" or "cold" with respect to the pro-inflammatory and anti-inflammatory immunologic state of the TME [127]. The combined tumor-TIL predictions were generated for the publicly available WSIs of the breast cancer study arm in the

FIGURE 10.1

"Hot" immune subtype of breast cancer visualized with a composite Tumor-TIL map, TCGA BRCA E2-A14X-01Z-00-DX1. Tumor-TIL analyses in primary ductal carcinoma of the breast identifies a predominantly diffuse spatial distribution of intratumoral TILs with focal peritumoral lymphoid aggregates. Composite Tumor-TIL map: (A) low-magnification H&E WSI, (B) automated lymphocyte detection displayed as a spatial probability map, (C) automated tumor detection displayed as a spatial probability map, and (D) Combined Tumor-TIL map with tumor (yellow), lymphocytes (red), and non-tumor tissues (gray). TILs, tumor infiltrating lymphocytes; WSI, whole-slide image; H&E, hematoxylin and eosin.

FIGURE 10.2

"Cold" immune subtype of breast cancer visualized with a composite Tumor-TIL map, TCGA BRCA GM-A2DB-01Z-00-DX1. Tumor-TIL analyses in primary infiltrating ductal carcinoma of the breast identifies a predominantly circumferential spatial distribution of peritumoral TILs at the invasive edge of the tumor with focal areas of intratumoral TILs. Composite Tumor-TIL map: (A) low-magnification H&E WSI, (B) automated lymphocyte detection displayed as a spatial probability map, (C) automated tumor detection displayed as a spatial probability map, and (D) Combined Tumor-TIL map with tumor (yellow), lymphocytes (red), and non-tumor tissues (gray). TILs, tumor infiltrating lymphocytes; WSI, whole-slide image; H&E, hematoxylin and eosin.

Cancer Genome Atlas (TCGA) project and have been made publicly available online in a web-based interface that allows the user to interactively navigate and evaluate the predictions of tumor-TIL maps with the corresponding H&E WSIs in 1015 WSIs of the TCGA Breast Cancer (BRCA) collection [128].

Le et al. have also developed a course-grained pancreatic cancer detection tool for invasive pancreatic ductal adenocarcinoma (PDAC) [129] that identifies image patches with malignant poorly formed glands and invasive nests of tumor cells within the context of normal pancreatic acinar tissue, pancreatic islet cells, stroma,

FIGURE 10.3

Tumor-TIL maps in Primary and Metastatic Pancreatic Cancer, TCGA PRAD XD-AAU1-01Z-00-DX1 and TCGA PRAD XD-AAU1-01Z-00-DX2, respectively. Top Row: Tumor-TIL analyses in primary PDAC. B*lue arrow* from Tumor-TIL map to ROI showing tumor cells admixed with TILs. Bottom Row: Tumor-TIL analyses in metastatic PDAC to the spleen. B*lue arrow* from Tumor-TIL map to ROI showing the interface between PDAC poorly formed malignant glands and splenic lymphocytes. [Composite images combine low-magnification H&E WSIs, automated lymphocyte detection probability, and automated tumor detection probability in order to generate combined Tumor-TIL spatial maps (tumor in yellow, lymphocytes in red, and non-tumor tissues in gray) as shown in Figures 10.1 and 10.2.] TILs, tumor infiltrating lymphocytes; WSI, whole-slide image; H&E, hematoxylin and eosin; PDAC, pancreatic ductal carcinoma, ROI, region of interest.

immune cells, nerves, and vessels. The histologic appearances and intrinsic features of pancreatic cancer are extremely diverse and represent a diagnostically challenging even for the most experienced pathologists. Nonetheless, preliminary work looks promising, and this method has been paired with existing lymphocyte detection methods [41,125], as shown in Fig. 10.3.

The definition and criteria for different types of architectural elements and regions of tissues can be developed and tuned to match a wide variety of scientific applications to aid the scientific interpretability of Pathomics within the appropriate histologic context. For example, different types of tissue regions may or may not be disjoint, so a tumor region that consists of cancer, tumor-associated stroma, and TILs can be subdivided in a data-driven manner with emerging artificial intelligence applications in digital pathology image analysis to specifically identify intratumoral and peritumoral TILs, which can be further subdivided to identify intraepithelial TILs and stromal TILs. To put this into context, if a pathologist or group of pathologists attempted to perform this type of task in multiple fields of view under the microscope for every tissue section for multiple slides per case across hundreds to thousands of glass slides, this would be prohibitive due to the amount of labor, time, and cost and almost impossible to realistically consider given the limited availability of practicing pathologist and intrinsic intra- and interobserver variability.

Multiplex immunohistochemistry with digital pathology and deep learning

Building on the exciting advances with computational detection of lymphocytes to identify TILs within the histologic landscape of the cancer, a conceptually straight-forward approach is to integrate insights from TIL maps and specifically identify the various types and subsets of aforementioned immune cells based on the expression of surface and cellular biomarkers and their in situ spatial distribution in the TME [42,130–133]. In routine diagnostic surgical pathology, consecutive serial sections of tissues are stained with one marker at a time and interpretation is based on the presence of a marker or a semiquantitative estimation of the number of positive cells of interest. Multiplexed chromogenic immunohistochemistry (mIHC) and immuno-fluorescence (mIF) have recently emerged to simultaneously detect multiple bio-markers in the same tissue section to perform molecular immune profiling in situ in formalin-fixed paraffin-embedded (FFPE) samples in order to preserve limited tissue in samples [133–141].

However, the manual evaluation and interpretation of the immunohistochemical (IHC) expression of a single marker is highly subjective and time-consuming due to the nuances in relationship between expression and stain intensity, as well as non-specific background staining, heterogeneous expression, subcellular localization, and variability in selecting appropriate ROIs to score [42,142], which can be heavily influenced by preanalytic variables intrinsic to the various differences in chemical methods, tissue fixation, and histology laboratory processing and staining protocols. Similarly, challenges still remain for computationally aligning or registering serial sections with companion H&E tissue sections, which can vary due to intrinsic architectural and texture differences in each section. There are also drawbacks with generating spatial molecular maps from serial sections that are related to the spatial resolution of molecular IHC biomarkers, as well as challenges associated to variations that are introduced into tissue samples during histologic sectioning and processing for sample preparation. Another overarching challenge that remains as a barrier to the analyses of spatial multiplex IHC and IF in WSIs is the need for training datasets.

Despite these challenges and variables, digital pathology image analysis tools can play a very important role to help pathologists routinely quantify the expression of IHC biomarkers in specific types of cells, differentiate various expression levels, and colocalize the expression of multiple markers. Future clinically adopted analytic methods for mIHC, mIF, and combined IHC/IF methods will have to label and classify different types of cells, distinguish morphologically similar but functionally distinct cells, and delineate tissue regions, which can be incredibly powerful and very helpful for pathologists. Similarly, the potential of integrated analytic methods for mIHC, mIF, and combined IHC/IF methods to identify, quantify, and classify different types of cells, distinguish morphologically similar but functionally distinct cells, and delineate tissue regions have tremendous potential to provide insight into tumor biology that can be transformative for immunotherapy.

Early clinical applications of digital pathology for semiquantitative analysis of IHC markers were focused on computationally scoring the expression of estrogen receptor (ER), progesterone receptor (PR), HER-2, and Ki67 in invasive breast cancer. The goals of these efforts were to reduce intra- and interobserver variability in IHC scoring by pathologists through the precise measurement of the subcellular localization and intensity of antigens [12,13,143]. Despite the potential of these methods, the utilization of digital pathology in the daily workflow of surgical pathology laboratories has not achieved widespread adoption due to the necessity for extensive validation, technical expertise, computational resources, and frequent calibration for IHC staining with positive and negative controls [12,13,143,144].

Whether it is a single marker or multiple markers that need histopathologic evaluation, there are over 100,000 cells in a typical tissue section or WSI of a glass slide, where IHC expression of specific cells of interest or multiple types of labeled cells need to be interpreted within the appropriate context. IHC expression of several markers have to be simultaneously interpreted within the histologic context of tumor cellularity, architectural distortion, tumor growth pattern, tumor-associated stromal responses, inflammatory responses, presence or absence of necrosis, and spatially induced differences of the nuanced expression of biomarkers in the central areas of tumor, infiltrative nests, invasive border, and interface with the adjacent surrounding normal tissues. In order to perform such a daunting task that evaluates, integrates, and interprets six or more markers simultaneously in a single section with these novel mIHC and mIF applications, a technological transition to digital pathology appears inevitable since pathologists are not trained to interpret sections or WSIs with multiple markers and colors.

Nonetheless, these challenges must be addressed since mIHC and mIF applications have the potential to transform the diagnostic evaluation of cancer through the simultaneous assessment of multiple immune and cancer-related pathways and their spatial relationships in the TME in order to elucidate cancer-immune interactions in tissue samples [133−141]. In terms of computer science and computer vision, the types of tasks that need to be developed for deep learning applications are categorized as semantic instance segmentation, which may surpass the limitations of traditional digital pathology image analysis tools without artificial intelligence. Within the context of spatial molecular pathology analyses, this translates to a need to segment cells and/or tissue regions, which are assigned one or more class labels for each cell and/or tissue region. Current work in digital pathology image analysis for mIHC and mIF is exploring unbiased, unsupervised, and semisupervised deep learning methods to perform automatic IHC analysis in order to isolate and detect the expression of individual markers and measure the extent of expression in tumor and immune cells through color deconvolution, optical density, and multispectral separation of chromogens [42,142].

Previous work in several studies have explored three immune biomarkers on a single tissue section in combination with an adjacent section stained by H&E or another biomarker to delineate the tumor [132]. Due to the availability of mIHC, mIF, and the variety of approaches to apply this advanced histologic technique, there have been several recent studies with multiple markers in NSCLC and cancer in other anatomic sites [131−133,135,137−139,145,146]. Novel multispectral approaches that can identify, segment, and evaluate more than three colors at a time have been developed to interpret mIHC within the context of the biological properties of the protein markers of tumor and immune cells by incorporating methods to assign each pixel with a collection of constituent signals from the chromogens in the color mixture [42,135,142,147−149]. This method can usefully address IHC co-expression in subsets of cell types with mIHC and mIF and represents a lot of progress since the maximum number of stains that could be unmixed was limited to three colors previously [42,142,147,149].

A prospective study has also been performed that explored the heterogeneous nature of metastatic melanoma using mIHC correlated with flow cytometry (FACS) to quantify immune subsets in the intratumoral, tumor-associated stromal compartments, and leading invasive edge of the tumor [150]. This study evaluated the association between intratumoral CD8+ T-cells and PDL1 expression in melanoma in combination with FACS to obtain data regarding the differentiation of T-cells and subsets, activation status, and expression of immune checkpoint molecules. mIHC identified significantly higher T_{reg} cells than FACS and showed preferential stromal CD4+ T-cells. This study proposed a model of the immune context of metastatic melanoma with respect to PDL1 expression in melanoma cells and/or macrophages, presence or absence of intratumoral CD8+ TILs, and intratumoral and peritumoral tumor location. This study also provided insight into treatment response with checkpoint inhibitor therapy because PDL1 expression was more prevalent in macrophages in this study [150]. A separate study in metastatic melanoma utilized a novel combination of quantitative IHC, quantitative mIF, and next-generation sequencing for T-cell antigen receptors (TCRs) to show that the proliferation of intratumoral CD8+ TILs was directly correlated with radiographic reduction in tumor size with Pembrolizumab therapy [151]. This study also identified that pretreatment samples had increased numbers of intratumoral and peritumoral cells that expressed CD8, PD-1, and PD-L1, as well as close proximity between PD-1 and PD-L1.

Deep learning methods have also been used to detect and classify cells in mIHC WSIs of breast cancer, where a recent approach [152] involved a two stage approach with an initial neural network to carry out cell detection and cell counting coupled to a second neural network to carry out cell classification, where the annotations required labeling cells with dots. Another recent approach that focuses on reducing the requirement for training data is the development of super-resolution methods that are designed to predict high-resolution labels by primarily utilizing low-resolution training data, generally augmented with sparse high-resolution training data [153]. Generating training data in these approaches involves a combination of labeling patches to indicate density of different cells in each patch that is supplemented with dot annotation.

The emergence of mIHC and mIF and their natural combination with digital pathology and deep learning methods for quantitative IHC interpretation has the potential to address the challenges that can enable this kind of rich information from multiple biomarkers to become routinely used to provide clinically useful prognostic and predictive information [29–31,42,136,142,148]. There appears to be much less doubt and increasing excitement about methods that interrogate and quantify the nature of the interactions among the different types of immune cells in the TME to provide useful prognostic information by identifying key immunoregulatory cells. The potential of identifying clinically actionable insights from using mIHC and artificial intelligence to stratify patients for targeted immunotherapy in the neoadjuvant and adjuvant settings are too important to ignore [42,130]. Thus, development of new methods are absolutely necessary if mIHC and mIF are clinically adopted. If, and when, these methods become full-fledged methods to enable clinical decision support to guide treatment and provide prognostic information, rigorous evaluation, testing, and validation will be undoubtedly required. Since several commercially available mIF and mIHC methods have emerged recently, the future appears very bright for the incorporation of these methods into mainstream translational cancer research.

Vendor platforms

Deep learning algorithms have also found their way into commercial platforms. Commercial software for analysis of the immune infiltrates include the Genie Spectrum (Aperio ePathology Solutions, Vista, CA) [154,155], Image-Pro Plus 3.0 (Media Cybernetics, Silver Spring, MD) [156], Halo (Indica Labs, Corrales, NM) [151], ImageJ [157], VMscope (VMscope GmbH, Berlin, Germany) slide explorer [2], Vectra/inForm (PerkinElmer, Waltham, MA, USA) [158], SlidePath (Leica Biosystems, Wetzlar, Germany) [159], Tissue Studio (Definiens, Munich, Germany) [146], Author AI (Visiopharm Corporation, Westminster, CO, USA), and many others. A commercially available image analysis software platform, Web-Microscope, has also been utilized to (1) identify tissue regions containing TILs and (2) count the number of lymphocytes in each region [160], where the authors observed that TIL density in seminomas had prognostic relevance regarding disease relapse. PaigeAI and PathAI are also examples of companies that advertise the ability to carry out combinations of region characterization and cell identification in H&E WSIs as part of their respective efforts to develop deep learning applications to deliver more accurate diagnosis.

Conclusion

Artificial intelligence is rapidly assuming a crucial role in the elucidation and characterization of tumor immune interactions. Deep learning driven computational algorithms that support the construction of detailed spatial maps appear to be a relatively straightforward way to characterize general tumor immune interactions in the tumor microenvironment, which may be very helpful to predict treatment response and clinical outcomes. Thus, the utilization of advanced digital pathology and deep learning applications will likely grow very quickly over the next few years. This chapter has focused primarily on describing methods behind rapid advances in our ability to generate cancer immune maps and emerging methods that can be used in combination to provide many different types of potentially useful information to deliver precision medicine. Currently, the interpretation of cancer immune dynamics with the complex TME is challenging, but disease site-specific correlations between predictions with digital pathology and deep learning methods, quantitative analyses of mIHC and mIF, clinical outcomes, and treatment response are being actively studied to discover biomarkers and elcuidate complex relationships between tumors and immunity in order to help advance our ability to treat cancer. Even though mapping patient-specific tumor-immune interactions are still at an early stage, the crucial next phase of research regarding the quantitative analysis of spatial morphologic and molecular patterns emerging from these methods is beyond fascinating and hopefully clinically applicable. Last but not least, the power of the digital pathology and deep learning methods also lies in the ability to perform these computational analyses of WSIs across thousands to hundreds of thousands of cases in parallel without the need for additional tissue, time, or resources. It is also quite conceivable that analyses of mIF and mIHC in small subsets of site-specific diseases can be used to identify generalizable relationships that can be correlated with more high-throughput standard Pathomics analyses in H&E WSIs in much larger collections in order to gain further insight into tumor biology. Hopefully, these developments can lead to workflows that can be implemented in pathology laboratories as practical clinical decision support tools for routine diagnostic surgical pathology. Thus, we hope the end of this chapter serves as a beginning to help imagine a future where WSIs of incoming tissue samples are analyzed with automated algorithms that perform diagnostic screening, quantify the expression of biomarkers in mIHC panels, provide prognostic information, help identify therapeutic targets, and predict treatment response.

References

[1] Denkert C, et al. Tumor-associated lymphocytes as an independent predictor of response to neoadjuvant chemotherapy in breast cancer. Journal of Clinical Oncology 2010;28(1):105−13.

[2] Denkert C, et al. Standardized evaluation of tumor-infiltrating lymphocytes in breast cancer: results of the ring studies of the international immuno-oncology biomarker working group. Modern Pathology 2016;29(10):1155−64.

[3] Hendry S, et al. Assessing tumor-infiltrating lymphocytes in solid tumors: a practical review for pathologists and proposal for a standardized method from the international immuno-oncology biomarkers working group: Part 2: TILs in melanoma, gastrointestinal tract carcinomas, non-small cell lung carcinoma and mesothelioma, endometrial and ovarian carcinomas, squamous cell carcinoma of the head and neck, genitourinary carcinomas, and primary brain tumors. Advances in Anatomic Pathology 2017;24(6): 311−35.

[4] Salgado R, et al. The evaluation of tumor-infiltrating lymphocytes (TILs) in breast cancer: recommendations by an International TILs Working Group 2014. Annals of Oncology 2015;26(2):259−71.

[5] Gurcan MN, et al. Histopathological image analysis: a review. IEEE Reviews in Biomedical Engineering 2009;2:147.

[6] Irshad H, et al. Methods for nuclei detection, segmentation, and classification in digital histopathology: a review—current status and future potential. IEEE Reviews in Biomedical Engineering 2014;7.

[7] Kothari S, et al. Pathology imaging informatics for quantitative analysis of whole-slide images. Journal of the American Medical Informatics Association: JAMIA 2013; 20(6):1099−108.

[8] Madabhushi A, Lee G. Image analysis and machine learning in digital pathology: challenges and opportunities. Medical Image Analysis 2016;33:170−5.

[9] Xing F, Yang L. Robust nucleus/cell detection and segmentation in digital pathology and microscopy images: a comprehensive review. IEEE Reviews in Biomedical Engineering 2016;9:234−63.

[10] Amgad M, et al. Structured crowdsourcing enables convolutional segmentation of histology images. Bioinformatics 2019;35.

[11] Amgad M, et al. Joint region and nucleus segmentation for characterization of tumor infiltrating lymphocytes in breast cancer. In: Medical imaging 2019: digital pathology. International Society for Optics and Photonics; 2019.

[12] Cooper L, et al. Feature-based registration of histopathology images with different stains: an application for computerized follicular lymphoma prognosis. Computer Methods and Programs in Biomedicine 2009;96(3):182−92.

[13] Cooper LA, et al. PanCancer insights from the Cancer Genome Atlas: the pathologist's perspective. The Journal of Pathology 2018;244(5):512−24.

[14] Cooper LA, et al. The tumor microenvironment strongly impacts master transcriptional regulators and gene expression class of glioblastoma. American Journal Of Pathology 2012;180(5):2108−19.

[15] Cooper LA, et al. Integrated morphologic analysis for the identification and characterization of disease subtypes. Journal of the American Medical Informatics Association 2012;19(2):317−23.

[16] Cooper LA, et al. Morphological signatures and genomic correlates in glioblastoma. IEEE International Symposium on Biomedical Imaging 2011:1624−7.

[17] Gajewski TF, Schreiber H, Fu YX. Innate and adaptive immune cells in the tumor microenvironment. Nature Immunology 2013;14(10):1014−22.

[18] Gurcan MN, et al. Developing the Quantitative Histopathology Image Ontology (QHIO): a case study using the hot spot detection problem. Journal of Biomedical Informatics 2017;66:129–35.

[19] Janowczyk A, et al. High-throughput biomarker segmentation on ovarian cancer tissue microarrays via hierarchical normalized cuts. IEEE Transactions on Biomedical Engineering 2012;59(5):1240–52.

[20] Janowczyk A, et al. A resolution adaptive deep hierarchical (RADHicaL) learning scheme applied to nuclear segmentation of digital pathology images. Computer Methods in Biomechanics and Biomedical Engineering: Imaging and Visualization 2018;6(3):270–6.

[21] Janowczyk A, Madabhushi A. Deep learning for digital pathology image analysis: a comprehensive tutorial with selected use cases. Journal of Pathology Informatics 2016;7.

[22] Kumar A, et al. Automated analysis of immunohistochemistry images identifies candidate location biomarkers for cancers. Proceedings of the National Academy of Sciences 2014;111(51):18249–54.

[23] Kumar H, Kawai T, Akira S. Pathogen recognition by the innate immune system. International Reviews of Immunology 2011;30(1):16–34.

[24] Madabhushi A, et al. Computer-aided prognosis: predicting patient and disease outcome via quantitative fusion of multi-scale, multi-modal data. Computerized Medical Imaging and Graphics 2011;35(7–8):506–14.

[25] Netea MG, et al. Trained immunity: a program of innate immune memory in health and disease. Science 2016;352(6284):aaf1098.

[26] Nordstrom RJ. The quantitative imaging network in precision medicine. Tomography: A Journal for Imaging Research 2016;2(4):239–41.

[27] Norton K-A, et al. Multiscale agent-based and hybrid modeling of the tumor immune microenvironment. Processes (Basel, Switzerland) 2019;7(1):37.

[28] Bindea G, et al. Natural immunity to cancer in humans. Current Opinion in Immunology 2010;22(2):215–22.

[29] Bindea G, et al. Spatiotemporal dynamics of intratumoral immune cells reveal the immune landscape in human cancer. Immunity 2013;39(4):782–95.

[30] Farkona S, Diamandis EP, Blasutig IM. Cancer immunotherapy: the beginning of the end of cancer? BMC Medicine 2016;14:73.

[31] Fridman WH, et al. The immune contexture in human tumours: impact on clinical outcome. Nature Reviews Cancer 2012;12(4):298–306.

[32] Galon J, et al. The continuum of cancer immunosurveillance: prognostic, predictive, and mechanistic signatures. Immunity 2013;39(1):11–26.

[33] Galon J, et al. Type, density, and location of immune cells within human colorectal tumors predict clinical outcome. Science 2006;313(5795):1960–4.

[34] Galon J, et al. Towards the introduction of the 'Immunoscore' in the classification of malignant tumours. The Journal of Pathology 2014;232(2):199–209.

[35] Galon J, et al. Cancer classification using the Immunoscore: a worldwide task force. Journal of Translational Medicine 2012;10:205.

[36] Kalra J, Baker J. Multiplex immunohistochemistry for mapping the tumor microenvironment. In: Kalyuzhny AE, editor. Signal transduction immunohistochemistry: methods and protocols. New York, NY: Springer New York; 2017. p. 237–51.

[37] Sharma P, Allison JP. Immune checkpoint targeting in cancer therapy: toward combination strategies with curative potential. Cell 2015;161(2):205–14.

[38] Sharma P, et al. Novel cancer immunotherapy agents with survival benefit: recent successes and next steps. Nature Reviews Cancer 2011;11(11):805–12.

[39] Wolchok JD, et al. Nivolumab plus ipilimumab in advanced melanoma. New England Journal of Medicine 2013;369(2):122–33.

[40] Saltz J, et al. Towards generation, management, and exploration of combined radiomics and Pathomics datasets for cancer research. AMIA Joint Summits on Translational Science Proceedings 2017;2017:85–94.

[41] Saltz J, et al. Spatial organization and molecular correlation of tumor-infiltrating lymphocytes using deep learning on pathology images. Cell Reports 2018;23(1):181.

[42] Koelzer VH, et al. Precision immunoprofiling by image analysis and artificial intelligence. Virchows Archiv 2019;474(4):511–22.

[43] Thorsson V, et al. The immune landscape of cancer. Immunity 2018;48(4):812.

[44] Calì B, Molon B, Viola A. Tuning cancer fate: the unremitting role of host immunity. Open Biology 2017;7(4):170006.

[45] Aras S, Zaidi MR. TAMeless traitors: macrophages in cancer progression and metastasis. British Journal of Cancer 2017;117:1583.

[46] Dykes SS, et al. Stromal cells in breast cancer as a potential therapeutic target. Oncotarget 2018;9(34):23761–79.

[47] Choi J, et al. Diagnostic value of peripheral blood immune profiling in colorectal cancer. Annals of Surgical Treatment and Research 2018;94(6):312–21.

[48] Lepone LM, et al. Analyses of 123 peripheral human immune cell subsets: defining differences with age and between healthy donors and cancer patients not detected in analysis of standard immune cell types. Journal of Circulating Biomarkers 2016;5:5.

[49] Loi S, et al. Tumor-infiltrating lymphocytes and prognosis: a pooled individual patient Analysis of early-stage triple-negative breast cancers. Journal of Clinical Oncology 2019;37(7):559–69.

[50] Ogino S, et al. Integrative analysis of exogenous, endogenous, tumour and immune factors for precision medicine. Gut 2018;67(6):1168–80.

[51] Drake CG, Jaffee E, Pardoll DM. Mechanisms of immune evasion by tumors. Advances in Immunology 2006;90:51–81.

[52] Finn OJ. Immuno-oncology: understanding the function and dysfunction of the immune system in cancer. Annals of Oncology: Official Journal of the European Society for Medical Oncology 2012;23(Suppl. 8):viii6–9.

[53] Hanahan D, Weinberg RA. Hallmarks of cancer: the next generation. Cell 2011;144(5):646–74.

[54] Diaz-Cano SJ. General morphological and biological features of neoplasms: integration of molecular findings. Histopathology 2008;53(1):1–19.

[55] Parish CR. Cancer immunotherapy: the past, the present and the future. Immunology and Cell Biology 2003;81(2):106–13.

[56] Burnet M. Cancer; a biological approach. I. The processes of control. British Medical Journal 1957;1(5022):779–86.

[57] Burnet FM. The concept of immunological surveillance. Progress in Experimental Tumor Research 1970;13:1–27.

[58] Thomas L. On immunosurveillance in human cancer. Yale J Biol Med 1982;55(3–4):329–33.

[59] Bonnans C, Chou J, Werb Z. Remodelling the extracellular matrix in development and disease. Nature Reviews Molecular Cell Biology 2014;15(12):786–801.

[60] Kaczorowski KJ, et al. Continuous immunotypes describe human immune variation and predict diverse responses. Proceedings of the National Academy of Sciences of the United States of America 2017;114(30):E6097—e6106.

[61] Li B, et al. Comprehensive analyses of tumor immunity: implications for cancer immunotherapy. Genome Biology 2016;17(1):174.

[62] Maecker HT, McCoy JP, Nussenblatt R. Standardizing immunophenotyping for the human Immunology project. Nature Reviews Immunology 2012;12(3):191—200.

[63] Mellman I, Coukos G, Dranoff G. Cancer immunotherapy comes of age. Nature 2011; 480(7378):480—9.

[64] Ribas A. Releasing the brakes on cancer immunotherapy. New England Journal of Medicine 2015;373(16):1490—2.

[65] Seager RJ, et al. Dynamic interplay between tumour, stroma and immune system can drive or prevent tumour progression. Convergent Science Physical Oncology 2017;3: 034002.

[66] Smyth MJ, et al. Combination cancer immunotherapies tailored to the tumour microenvironment. Nature Reviews Clinical Oncology 2016;13(3):143—58.

[67] Curran MA, et al. PD-1 and CTLA-4 combination blockade expands infiltrating T cells and reduces regulatory T and myeloid cells within B16 melanoma tumors. Proceedings of the National Academy of Sciences of the United States of America 2010;107(9): 4275—80.

[68] Grosso JF, Jure-Kunkel MN. CTLA-4 blockade in tumor models: an overview of preclinical and translational research. Cancer Immunity 2013;13:5.

[69] Hodi FS, et al. Improved survival with ipilimumab in patients with metastatic melanoma. New England Journal of Medicine 2010;363(8):711—23.

[70] Patel SP, Kurzrock R. PD-L1 expression as a predictive biomarker in cancer immunotherapy. Molecular Cancer Therapeutics 2015;14(4):847—56.

[71] Topalian SL, et al. Survival, durable tumor remission, and long-term safety in patients with advanced melanoma receiving nivolumab. Journal of Clinical Oncology 2014; 32(10):1020—30.

[72] Carbognin L, et al. Differential activity of nivolumab, Pembrolizumab and MPDL3280A according to the tumor expression of programmed death-ligand-1 (PD-L1): sensitivity analysis of trials in melanoma, lung and genitourinary cancers. PloS One 2015;10(6):e0130142.

[73] Parry RV, et al. CTLA-4 and PD-1 receptors inhibit T-cell activation by distinct mechanisms. Molecular and Cellular Biology 2005;25(21):9543—53.

[74] Robert C, et al. Ipilimumab plus dacarbazine for previously untreated metastatic melanoma. New England Journal of Medicine 2011;364(26):2517—26.

[75] Spill F, et al. Impact of the physical microenvironment on tumor progression and metastasis. Current Opinion in Biotechnology 2016;40:41—8.

[76] Versteven M, et al. A versatile T cell-based assay to assess therapeutic antigen-specific PD-1-targeted approaches. Oncotarget 2018;9(45):27797—808.

[77] Brahmer JR, et al. Safety and activity of anti-PD-L1 antibody in patients with advanced cancer. New England Journal of Medicine 2012;366(26):2455—65.

[78] Keir ME, et al. PD-1 and its ligands in tolerance and immunity. Annual Review of Immunology 2008;26(1):677—704.

[79] Passiglia F, et al. PD-L1 expression as predictive biomarker in patients with NSCLC: a pooled analysis. Oncotarget 2016;7(15):19738—47.

[80] Roma-Rodrigues C, et al. Targeting tumor microenvironment for cancer therapy. International Journal of Molecular Sciences 2019;20(4):840.

[81] Topalian SL, et al. Safety, activity, and immune correlates of anti-PD-1 antibody in cancer. New England Journal of Medicine 2012;366(26):2443−54.

[82] Ung C, Kockx M, Waumans Y. Digital pathology in immuno-oncology − a roadmap for clinical development. Expert Review of Precision Medicine and Drug Development 2017;2(1):9−19.

[83] Cooper WA, et al. Intra- and interobserver reproducibility assessment of PD-L1 biomarker in non-small cell lung cancer. Clinical Cancer Research 2017;23(16): 4569−77.

[84] Troncone G, Gridelli C. The reproducibility of PD-L1 scoring in lung cancer: can the pathologists do better? Translational Lung Cancer Research 2017;6(Suppl. 1): S74−s77.

[85] Hendry S, et al. Assessing tumor-infiltrating lymphocytes in solid tumors: a practical review for pathologists and proposal for a standardized method from the international immunooncology biomarkers working group: Part 1: assessing the host immune response, TILs in invasive breast carcinoma and ductal carcinoma in situ, metastatic tumor deposits and areas for further research. Advances in Anatomic Pathology 2017;24(5):235−51.

[86] Mascaux C, et al. Immune evasion before tumour invasion in early lung squamous carcinogenesis. Nature 2019;571(7766):570−5.

[87] Coulie PG, et al. Tumour antigens recognized by T lymphocytes: at the core of cancer immunotherapy. Nature Reviews Cancer 2014;14(2):135−46.

[88] Donnem T, et al. Strategies for clinical implementation of TNM-Immunoscore in resected nonsmall-cell lung cancer. Annals of Oncology 2016;27(2):225−32.

[89] Mlecnik B, et al. Tumor immunosurveillance in human cancers. Cancer and Metastasis Reviews 2011;30(1):5−12.

[90] Angell H, Galon J. From the immune contexture to the Immunoscore: the role of prognostic and predictive immune markers in cancer. Current Opinion in Immunology 2013;25(2):261−7.

[91] Broussard EK, Disis ML. TNM staging in colorectal cancer: T is for T cell and M is for memory. Journal of Clinical Oncology 2011;29(6):601−3.

[92] Mlecnik B, et al. Histopathologic-based prognostic factors of colorectal cancers are associated with the state of the local immune reaction. Journal of Clinical Oncology 2011;29(6):610−8.

[93] Savas P, et al. Clinical relevance of host immunity in breast cancer: from TILs to the clinic. Nature Reviews Clinical Oncology 2016;13(4):228.

[94] Gu J, Wang Z, et al. Recent advances in convolutional neural networks. Pattern Recognition 2018;77:354−77.

[95] Dai Y, Wang G. A deep inference learning framework for healthcare. Pattern Recognition Letters 2018;103.

[96] Xing F, et al. Deep learning in microscopy image analysis: a survey. IEEE Transactions on Neural Networks and Learning Systems 2017:1−19.

[97] Suzuki K, Zhou L, Wang Q. Machine learning in medical imaging. Pattern Recognition 2017;63:465−7.

[98] Kokkinos I. UberNet: training a universal convolutional neural network for low-, mid-, and high-level vision using diverse datasets and limited memory. 2017. p. 6129−38.

[99] Khatami M, et al. BundleMAP: anatomically localized classification, regression, and hypothesis testing in diffusion MRI. Pattern Recognition 2017;63:593—600.

[100] Chen H, et al. DCAN: deep contour-aware networks for object instance segmentation from histology images. Medical Image Analysis 2017;36:135—46.

[101] Radford A, Metz L, Chintala S. Unsupervised representation learning with deep convolutional generative adversarial networks. 2016.

[102] Graham B. Spatially-sparse convolutional neural networks. 2014. p. 1—13. arXiv preprint arXiv:1409.6070.

[103] Hou L, et al. Patch-based convolutional neural network for whole slide tissue image classification. Proceedings of the IEEE Conference on Computer Vision and Pattern Recognition (CVPR) 2016:2424—33.

[104] Murthy V, et al. Center-focusing multi-task CNN with injected features for classification of glioma nuclear images. IEEE Winter Conference on Applications of Computer Vision (WACV) 2017:834—41.

[105] Hou L, et al. Sparse autoencoder for unsupervised nucleus detection and representation in histopathology images. Pattern Recognition 2019;86:188—200.

[106] Schmidhuber Jr. Deep learning in neural networks: an overview. Neural Networks 2015;61:85—117.

[107] Russakovsky O, et al. Imagenet large scale visual recognition challenge. International Journal of Computer Vision 2015;115(3):211—52.

[108] Ronneberger O, Fischer P, Brox T. U-net: convolutional networks for biomedical image segmentation. In: International conference on medical image computing and computer-assisted intervention; 2015. p. 234—41.

[109] Makhzani A, Frey B. k-Sparse Autoencoders. In: International conference on learning representations (ICLR); 2014 (available as arXiv preprint arXiv:1312.5663).

[110] Ng A. Sparse autoencoder. In: CS294A Lecture notes 72. Stanford University; 2011. p. 1—19.

[111] Basavanhally AN, et al. Computerized image-based detection and grading of lymphocytic infiltration in HER2+ breast cancer histopathology. IEEE Transactions on Biomedical Engineering 2009;57(3):642—53.

[112] Panagiotakis C, Ramasso E, Tziritas G. Lymphocyte segmentation using the transferable belief model. In: International conference on pattern recognition. Springer; 2010.

[113] Yuan Y, et al. Quantitative image analysis of cellular heterogeneity in breast tumors complements genomic profiling. Science Translational Medicine 2012;4(157): 157ra143.

[114] Sirinukunwattana K, et al. Locality sensitive deep learning for detection and classification of nuclei in routine colon cancer histology images. Medical Imaging 2016;35: 1196—206.

[115] Zhou Y, et al. Nuclei segmentation via sparsity constrained convolutional regression. In: 2015 IEEE 12th international symposium on biomedical imaging (ISBI). IEEE; 2015.

[116] Xu J, et al. Stacked sparse autoencoder (SSAE) for nuclei detection on breast cancer histopathology images. IEEE Transactions on Medical Imaging 2015;35(1):119—30.

[117] Vu QD, et al. Methods for segmentation and classification of digital microscopy tissue images. Frontiers in Bioengineering and Biotechnology 2019;7.

[118] Goodfellow I, et al. Generative adversarial nets. In: Advances in neural information processing systems; 2014.

[119] Mahmood F, et al. Deep adversarial training for multi-organ nuclei segmentation in histopathology images. 2018.

[120] Hou L, et al. Robust histopathology image analysis: to label or to synthesize? Proceedings of the IEEE Conference on Computer Vision and Pattern Recognition 2019:8533—42.

[121] Foran DJ, et al. Computer-assisted discrimination among malignant lymphomas and leukemia using immunophenotyping, intelligent image repositories, and telemicroscopy. IEEE Transactions on Information Technology in Biomedicine 2000;4(4):265—73.

[122] Sertel O, et al. Histopathological image analysis using model-based intermediate representations and color texture: follicular lymphoma grading. Journal of Signal Processing Systems 2009;55(1—3):169.

[123] Corredor G, et al. Spatial architecture and arrangement of tumor-infiltrating lymphocytes for predicting likelihood of recurrence in early-stage non—small cell lung cancer. Clinical Cancer Research 2019;25(5):1526—34.

[124] Heindl A, et al. Relevance of spatial heterogeneity of immune infiltration for predicting risk of recurrence after endocrine therapy of ER+ breast cancer. Journal of the National Cancer Institute 2017;110(2):166—75.

[125] Abousamra S, et al. Learning from thresholds: fully automated classification of tumor infiltrating lymphocytes for multiple cancer types. arXiv e-prints; 2019.

[126] Le H, et al. Utilizing automated breast cancer detection to identify spatial distributions of tumor infiltrating lymphocytes in invasive breast cancer. arXiv e-prints; 2019.

[127] Bonaventura P, et al. Cold tumors: a therapeutic challenge for immunotherapy. Frontiers in Immunology 2019;10(168).

[128] Tumor-TIL maps for TCGA Breast WSIs. Available from: https://mathbiol.github.io/tcgatil/. [Accessed 12 July 2019].

[129] Le H, et al. Pancreatic cancer detection in whole slide images using noisy label annotations. In: Medical image computing and computer assisted intervention — MICCAI. Shenzhen, China: Springer International Publishing; 2019.

[130] Blank CU, et al. Cancer immunology. The "cancer immunogram". Science 2016; 352(6286):658—60.

[131] Barua S, et al. Spatial interaction of tumor cells and regulatory T cells correlates with survival in non-small cell lung cancer. Lung Cancer 2018;117:73—9.

[132] Ma Z, et al. Data integration from pathology slides for quantitative imaging of multiple cell types within the tumor immune cell infiltrate. Diagnostic Pathology 2017;12(1): 69.

[133] Hofman P, et al. Multiplexed immunohistochemistry for molecular and immune profiling in lung cancer-just about ready for prime-time? Cancers 2019;11(3):283.

[134] Levenson RM, Borowsky AD, Angelo M. Immunohistochemistry and mass spectrometry for highly multiplexed cellular molecular imaging. Laboratory Investigation 2015; 95(4):397—405.

[135] Parra ER, Francisco-Cruz A, Wistuba II. State-of-the-Art of profiling immune contexture in the era of multiplexed staining and digital analysis to study paraffin tumor tissues. Cancers (Basel) 2019;11(2).

[136] Blom S, et al. Systems pathology by multiplexed immunohistochemistry and whole-slide digital image analysis. Scientific Reports 2017;7(1):15580.

[137] Gorris MAJ, et al. Eight-color multiplex immunohistochemistry for simultaneous detection of multiple immune checkpoint molecules within the tumor microenvironment. The Journal of Immunology 2018;200(1):347—54.

[138] Ilie M, et al. Automated chromogenic multiplexed immunohistochemistry assay for diagnosis and predictive biomarker testing in non-small cell lung cancer. Lung Cancer 2018;124:90—4.

[139] Remark R, et al. In-depth tissue profiling using multiplexed immunohistochemical consecutive staining on single slide. Science Immunology 2016;1(1):aaf6925.

[140] Tsujikawa T, et al. Quantitative multiplex immunohistochemistry reveals myeloid-inflamed tumor-immune complexity associated with poor prognosis. Cell Reports 2017;19(1):203—17.

[141] Gibney GT, Weiner LM, Atkins MB. Predictive biomarkers for checkpoint inhibitor-based immunotherapy. The Lancet Oncology 2016;17(12):e542—51.

[142] Seyed Jafari SM, Hunger RE. IHC optical density score: a new practical method for quantitative immunohistochemistry image analysis. Applied Immunohistochemistry and Molecular Morphology 2017;25(1):e12—3.

[143] Farris AB, et al. Whole slide imaging for analytical anatomic pathology and telepathology: practical applications today, promises, and perils. Archives of Pathology and Laboratory Medicine 2017;141(4):542—50.

[144] Aeffner F, et al. Digital microscopy, image analysis, and virtual slide repository. Institute for Laboratory Animal Research (ILAR) 2018;59(1):66—79.

[145] Koh J, et al. High-Throughput multiplex immunohistochemical imaging of the tumor and its microenvironment. Journal of the Korean Cancer Association 2019;52(1):98—108.

[146] Steele KE, et al. Measuring multiple parameters of CD8+ tumor-infiltrating lymphocytes in human cancers by image analysis. Journal for ImmunoTherapy of Cancer 2018;6(1):20.

[147] Chen T, Srinivas C. Group sparsity model for stain unmixing in brightfield multiplex immunohistochemistry images. Computerized Medical Imaging and Graphics 2015; 46(Pt 1):30—9.

[148] Parra ER, et al. Image analysis-based assessment of PD-L1 and tumor-associated immune cells density supports distinct intratumoral microenvironment groups in non-small cell lung carcinoma patients. Clinical Cancer Research 2016;22(24):6278—89.

[149] Ruifrok AC, Johnston DA. Quantification of histochemical staining by color deconvolution. Analytical and Quantitative Cytology and Histology 2001;23(4):291—9.

[150] Halse H, et al. Multiplex immunohistochemistry accurately defines the immune context of metastatic melanoma. Scientific Reports 2018;8(1):11158.

[151] Tumeh PC, et al. PD-1 blockade induces responses by inhibiting adaptive immune resistance. Nature 2014;515(7528):568—71.

[152] . Hagos YB, et al. ConCORDe-net: cell count regularized convolutional neural network for cell detection in multiplex immunohistochemistry images.

[153] Malkin K, et al. Label super-resolution networks. 2018.

[154] Angell HK, et al. Digital pattern recognition-based image analysis quantifies immune infiltrates in distinct tissue regions of colorectal cancer and identifies a metastatic phenotype. British Journal of Cancer 2013;109(6):1618—24.

[155] Degnim AC, et al. Immune cell quantitation in normal breast tissue lobules with and without lobulitis. Breast Cancer Research and Treatment 2014;144(3):539—49.

[156] Johansson AC, et al. Computerized image analysis as a tool to quantify infiltrating leukocytes: a comparison between high- and low-magnification images. Journal of Histochemistry and Cytochemistry 2001;49(9):1073—9.

[157]   Lopez C, et al. Development of automated quantification methodologies of immuno-histochemical markers to determine patterns of immune response in breast cancer: a retrospective cohort study. BMJ Open 2014;4(8):e005643.

[158]   Huang W, Hennrick K, Drew S. A colorful future of quantitative pathology: validation of Vectra technology using chromogenic multiplexed immunohistochemistry and prostate tissue microarrays. Human Pathology 2013;44(1):29–38.

[159]   Ribas A, et al. Oncolytic virotherapy promotes intratumoral T cell infiltration and improves anti-PD-1 immunotherapy. Cell 2017;170(6). 1109–1119.e10.

[160]   Linder N, et al. Deep learning for detecting tumour-infiltrating lymphocytes in testicular germ cell tumours. Journal of Clinical Pathology 2019;72(2):157–64.

CHAPTER

Overview of the role of artificial intelligence in pathology: the computer as a pathology digital assistant

11

John E. Tomaszewski, MD

SUNY Distinguished Professor and Chair, Pathology and Anatomical Sciences, University at Buffalo, State University of New York, Buffalo, NY, United States

Introduction

As this chapter goes to press, two great waves of change are sweeping through the science and the practice of medicine. These are the molecular revolution and computational analytics. These two scientific movements are radically altering the ways in which we approach all aspects of human biology. Previous chapters have discussed machine learning strategies in detail, with an emphasis on deep learning via various kinds of neural networks, ranging from basic convolutional models to advanced architectures such as graphic and capsule networks. In this chapter, I will describe the overall framework in which digital and computational pathologies are embedded, summarize these various strategies, and provide examples from the literature that illustrates many of the topics covered. This overview is designed to show how pathology is evolving and will continue to evolve in the age of artificial intelligence (AI). One major thesis is that human pathologists will not be replaced by computers. Instead, the computer will serve as a highly capable "digital assistant," and this synergistic pairing of human intelligence (HI) and AI will ensure that pathology will be a major driver of personalized medicine.

Computational pathology: background and philosophy
The current state of diagnostics in pathology and the evolving computational opportunities: "why now?"

Diagnostic pathology in the early 21st century is still very much an analog enterprise which uses a work process that was developed in the early 20th century and which has been substantially carried forward into the early 21st century. The processes of chemically treating and processing tissue, microtomy, staining, and the creation of

Artificial Intelligence and Deep Learning in Pathology. https://doi.org/10.1016/B978-0-323-67538-3.00011-7

glass slides which are viewable with a wide-field optical instrument (the micro-scope) are essentially the same processes established by early surgical pathologists. The data obtained from these processes yield continuous variables which a human pathologist diagnostician uses to drive classification systems. The output of these classifiers is in turn used by clinicians to support therapeutic decisions. This analog process is cost-effective in that it yields core actionable information in many cases and consumes only a very small fraction of total healthcare costs. These processes, however, have been fundamentally the same for 100 years and are not adapted to the rapidly changing diagnostic environment. There is a growing need for precision diagnostics. High-cost, high-risk therapeutic interventions require diagnostic and theranostic systems which model the most effective therapeutic choices with a high degree of precision and accuracy. The efficiency of the diagnostic/theranostic system has a direct and major impact on the global cost-effectiveness of the entire clinical care system.

Several new opportunities are now converging to make precision diagnostics a 21st century reality. Big data is becoming available in multiple modes. The molec-ular revolution which entered the practice of pathology and laboratory medicine in the 1980s is now becoming routinely available. Genomics, epigenomics, transcrip-tomics, proteomics, metabolomics, and microbiomics all offer digital "multi-omic" big data opportunities in research and practice [1]. Likewise, the extension of the electronic medical record to all aspects of medical practice through the US federal "meaningful use" programs in health information technology has opened digital access to the big data of the clinical record through synoptic reporting and natural language processing. Whole slide images of tissue sections are typically multigiga-pixel in size and as such are a third modal window providing digital access to the big data of complex medical conditions. In tissue-based diagnostics, advances in whole slide imaging (WSI) technology are poised to cross the threshold from purely edu-cation and research use to diagnostics. The recent FDA approval of WSI systems opens up enormous opportunities for computer-aided pathological diagnosis. WSI and image analytics are poised to become mainstream methods of histopathological interpretation yielding faster, more accurate, and cheaper diagnoses, prognoses, and theranostic predictions of important diseases including cancer.

Access to high-performance computing in the medical field has also dramatically increased over the past decade. Graphical processing units and tensor processing units are now available in medical settings. Computing jobs which would previously take days or even weeks to perform in a research setting are now available through cloud computing or even at the desktop. Storage costs have seen dramatic reductions over the past 5 years.

Most importantly, our approaches to and understanding of machine learning have made a dramatic turn since 2012 when AlexNet won the ImageNet Large Scale Visual Recognition Challenge by a large margin using a convolutional neural network (CNN) [2]. With the resurgence of interest in and the success of modern neural networks and data-driven deep learning approaches, the current decade has seen a dramatic acceleration in our opportunities to learn from massive quantities of data with limited labels. The analytics which can be applied is now beginning to match the big data of biology and medicine.

Digital pathology versus computational pathology

It is important to distinguish between the terms *digital pathology* and *computational pathology.*

Digital pathology is best understood as the digital workflow tools which are more focused on the front end of the process. Digital pathology is a dynamic, image-based environment that enables the acquisition, management, and interpretation of pathology information generated from a digitized glass slide. Healthcare applications include primary diagnosis, diagnostic consultation, intraoperative diagnosis, medical student and resident training, manual and semiquantitative review of immunohistochemistry (IHC), clinical research, diagnostic decision support, peer review, and tumor boards. Digital pathology is an innovation committed to the reduction of laboratory expenses, an improvement of operational efficiency, enhanced productivity, and improving treatment decisions and patient care.

Broadly written, the approaches to the computational modeling of complex systems of human disease from big data are termed "*computational pathology.*" In 2011, Fuchs and Buhmann [3] opined that "Computational Pathology investigates a complete probabilistic treatment of scientific and clinical workflows in general pathology, i.e., it combines experimental design, statistical pattern recognition, and survival analysis within a unified framework to answer scientific and clinical questions in pathology." Computational pathology focuses on the analytics of extracting data from the output of sensors and turning those data into information and knowledge. This might include both prognostics and outcome prediction or simply a quantitative cataloging of tissue morphologies represented by computation.

Data on scale

The scientific understanding of human structure has stagnated as a largely descriptive endeavor for many decades. Structural science learning related to cells, organelles, and tissues is central to the disciplines of cell biology and pathology. With the advent of machine vision and machine learning, major advances in computing and network power, and the rapid evolution of advanced biophysical systems for cellular imaging, these disciplines are poised to embrace a quantitative paradigm for their work. The data embedded in a cellular or tissue image are deep and full of complex relationships. Thousands of image metrics derived by machine vision can be captured from a field of view and used in the modeling of complex biological or disease system outcomes. Computational advances now offer the promise of enabling the quantitative analysis of human structural data.

Biological data lives on scale. Modern imaging, image analytics, and computational methods provide tools with which to quantitatively mine the data within macroscopic (10^1), microscopic (10^{-7}), and submicroscopic (10^{-10}) images. The ability to mine "subvisual" image features from digital pathology images using machine vision can develop feature data which may not be visually discernible by a pathologist.

There has also been recent substantial interest in combining and fusing radiologic imaging, and proteomics and genomics-based measurements with features extracted from digital pathology images for better prognostic prediction of disease aggressiveness and patient outcome. *Data fusion* is accomplished by computationally combining image data at these levels of scale with data from other modes of examination such as cell and molecular biological, biomechanical, and biophysical analyses. Data fusion offers the opportunity to quantitatively model complex human systems from massive multivariable statements.

We assert that *in the future, medical decision-making will rely on large datasets, collected across scale from molecular and imaging analyses, integrated by machine vision and machine learning, and that these integrated data will be used to model complex biological and disease systems. These complex computationally supported systems of data collection, integration, and modeling will be vetted by teams of humans with domain knowledge expertise.*

Machine learning tools in computational pathology: types of artificial intelligence

AI is not really a new concept. The term AI was first used by John McCarthy in 1955 [4]. He subsequently organized the Dartmouth conference in 1956 which started AI as a field. The label "AI" means very different things to different observers. For example, some commenters recognize divisions of AI as "statistical modeling" (calculating regression models and histograms) versus machine learning (Bayes, random forests, support vector machines [SVMs], shallow neural networks, or artificial neural network) versus deep learning (deep neural networks and CNNs). Others recognize categories of *traditional AI* versus *data-driven deep learning AI*. In this comparison, *traditional AI* starts with a human understanding of a domain and seeks to condition that knowledge into models which represent the world of that knowledge domain. When current lay commentators refer to "AI," however, they are usually referring to *data-driven deep learning AI*, which removes the domain knowledge inspired feature extraction part from the pipeline and develops knowledge of a domain by observing large numbers of examples from that domain.

The design approaches of traditional AI versus data-driven deep learning AI are quite different. The architects of *traditional AI learning systems* focus on building generic models. They often begin with a human understanding of the world through the statement of a prior understanding of the domain (see Fig. 11.1), develop metrics representing that prior, extract data using those metrics, and ask humans to apply class labels of interest to these data. These labels are then used to train the system to learn a hyperplane which separates one class from another. Traditional AI learning

FIGURE 11.1 Traditional AI Learning Pipeline

Traditional AI machine learning in image analytics begins with the creation of a hypothesis about the structures under study. The investigators, using domain knowledge, craft their prior understanding about the structures and develop computational metrics to examine that prior understanding. Features are extracted from the image using these metrics and labeled as coming from disease vs. not-disease. A machine classifier (e.g. support vector machines) is then used to create the best hyperplane separating the classes of disease vs. non-disease.

systems will often be ineffective in capturing the granular details of a problem, and if those details are important, a traditional AI learning system may model poorly.

A *data-driven deep learning machine learning system* on the other hand can capitalize on the capture of fine details of a system, but it may not illuminate an understanding of the big picture of the problem. Data-driven models are sometimes characterized as "black box" learning systems which produce classifications or transformed representations of real-world data but without an explanation of the factors that influence the decisions of the learning system. Traditional and deep learning models are compared in Table 11.1.

Data-driven deep learning AI approaches have limited human—machine interactions constrained to a short training period from human annotated data and human verification of the classifier output of the learning system. In contrast, in traditional AI learning systems, human experts can provide actionable insights and bring these

Table 11.1 A comparison of traditional artificial intelligence (AI) versus data-driven deep learning AI.

	Traditional AI	**Data-driven deep learning AI**
Positives	Traditional AI is focused on conditioning the knowledge possessed by humans into models representing the real world.	Data-driven AI involves abstracting knowledge of a target domain simply by observing a large number of examples from the domain.
	Human experts can provide actionable insights and may bring these rich understandings in the form of a "prior" understanding, which can function as an advanced starting point for an AI system.	Data-driven models capitalize on capturing the fine details from the data samples including important latent variables.
Negatives	Traditional AI, with its focus on building generic models, may be ineffective in capturing fine-grained details of the problem from important unrecognized features.	Human interaction with data-driven AI models is often limited to training or verifying predicted outcomes.
		Data-driven AI may function as a black box and sacrifice an understanding of the factors which influence decisions.

rich understandings to the learning system in the form of a "prior" understanding of the domain. A prior can function as an advanced starting point for a deep learning AI system. The broad understanding of the world that humans possess with their reasoning and inferencing abilities, efficiency in learning, and the ability to transfer knowledge gained from one context to other domains is not very well understood. Framing data-driven deep learning systems with the human understanding of "what is" offers a way forward for creating partnerships between HI and AI in advanced learning systems. There is need for "explainable AI (XAI)" which can explain the inferences, conclusions, and decision processes of learning systems. There is much work that needs to be done to bridge the gap between machine and HI.

The need for human intelligence—artificial intelligence partnerships

Pathologists, confronted with a future filled with massive and ever-expanding computing power, properly ask the question "…will a machine diagnostician replace a human diagnostician and if so when?". No one knows the answer to this question but a glimpse into the world of chess offers some useful guideposts.

The chess grandmaster Garry Kasparov describes his years as a grandmaster as a time when computational chess was quickly developing and challenging human player expertise [5]. In the 1970s and 80s, grandmasters successfully outplayed the computers of the day. In the 90s, the competitions were more matched. Kasparov noted that the things that computers do well are often the tasks where humans are weak and that the converse is also true. This concept caused Kasparov to ask whether the goal of computational chess play was to pit man against computer or rather was it to play the highest level of chess possible as a partnership of man and machine? Kasparov went on to observe a chess playing experiment in which the types of machine—human pairings varied. He saw that a weak human player paired with a machine with a better process was superior to a strong computer alone, and remarkably, also superior to a strong human player working with a machine which had an inferior process.

In the evolving world of computational pathology, the fear of artificial machine diagnostic intelligence displacing HI must be balanced with the opportunity of providing patients with more precise and accurate diagnostic, prognostic, and theranostic statements. What if, as in Kasparov's chess playing experience, that in computational pathology, a partnership of weak human diagnosticians + machines + better processes were better than strong human diagnosticians + machines + worse processes? The field of computational pathology would be immeasurably extended in its global availability and somewhat more democratized in its practice. The key to next generation diagnostics may, in fact, be getting machines and humans to interact using the best processes. I would opine that this system approach is native to the practice of pathology and laboratory medicine and that our specialty is the best positioned in all of medicine to explore the AI revolution by developing robust HI—AI partnerships in the domains of diagnostics, prognostics, and theranostics. Dr. Scott Doyle a computational pathology investigator at the University at Buffalo, State University of New York opines that "The true value of human diagnosticians is not that they are valuable because of their ability to do poorly what artificial intelligence robots can do easily. In fact, they are valuable because of all the things they can do that robots cannot do such as disparate data integration, ingenuity, serendipity, learning, experimentation, and value judgments. These are all central parts of the practice of pathology and laboratory medicine. In the end pathologists should/will focus on these things and leave the robotic tasks to the robots" (unpublished communication).

Human transparent machine learning approaches

Human transparent machine learning systems seek to have humans understand AI cognition. This means that humans must be able to understand the dynamics of the machine learning system. In human transparent machine learning, the machine learning system may have human-like sensing inputs. Most importantly, humans are able to trust the AI output of human transparent learning systems. In the computational pathology domain, this means that the outputs of machine learning systems must be vetted against the big 360′ view of the complete clinical context. In this construct, the digital assistance which results from any computational pathology systems is used only after cross referencing them with all of the meaning understood by human sensors. These human understandings are gleaned from the history, physical examination, clinical laboratory, radiology, surgical pathology, cytopathology, molecular pathology, and quality assurance information systems. In other words, pathologists will need to learn how to work with machine learning systems as senior partners who understand the big picture of patient care diagnostics.

Explainable artificial intelligence

The concept of XAI is that machine learning is understood by human operators and that through this understanding, a bilateral trust relationship is established between humans and machines. XAI contrasts sharply with the "black box criticism" of deep learning. XAI is very important when machine learning systems impact social systems. As diagnostics is a central function of medicine, which in turn impacts all aspects of the societal good of health and wellness, XAI is a particularly desirable form of AI in computational pathology. Regulators of clinical laboratories and the diagnostic process should have a strong interest in XAI as it offers the transparency and real-world rationales which make algorithmic outputs testable and subject to quality assurance processes. XAI guards against AI "cheating," in which a learning system tracks surrogate labels but is not truly informative. For example, a data-driven deep learning AI system that used histological images tagged with ICD10 codes could never be relied on to distinguish cancer from noncancer using pixel data from digital virtual slides. Or even more simply, if the slides with cancer in a training dataset had been marked with a red dot by a previewer and the machine learning system learned to look for a "red dot" to classify the dataset into cancer versus not-cancer, the resulting classifier might be 100% effective in the training data but 0% extensible to other test datasets.

Deep learning systems may be adapted to XAI through a technique called layer-wise relevance propagation, which determines the features in an input vector which contribute most strongly to a neural network's output [6]. Exposing the output layers or even the early activation layers of neural networks to human observers for error correction or other annotations may also be used to support XAI (Fig. 11.2).

Cognitive artificial intelligence

Cognitive computing seeks to simulate the functioning of the human brain with software and hardware which senses, responds to stimulus, and reasons. Cognitive AI systems stimulate human thought in finding solutions to broad and complex problems. Cognitive AI systems should be adaptive, interactive, iterative, and contextual. Cognitive learning systems are adaptive in that they learn in real time or near real time and they learn as information changes. Cognitive systems are interactive with users. Cognitive systems help define problems by asking multiple questions or finding additional sources of information to make the statement of a problem less ambiguous. Cognitive learning systems understand, identify, and extract contextual elements such as meaning, syntax, time, location, appropriate domain,

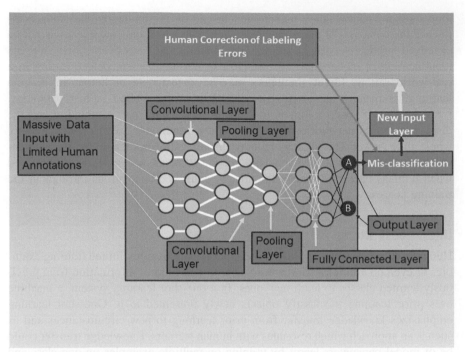

FIGURE 11.2 Opportunities for Human Interaction with Deep Learning Systems

In data driven deep learning systems the output classifications of images are derived from numerous calculations within "hidden" layers often without an explanation of the factors which influence the decisions of the learning system. Deep learning AI systems such as this convolutional neural network input large amounts of data with limited human labels. Convolutional and pooling layers may feed fully connected layers which in turn drive an output classifier. Errors in the output classifier are opportunities for human intelligence to correct the system and feed these new labels back into the input of the system. Other opportunities for human interaction with the learning system may exist in the human understanding and annotation of the activation layers of the convolutional neural network.

regulations, user's profile, process, task, and goals. Cognitive systems utilize multiple types of input data including human perceived sensory data. Cognitive AI self-learning systems weight context and conflicting evidence by using tools such as data mining, pattern recognition, and natural language processing. Cognitive AI systems in healthcare are thought of by some to be a tool for physicians to bridge the machine—doctor—patient chasm [7]. An example of cognitive computing is IBM Watson for Oncology, which has been used to derive ranked options for treatment of cancer.

Human in the loop

Human-in-the-loop learning models require human interaction. Human-in-the-loop systems allow humans to change the output of the learning systems. Human-in-the-loop simulators always have human input as part of the simulation, and humans influence the outcomes of the simulation exercise such that the outcomes may not be exactly reproducible. Human-in-the-loop simulations, however, allow for the identification of model shortfalls which may not be apparent before testing in a real-world setting. Flight simulators may be an example of human-in-the-loop learning. Human in the loop approaches have been applied to histopathology. Lutnick et al. [8] used a human-in-the-loop strategy for data annotation and the display of neural network predictions within a commonly used digital pathology whole slide viewer. This strategy reduced the annotation burden in that the segmentation of human and mouse renal microcompartments was repeatedly improved when humans interacted with automatically generated annotations throughout the training process.

One-shot learning

Humans have the capacity to learn object classifications from limited training examples or even no examples. Humans are able to make use of information from previously learned classes to learn new ones. In a one-shot learning system, a machine uses prior learning to classify objects newly presented to it. One-shot learning emphasizes knowledge transfer from prior learning to new circumstances and as such is an approach which resonates with human learners. Knowledge transfer could be of model parameters learnt by training on multiple examples on one class and then applying them to a new object class. Knowledge transfer may be done by sharing features across classes. Mutual information among learned objects could be applied to learning a new class of object. Knowledge transfer may also occur through the transfer of context. For example, knowing the context of camera geometry used to classify one object may help classify a new object.

The computational approaches described above can be applied to any laboratory data used in the clinical setting, and these methods are opportunities to innovate in all of the disciplines in pathology and laboratory medicine. Cabitza et al. [9] outlined the opportunities of machine learning in laboratory medicine, and these authors anticipate a flood of applications in the near future. In the following sections, however, we will mostly focus on the use cases of computational pathology in cellular and tissue-based image data.

Image-based computational pathology
Core premise of image analytics: what is a high-resolution image?

A foundational hypothesis supporting the concept of cell and tissue image—based computational pathology is that a high-resolution image is *a self-organizing set of data* which uniquely represents all of the genes, and all of the molecules, and all of the cells in that scene at one point in time. As a self-organizing piece of data, the image can only uniquely have the phenotype which it presents. An *image is what it is for very specific reasons*. Those reasons are the relationships among the genomics, epigenomics, proteomics, metabolomics, and all the "omics" which go into making that image. A high-resolution image is a window onto the *relationships* among all of the genes, and all of the molecules, and all of the cells in the scene at one particular point in time.

The targets of image-based calculations

The targets for algorithmic computation in image-based pathology include (1) the pixels in the image; (2) cells and organelles; (3) tissues and tissue elements and the complex relationships among pixels and cellular/tissue elements. Each of these targets may be amenable to many image analytic approaches, but some approaches are better suited for one or another of the targets. Machine learning systems driving decisions can be applied to the data extracted from any of these targets. The following are some examples of computational schemes for examining each of these targets.

Pixels: Pixels are the basic building blocks of digital images. They are a rich source of information in the color and intensity domains. Image texture features are metrics calculated from pixels that contain information about colors or intensities. Texture features can be viewed across an entire slide and leveraged as input data for machine learning systems, or they may be sorted into feature representations of cellular and tissue objects (as below). Thousands of texture features can be calculated from a histopathological image. The features can be extracted in cost-efficient unsupervised ways. Texture features data can be approached statistically. For example, an edge detection algorithm could examine the gradient magnitude and the gradient direction of the pixels and yield an "edgeness" metric for an entire image or segments of an image.

Cells and organelle segmentation: Cells and organelles are obvious biological units of interest to pathologists. Gathering quantitative information about cells is central to a computational pathologist's modern exploration of Virchow's cellular theory of disease. Segmentation of cells, nuclei, membranes, and organelles from image metrics can be accomplished by a variety of whole scene segmentation approaches, some of which include texture features, size and shape features, densitometric features, and chromatin-specific features [10].

Tissue and tissue elements and the complex relationships among pixels and cellular/tissue elements: The grand challenge for analytic approaches to computational pathology is to capture the image embedded information which is informative in modeling complex disease systems such as disease progression and the predictive modeling supporting therapeutic choices. Much of this information is embedded in the spatial relationships between cells. Spatial arrangement features can either be explicitly harvested or discovered with deep learning systems. Graph embedding theory is an example of a method which is well-adapted for exploring the relationships among pixels and cellular and tissue elements in high-resolution histopathological image data [10]. Graphs can be constructed for modeling different states of tissue and to distinguish these different states from others by calculating metrics on the graphs and classifying their values.

First fruits of computational pathology: *the evolving digital assistant*

The concepts of AI—HI partnerships and human transparent machine learning approaches raise an aspiration for a *digital assistant* to help pathologists in their daily work. Such an assistant would reduce repetitive tasks which are subject to error and free up pathologist time for complex medical decision-making. A *digital assistant* would reduce the organization and triage work, search and identify functions, and make data quantification (particularly from images) more accessible. The *digital assistant* would generally help pathologists to practice at "the top of their licenses." This vision does not yet exist in the reality of current state clinical practice, but it is on the way. The following are just some of the anticipated facilitating functions projected from the research literature into which the *digital assistant* may evolve.

The digital assistant for quality control

All laboratories have robust and active quality control and quality assurance at the core of their workflow. In modern-day clinical chemistry and hematology laboratories, for example, the information transfer about individual or batch value comparisons to both internal and external reference values is continuous and real time. There is a conversation between instruments and the laboratory professional human operators, which is always engaged and bidirectional. Heuristics are used to flag significant deviations from acceptable norms.

In the current state, anatomical pathology, laboratory quality control, and quality assurance are much more qualitative and discontinuous. As anatomical pathology moves to a digital pathology workflow, the need for precise quantitative quality control and quality assurance systems is becoming apparent. Computational pathology algorithms, particularly in unsupervised architectures, are susceptible to interpreting the noise of artifacts as true biological signal. Quality parameters which matter can be subtle and easily overlooked. Artifacts can adversely affect the performance of computational pathology machine learning systems [11,12]. In an integrated digital pathology workflow, using WSI, continuous, real-time, and precise quality image metrics are needed to understand and normalize the preanalytic variance inherent in glass slide preparation.

Lab accreditation organizations are keenly aware of the need to address quality assurance in digital and computational pathology. The College of American Pathologists has recently performed a metaanalysis of the literature and published guidelines on the Quantitative Image Analysis (QIA) of Human Epidermal Growth Factor Receptor 2 Immunohistochemistry for Breast Cancer [13]. They recommend that "to improve accurate, precise, and reproducible interpretation of HER2 IHC results for breast cancer, QIA and procedures must be validated before implementation, followed by regular maintenance and ongoing evaluation of quality control and quality assurance. HER2 QIA performance, interpretation, and reporting should be supervised by pathologists with expertise in QIA."

Vendors of whole slide scanning devices have also recognized that the quality of the rendered whole slide images impacts on the ability of pathologists to diagnose. When scanning the same slide on the same scanner at different times, the WSI appearance may contain subtle differences even when viewed on the same display because of variances in the scanner characteristics and/or other factors such as temperature or mechanical shifts.

Color reproduction has been approached by commercial developers through the construction of standardized slide phantoms matching the colors in the scanned images to the actual slide color [14]. The colors observed in phantoms are, however, not the same as those viewed in tissue matrix. Alternatively, commercial systems have used quantitative image quality assessment based on parameters such as sharpness, contrast, brightness, uniform illumination, and color separation to evaluate the scanner performance. In a study on HercepTest slides [15], the authors note that this computational approach is independent of image content or test specimen.

Open source approaches to the development of the digital assistant for quality assurance (QA) processes in computational pathology are also evolving. Janowczyk et al. have recently proposed an open source quality control tool for digital pathology slides which they call "HistoQC" [11]. Their system offers a modular QC application, which employs a suite of image metrics (such as color histograms, brightness, and contrast), images features detectors (for example, edge and smoothness), and supervised classifier systems (i.e., a drawing tablet with pen annotation) to facilitate QA work. The user interacts with the system through a python-based pipeline. Relevant output images of artifacts are created and presented with metadata and then sent to a data analytic tool. These authors have developed an HTML-5 user interface that allows for real-time visualization.

The digital assistant for histological object segmentation

The segmentation of histological objects by computational methods is an active area of research in pathology. The following describes some of the ways in which a variety of approaches have been employed to support clinically relevant image interpretation in pathology.

Nuclei

The enumeration and categorization of nuclei and nuclear features is a central task in many types of histopathological diagnoses. Nuclear detection methods are numerous. Xu et al. in a paper describing a deep learning strategy compiling examples of 23 different handcrafted feature-based approaches include color-based, edge-based, contextual information—based, and texture-based designs for nuclear segmentation [16]. Nuclear shape and orientation as measured predominantly by tensor information have been used in tissue microarray images to model nuclear pleomorphism and to be independently predictive of poorer survival in breast cancer [17]. The challenge with most of these approaches is in their ability to generalize across multiinstitutional datasets encompassing the loud "noise" of the preanalytic variance which is resident in slide preparation and scanning. Recently, deep learning techniques have been applied to the problem of nuclei segmentation, feature extraction, and classification. Breast cancer nuclei classification in histopathology has been examined by comparing several supervised learning methods with deep learning systems. The deep learning systems all outperformed the supervised machine classifier algorithms [18]. Other examples of deep learning strategies applied to nuclei detection cancer images have included (1) stacked sparse autoencoders used to learn high-level features from just pixel data of nuclei in breast cancer [16]; (2) a deep contour aware network (DCAN) using multilevel contextual features in a fully CNN with an auxiliary supervision scheme in the segmentation of nuclei from glioblastoma [19]; and (3) the use of cycle generative adversarial networks (cycleGANs) deep learning to improve multiorgan nuclei segmentation to almost 95% [20].

Mitoses

The recognition, enumeration, and classification of mitotic figures in histopathological images are central tasks in many histopathological grading systems. Pathologists often use the data from multiple z planes of focus in combination to distinguish mitotic figures from other condensed chromatin structures. As WSI often does not provide data from multiple z planes, the detection of mitotic figures in standard 2D whole slide images has become a high profile contest among investigative groups in digital pathology. Many competitive grand challenges have compared the effectiveness among a variety of computational approaches to the detection of mitoses. The winner of one of these grand challenges captioned in the paper by Ciresan [21] used a patch approach at 40× resolution with deep neural network learning. Janowczyk and Madabhushi [22] have adapted this approach, used a smaller patch size at 20× resolution, and leveraged segmentation of region of interests (ROIs) using a blue ratio segmentation protocol to enrich for ROIs containing mitotic figures. Wang et al. [23] have sought to address mitosis detection by presenting a convergent approach to combine domain-inspired features with deep learning features to detect mitoses. They showed that this integrated approach yielded superior detection accuracy compared to deep learning or handcrafted feature-based strategies alone.

The recognition, enumeration, and classification of mitotic figures are likely to be important tasks in diagnostic histopathology which will require the partnership of AI and HI to bring an efficient and safe computational tool to the clinical diagnostic market.

Tumor-infiltrating lymphocytes

In a previous chapter, Saltz and colleagues provided a detailed rationale for the importance of tumor-infiltrating lymphocytes (TILs) and gave examples involving the classification characterization of functionally relevant subpopulations of these lymphocytes and their positive and/or negative roles. For the reasons described, the detection, enumeration, and relationships among TILs are topics of great interest, particularly, for investigators interested in immuno-oncology. Klauschen et al. [24] have recently reviewed many computational approaches, which have been used to analyze TILs. TILs have been most commonly enumerated using semiquantitative scoring systems. Standardized TIL scoring has been used to good effect in clinical trials of breast cancer. Scoring systems, however, are subject to interobserver variance. The precise and time-efficient quantification of TILs is a needed tool for both research and clinical work. Computational approaches to the tasks of TIL characterization are required to enable the conduct of precision medicine clinical trials in oncology and autoimmune disease.

Traditional image analysis approaches to TIL identification rely on supervised or semisupervised systems. Through the identification of edges, cellular objects of interest are segmented and features are extracted from these objects which allow for the classification into different cell types. Thresholding, watershed, level set, color-space clustering, and morphological shape—based algorithms have all been used for the identification of TILs. These computations often require a priori knowledge of lymphocyte morphological variance, but their workings are explainable to the investigators. Relatively small datasets are used to train these handcrafted systems. Tuning the algorithmic parameters of these computational systems to handle the many cell types which need to be separated from lymphocytes, however, can be a daunting task.

Deep learning has recently been used in the detection of TILs. Janowczyk and Madabhushi [22] have used CNNs and patch classification schemes to identify lymphocytes in standard H&E histology. Larger training sets are needed to subsume the morphological variance of scenes and preparative variance, but the deep learning system in essence tunes itself. The exact nature and biological significance of the learned features may, however, be opaque. The understanding of the immune subtypes resident in host response networks may be critical to choosing effective immune therapies. Other studies have employed deep learning methods using different patch classification, boundary detection, and segmentation algorithms on tissue sections labeled immunohistochemically for lymphocytes and lymphoid subsets. The combination of molecular labels with deep learning systems offers the potential for the understanding of biologically explainable networks. Such methods could be adapted to assays designed for the examination of clinically relevant immune networks such as the relationships of immune checkpoint inhibitor molecules on host response and tumor cells.

Glands and acini

The histopathological definition of "gland" varies with the organ. Morphological deviation from normal gland structure is used by pathologists to define reactive conditions, dysplastic precancer, cancer, and cancer grade. Obviously, the segmentation of glandular objects is the first step when considering the computational analysis diseases which are defined by gland disorganization.

Gland segmentation in colon histopathology has a significant literature. The gland segmentation in colon histology images (GlaS) grand challenge [25] in computational pathology asked participants from the computer vision and medical imaging research communities to develop and compare gland segmentation algorithms of benign colonic glands and colon cancer glands. Accuracy of the detection of individual glands; volume-based accuracy of the segmentation of individual glands; and the boundary-based similarity between glands and their corresponding segmentations were the metrics for comparisons. Gland detection accuracy was performed using the F1 score ($2\times$ precision $\times$ recall/precision + recall). Volume-based segmentation accuracy was evaluated using the dice index which is a measure of agreement or similarity between two sets of samples. In this competition, these sample sets included a set of pixels corresponding to a ground truth object (G) and a set of pixels belonging to a segmented object (S). Boundary-based segmentation accuracy between ground truth (G) and segmented object (S) was evaluated using object-level Hausdorff distances. In general, two broad approaches to gland segmentation were employed by the competitors. The first approach was to start by identifying pixels belonging to glands which were then grouped to form a separate spatial glandular object. The second approach began with candidate objects which were then classified as glands or nonglands. All of the methods which were based on CNNs used the first approach. Only one method followed the second approach whereby candidate objects forming part of the gland, namely lumens or epithelial boundaries, were identified first and then classified into different types followed by full gland segmentation. Overall, the pixel-based CNN entries had the strongest performances. A novel DCAN [19] (Chen et al., read also below) was the overall winner of the challenge.

The segmentation of prostatic acini is a problem analogous to that of colonic gland identification. Traditional handcrafted image analysis techniques begin with a prior concept of acinar structure. Monaco et al. [26] conceived of a prostatic acinus as a lumen surrounded by a collar of epithelium. To distinguish between benign prostatic glands and prostatic adenocarcinoma, a Markov iteration was used to group and separate microacini from benign glands. Separation of Gleason patterns 3 versus 4 was facilitated by this schema. Singh et al. [27] used a combination of pixel and object-level classifiers which incorporated local and spatial information for consolidating pixel-level classification results into object-level segmentation of acini. As alluded to above, Chen et al. [19] have described a DCAN which provides a unified multitask learning framework examining contextual features by using a fully convolutional network. The fully convolutional network takes an image as input and outputs a probability map in one forward propagation. In this system, object features (for example, texture and color) are integrated with contour information. The result is a system which addresses the difficult problem of separating touching objects. The system is extensible to many types of objects including benign and malignant colonic glands and nuclei.

The digital assistant in immunohistochemistry

The in situ IHC analysis of tissues for molecular markers is central to the moderate practice of pathology. IHC biomarkers are used for tissue classification tasks, as grading tools and as predictive markers. The qualitative/semiquantitative analysis of IHC markers can have significant gaps in precision (TP/TP + FP) and recall (TP/TP + FN). Computational methods have been explored for many years as possible tools for improving the operating characteristics of IHC tests. Gavrielides et al. [28] examined the use of computationally assisted image evaluation in the scoring of HER-2 IHC. These authors found that a computer-assisted mode which provided a HER-2 reference image along with a corresponding feature plot of membrane staining intensities and membrane staining completeness improved both interobserver and intraobserver agreement when scoring HER-2.

Machine learning systems are being developed to analyze IHC labels. Chang et al. [29] have addressed image cytometry multiplex IHC data by comparing manual gating of lymphoid subsets to clustering algorithms and sparse representations to yield biologically interpretable subset populations.

Vandenberghe et al. [30] compared handcrafted features and machine classifiers (SVMs and random forest) to a deep learning CNN (ConvNets) in the analysis of HER-2/neu staining in breast cancer. Overall the accuracy of the neural network deep learning methods was somewhat better than the handcrafted feature classifiers. Interestingly, none of the methods were particularly good in their accuracy of scoring 2+ cells, where interobserver variance and clinical significance are known to be great.

Khosravi et al. [31] have compared six different deep learning systems using transfer learning for the scoring of IHC biomarkers in bladder and breast cancer. Transfer learning is the pretraining of a network architecture on a very large dataset and the use of that trained model for new classification tools for a data asset with limited size. In this study, the transfer learning strategies included pretraining of the network as a feature extractor and the fine-tuning of a pretrained network. The accuracy retrieval curves for the prediction of biomarker score ranged from 72% to 99%.

The digital assistant in tissue classification

The identification of cancer and its separation from reactive conditions are fundamental high-order functions of histopathologists. The two sequential activities of the pathologist workflow in executing these functions are the identification of candidate regions of interest and the subsequent classification of those regions into meaningful clinicopathological classes. These processes are true in any subspecialty of oncological surgical pathology. Breast cancer has been of particular interest to investigators studying computational pathology approaches to cancer diagnosis.

Fondon et al. [32] reviewed the use of traditional machine learning in breast cancer diagnosis. These authors approached the problems of automatically identifying and classifying breast histopathological digital images into one of the four classes: normal, benign lesion, in situ carcinoma, and invasive carcinoma. The functions of preprocessing, feature extraction from nuclei, regions, textures, and the use of these features to drive a variety of machine classifier tools are described. The SVM classifiers were most efficient with accuracy of up to 76%.

Deep learning approaches to breast cancer diagnosis using CNNs are being vigorously explored. Araujo et al. [33] have used CNNs on digital images from the Bioimaging 2015 breast histology classification challenge to separate into the same four classes of normal, benign lesion, in situ carcinoma, and invasive carcinoma. The overall sensitivity of the CNN in finding the carcinoma classes was 80%.

Cruz-Roa et al. [34] have used CNN deep learning to automatically identify invasive breast cancer on whole slide images from the Cancer Genome Atlas and from whole slide images collected from three contributing institutions. They found a positive predictive value of 72% and a negative predictive value of 97% for identifying invasive breast cancer. CNN classifiers outperformed visual feature classifiers (color and intensity, color histograms, shape index histograms, Haralick features, and graph-based features) in this study. Bejnordi et al. [35] have extended the CNN approach on whole slide breast images by using context-aware stacked CNNs for a similar task of separation of the classes normal/benign, ductal carcinoma in situ, and invasive carcinoma. In their "context-aware" approach, these authors first trained a CNN using high-pixel resolution information to classify the tissue into different classes. To incorporate more context, they fed much larger patches to this model at the time of testing. The output of this first system is then the input to a second stacked system, which uses the compact informative representations of the first model together with the information of the surrounding context to learn global independence of structures in different lesion categories. In this 3 class task, they achieved an accuracy of 0.812.

The digital assistant in finding metastases

The tasks of searching for and identifying cancer metastases in lymph nodes are critical but time-consuming work for diagnostic pathologists. In breast cancer, the definition of nodal status by histopathology is ground truth for the assignment of nodal status. Current clinical guidelines codify the sizing of lymph node metastases into pN 0 (i-): No regional lymph node metastases histologically, negative IHC; pN0 (i-): Malignant cells in regional lymph node(s) no greater than 0.2 mm and no more than 200 cells (detected by H&E or IHC including isolated tumor cells [ITCs]); pN1mi: Micrometastases (greater than 0.2 mm and/or more than 200 cells, but none greater than 2.0 mm); and pN1 macrometastases at least 1 tumor deposit greater than 2.0 mm. Steiner et al. [36] have used a scoring system for gauging how difficult it is for a pathologist to distinguish among these classes which they term "obviousness scores." In their study, it was found, not surprisingly, that the obviousness score is high for macrometastases and low for identifying isolated tumor cells. These authors also examined the impact of deep learning algorithmic assistance, which they named the Lymph Node Assistant (LYNA), on the obviousness score. LYNA improved the obviousness score for micrometastasis detection. The impact on assignment of the other classes is was less apparent. The average review time was also decreased for micrometastasis detection with LYNA, marginally improved for a negative class assignment, and not significantly impacted for the assignment of macrometastases or isolated tumor cells.

A recent competition (CAMELYON16) [37] to develop algorithmic solutions for the automated detection of sentinel lymph node metastases had 32 algorithms submitted. The areas under the curves (AUCs) for the receiver operating characteristic curves ranged from 0.556 to 0.994. The top five algorithms had a mean AUC comparable to the study pathologists' interpretations in the absence of time constraints.

Such studies offer the real possibility that the algorithmic digital assistant may provide a valuable prescreening function in histopathology in future diagnostic workflows.

The digital assistant in predictive modeling and precision medicine

Apart from substantially aiding the pathologists in decision-making, the use of computational imaging tools could enable the creation of digital imaging—based companion diagnostic assays that would allow for improved disease risk characterization. Unlike expensive molecular-based assays that involve destroying the tissue and invariably capture genomic or proteomic measurements from a small part of the tumor, these digital imaging—based companion diagnostic tests could be offered for a fraction of the price and could enable characterization of disease heterogeneity across the entire landscape of the tissue section. Both traditional AI and deep learning approaches for the modeling of patient outcomes and response to therapy have been explored in a variety of neoplastic and nonneoplastic conditions.

Lu et al. [17] have studied the prediction of survival in early stage estrogen-positive breast cancers using a traditional AI approach. These authors examined tissue microarrays for 615 features related to nuclear shape, texture, and orientation. They identified the top 15 quantitative history morphometric features which in combination modeled, using a linear discriminate analysis classification, the probability of long-term versus short-term disease-specific survival. Features relating to the heterogeneity of nuclear orientation dominated in this model. The authors in multivariate analysis controlled for tumor stage found that their model was strongly independently predictive of patient's survival in estrogen receptor (ER)—positive and lymph node—negative breast carcinomas.

Bychkov et al. [38] took a deep learning approach to the prognostic modeling of colon cancer outcomes from standard histopathology. These authors used an image analysis pipeline which included long short-term memory (LSTM) networks that allow the learning system to detect and memorize image tiles, which encode relevant and contributory morphologic information and disregard irrelevant image titles.

Through this architecture, the authors attempted to find units which performed biologically meaningful discriminations of tissue patterns. They hypothesized that if the system observed tiles which contained information regarding disease, then some memory cells within the network will learn this pattern, aggregate it into memory, and propagate the understanding through the network. The authors used LSTM networks to examine tissue microarrays of colorectal carcinoma. They found that the LSTM model provided a strong hazard ratio for disease prognosis as compared to visual scoring, but that their LSTM system did not outperform the Dukes staging system for colorectal carcinoma prognosis.

Deep learning classifiers have also been used in predicting outcomes of nonneoplastic conditions. For example, in the arena of cardiac pathology, Nirschl et al. [39] used deep CNNs to predict clinical heart failure from H&E-stained whole slide images with 99% sensitivity and 94% specificity.

The clinical pathology laboratories of health systems offer robust data basis of well-organized quantitative data representing the chronological patient record. Cabitza and Banfi [9] review multiple applications of machine learning to clinical laboratory data for the diagnosis, prognosis, and predictive modeling of a variety of conditions. These authors predict a deluge of investigations using clinical laboratory data and machine learning in the near future.

The digital assistant for anatomical simulation learning

Just as the digital revolution has required a robust infrastructure, so also does the learning from and teaching of complex 3D subjects like anatomy. Pedagogically relevant programs to develop, test, and scale a data-intensive, bandwidth-heavy, digitally enhanced, collection and visualization systems for anatomical data are critical to UME, GME, and CME training in radiology, surgery, and pathology. Simulation learning depends on computational approaches to the 3D structure of human gifts, large animal models, radiological images, and pathological specimens. 3D Slicer (http://www.slicer.org) is an open source software platform for the registration, interactive segmentation, visualization, and volume rendering of medical images and for research in image-guided therapy [40]. This sort of computational analysis of structure can integrate biological and digital phantoms within the pedagogic experience. This juxtaposition can allow for robust surgical simulation programs, which integrates the use of artificial phantoms, digital phantoms, and biological phantoms in preclinical surgical investigation, teaching, and training. This combination of the core activities of teaching and investigation in the structural sciences can offer a laboratory where students can learn in the new environment of quantitative structural science.

The digital assistant for image-omics data fusion

When trying to understand the cell biology systems which underpin all pathological interpretations, the data from different modes of examination are best not considered in isolation. Rather, these data are streams (or perhaps torrents) which integrate and literally "fuse" into robust representations of these complex cell and tissue systems. Both image and molecular 'omic (genomic, proteomic, metabolomics, etc.) data are dense and heterogeneous. Image data are strong at probing the relationships among features. Reductionist 'omic data are strong at probing causal pathways. The frameworks in which image data and 'omic data are represented are often quite different. We know digital image data as pixels features and values and 'omic data as molecular structures, molar quantities, and frequencies. It is not intuitively evident that these very different modes of data can live in the same space. Computational pathology and AI approaches, however, now allow for the quantitative fusion of these diverse cross-modal data streams in support of the modeling of complex biological systems.

There are several approaches to combining data. One is that of combining interpretations. In this method, there is an aggregation of the decisions made from classifiers. Each classifier corresponds to one particular data stream. This is quite common in biology and medicine. A combination of interpretations may, however, not be able to leverage all the power of the combined data streams because information is often lost in the process of converting from feature vectors to class labels.

A concatenation of high-dimensionality feature vectors is an inclusive approach, which subsumes all the available features; however, this approach invokes the "curse of multidimensionality," whereby the excess of features compared to patients may result in a classifier system which is overfit. Dimensionality reduction approaches such as principle component analysis (PCA) project feature vectors into a unified low-dimensionality eigenvector space. PCA assumes that the system data are contained within a linear space. Most biological systems, however, are nonlinear. Nonlinear dimensionality reduction approaches can be of assistance in addressing such complex systems. There are numerous algorithms for manifold learning and nonlinear dimensionality reduction. Some of these algorithms simply function as visualization tools, while others map data from high-dimensionality space to low-dimensionality spaces. Data may be combined by creating transformed representations of each data stream before combining the transformed representations. Data streams are projected (embedded) into a homogeneous metaspace, where all data are represented at the same scale. Embeddings may be combined in many ways. For example, one strategy is to combine embeddings by using high-dimensionality kernels. Kernels are dot product representations of each modality, which can be combined to create a fused representation of heterogeneous data. Using another method, Lee et al.[41] examined the effectiveness of fused data to predict biochemical recurrent of prostate cancer after radical prostatectomy. These authors employed a novel technique which they termed supervised multiview canonical correlation analysis (sMVCCA). Canonical correlation analysis (CCA) is a multivariate statistical method which seeks to find a linear subspace in which correlation between two sets of variables is maximized. Using sMVCCA, Lee et al. created an integrated feature vector composed of quantitative histopathological features and proteomic features obtained from tandem mass spectrometry of prostate cancer from radical prostatectomies. Kaplan–Meier analysis showed improved biochemical recurrence free survival prediction using the sMVCCA fused data classifier as compared to histology or proteomic features alone.

In another example, Savage and Yuan [42] presented a new tool for selecting informative features from heterogeneous data types and predicting treatment response and prognosis which they have named FusionGP. This is a Bayesian nonparametric method for integrating multiple data types. The relationships between input features and outcomes are modeled through a set of (unknown) latent functions. The latent functions are constrained using a set of Gaussian priors, and sparse feature selection is applied. The most strongly selected molecular features were evaluated in gene ontology for dominant core processes at work. These authors examined a cohort of 119 ER-negative and 345 ER-positive breast cancers to predict two important clinical outcomes: death and chemoinsensitivity by combining gene expression, copy number alteration, and digital pathology image data. For the prediction of disease-specific death, the molecular data were most informative for the ER-negative tumors. Interestingly, image features outperformed the molecular data in ER-positive tumors.

The digital assistant of the future might present the diagnostician with a variety of data fusion options to assist the HI–AI partnership team seeks in identifying the best precision diagnostic, prognostic, and predictive statements for a given patient.

Artificial intelligence and regulatory challenges

The adoption of computational methods into the diagnostic workflow will require an aligned combination of technology, economic value, and regulatory oversight to insure a safe process. The FDA employs a risk-based paradigm for medical device classification. "Premarket approval" (PMA) is required for Class III devices, which have no comparison to a predicate. A "510(K) Premarket notification" is a path to market for new devices which are substantially equivalent to predicate devices. In certifying image-based pathology systems, the FDA has broad experience in the regulation of image-based instrumentation driven by algorithms. The clinical use of algorithms in image-based assays in pathology already exists in several domains including automated hematology analyzers, chromosome analysis, FISH enumeration systems, urine sediment analysis, gynecological cytology, and IHC for predictive markers such as HER2/neu, ER, and progesterone receptor (PR).

When considering the regulation of market entry for deep learning AI systems in image-based pathology, the new regulatory challenge is to provide access to these powerful systems and yet constrain their application to use cases, where patient safety can be assured. Clearly, new approaches to the regulatory evaluation of machine learning systems are required.

The understanding of the relationship between digital image data and the human perception of image data in pathology is one challenge. Gallas and

Gravrielides [43] from the FDA are creating an evaluation program which develops information regarding which technical characteristics of an image-based system are important; learning how these technical characteristics impact pathologists' interpretations; and understanding how these technical characteristics can be measured. These authors and their colleagues have created an "evaluation environment for digital and analog pathology (eeDAP)." They anticipate that this be used as a "Clinical Outcome Assessment tool used in reader studies for A premarket submissions (PMA or 510k deNovo) to compare the accuracy or reproduce ability of pathologist evaluations of digital images on a display to those of glass slides on a microscope. The pathologist evaluations of outpatient tissue are the clinical outcomes. The accuracy or reproducibility is the clinical outcome assessment; this assessment reflects image quality." Such tools will be important in examining sources of discrepancies between pathologists for classifying different types of diseases, for developing a panel of histopathological patterns and related decision support tools for improving pathologist performance for these classification tasks, and in assessing pathologist performance with whole slide images versus traditional optical microscopy.

A second challenge is fixing on the target of regulation. Machine learning systems are endlessly changing. With each epoch, a machine learning system understands or "sees" a set of images differently and can output a different understanding of class assignments. The fundamental regulatory challenge for harnessing image-based machine learning systems as clinical decision tools is to constrain the questions asked to clinically meaningful outputs which can be tested against other forms of understanding. For example, if a machine learning system outputs an interpretation of Her2/neu IHC that seeks to classify a breast cancer as having amplification of this gene, the output of the image-based test can be validated with other modes of analysis such as PCR or FISH for Her2/neu amplification. This validation is only possible after some training and testing time of the machine learning system and during a period when the learning system is locked down and not changing. The qualification(s) of image-based machine learning systems as clinical laboratory tools are likely to address newly proposed machine learning systems in a series of locked down versions, each of which will have to be validated. Functionally, what will need to be developed are rapid validation programs with which regulatory agencies such as the FDA can quickly compare the outputs of locked down machine learning system versions against predicate testing systems.

The current literature on the use of image-based machine learning systems as clinical laboratory testing tools is primordial. It is apparent from a quick inspection that most of the studies cited above are investigational and not yet ready for use in clinical practice. The tremendous opportunities promised by machine learning technologies are, however, likely to soon propel these tools into 510(k) approval pathways. Humans in the loop architectures are likely to be deemed safer approaches for the early application of machine learning systems in pathology and laboratory medicine.

Educating machines—educating us: learning how to learn with machines

Pathological diagnostics, prognostics, and theranostic statements of cell and tissue samples are not just application spaces for AI, but they offer tremendous opportunities to learn more about HI—machine intelligence partnerships in unique ways. Researchers at the University at Buffalo, State University of New York (Doyle S, unpublished communications) are developing a novel approach to building machine learning—based systems, where classifier training is recast as a problem of pedagogy. In this approach, termed the "**AI School for Pathology**," AI agents are treated as students in a school where human agents are instructors and the learning context is that of higher order clinical phenotypes and clinical outcomes. Both AI and human agents learn the biological/medical realities and the meaning of data from tissue imaging, 'omics, electronic medical record (EMR), and their fused data products. Within this paradigm, learning researchers propose to examine various portals for AI—human agent interactions analogous to those of teachers and students in a traditional learning setting. The understandings generated from this project will help advance research in one of the key challenge areas for AI today, namely, enabling AI systems to learn as humans learn.

References

[1] Hasin Y, Seldin M, Lusis A. Multi-omics approaches to disease. Genome Biology 2017; 18:83. https://doi.org/10.1186/s13059-017-1215-1.

[2] Krizhevsky A, Sutskever I, Hinton GE. ImageNet classification with deep convolutional neural networks. Advances in Neural Information Processing Systems 2012:1—9.

[3] Fuchs T, Buhmann JM. Computational pathology: challenges and promises for tissue analysis. Computerized Medical Imaging and Graphics 2011;35:515—30.

[4] Website: John McCarthy Available from: https://en.wikipedia.org/wiki/John_McCarthy_(computer_scientist). [Accessed 14 September 2019].

[5] Rasskin-Gutman D. Chess metaphors: artificial intelligence and the human mind, 2009, MIT Press, ISBN: 9780262182676.

[6] Bach S, et al. On pixel-wise explanations for non-linear classifier decisions by layer-wise relevance propagation. PLoS One 2015;10(7):e0130140.

[7] Website: Robinson S. Cognitive computing in healthcare mends doctor-patient gap. 2018. Available at: https://searchenterpriseai.techtarget.com/opinion/Cognitive-computing-in-healthcare-mends-doctor-patient-gaps. [Accessed 14 September 2019].

[8] Lutnick B, et al. An integrated iterative annotation technique for easing neural network training in medical image analysis. Nature Machine Intelligence 2019;1(2):112—9.

[9] Cabitza F, Banfi G. Machine learning in laboratory medicine: waiting for the flood? Clinical Chemistry and Laboratory Medicine 2018;56(4):516—24.

[10] Gurcan MN, et al. Histopathological image analysis: a review. IEEE reviews in biomedical engineering 2009;2:147—71.

[11] Janowczyk A, et al. HistoQC: an open-source quality control tool for digital pathology slides. JCO Clinical Cancer Informatics 2019;3:1—7.

[12] Leo P, et al. Stable and discriminating features are predictive of cancer presence and Gleason grade in radical prostatectomy specimens: a multi-site study. Scientific Reports 2018;8:14918.

[13] Bui MM, et al. Quantitative image analysis of human epidermal growth factor receptor 2 immunohistochemistry for breast cancer: guideline from the College of American Pathologists. Archives of Pathology & Laboratory Medicine 2019:1−16.

[14] Shrestha P, Hulsken B. Color accuracy and reproducibility in whole slide imaging scanners. Journal of Medical Imaging 2014;1:027501.

[15] Shrestha P, et al. A quantitative approach to evaluate image quality of whole slide imaging scanners. Journal of Pathology Informatics 2016;7:56.

[16] Xu J, et al. Stacked sparse autoendoder (SSAE) for nuclei detection on breast cancer histopathology images. IEEE Transactions on Medical Imaging 2016;35(1):119−30.

[17] Lu C, et al. Nuclear shape and orientation features from H&E images predict survival in early-stage estrogen receptor-positive breast cancers. Laboratory Investigation 2018; 98(11):1438−48.

[18] Feng Y, Zhang L, Yi Z. Breast cancer cell nuclei classification in histopathology images using deep neural networks. International Journal for Computer Assisted Radiology and Surgery 2018;13:179−91.

[19] Chen H, et al. DCAN: Deep contour-aware networks for object instance segmentation from histology images. Medical Image Analysis 2017;36:135−46.

[20] Mahmood F, et al. Adversarial U-net with spectral normalization for histopathology image segmentation using synthetic data. Proceedings of SPIE 2019;10956. Medical Imaging.

[21] Ciresan DC, et al. Mitosis detection in breast cancer histology images with deep neural networks. Medical Image Computing and Computer-Assisted Intervention 2013; 16(Pt2):411−3.

[22] Janowczyk A, Madabhushi A. Deep learning for digital pathology image analysis: a comprehensive tutorial with selected use cases. Journal of Pathology Informatics 2016;7:29.

[23] Wang H, et al. Mitosis detection in breast cancer pathology images by combining hand-crafted and convolutional neural network features. Journal of Medical Imaging 2014; 1(3):034003.

[24] Klauschen F, et al. Scoring of tumor-infiltrating lymphocytes: from visual estimation to machine learning. Seminars in Cancer Biology 2018;52:151−7.

[25] Sirinukunwattana K, et al. Gland segmentation in colon histology images: the GlaS challenge contest. Medical Image Analysis 2017;35:489−502.

[26] Monaco JP, et al. High-throughput detection of prostate cancer in histological sections using probabilistic pairwise Markov models. Medical Image Analysis 2010;14(4): 617−29.

[27] Singh M, et al. Gland segmentation in prostate histopathological images. Journal of Medical Imaging 2017;4(2). 027501-1-02750125.

[28] Gavrielides MA, et al. Observer variability in the interpretation of HER2/neu immunohistochemical expression with unaided and computer-aided digital microscopy. Archives of Pathology & Laboratory Medicine 2011;135:233−42.

[29] Chang YH, et al. Multiplexed immunohistochemistry image analysis using sparse coding. In: Conference proceedings: annual international conference of the IEEE engineering in medicine and biology society. IEEE engineering in medicine and biology society. Annual conference 2017; 2017. p. 4046−9.

[30] Vandenberghe ME, et al. Relevance of deep learning to facilitate the diagnosis of HER2 status in breast cancer. Scientific Reports 2017;7:45938.

[31] Khosravi P, et al. Deep convolutional neural networks enable discrimination of heterogeneous digital pathology images. EbioMedicine 2018;27:317−28.

[32] Fondon I, et al. Automatic classification of tissue malignancy for breast carcinoma diagnosis. Computers in Biology and Medicine 2018;96:41−51.

[33] Araujo T, et al. Classification of breast cancer histology images using convolutional neural networks. PLoS One 2017;12(6):e0177544.

[34] Cruz-Roa A, et al. Accurate and reproducible invasive breast cancer detection in whole slide images: a deep learning approach for quantifying tumor extent. Scientific Reports 2017;7:46450.

[35] Bejnordi BE, et al. Context-aware stacked convolutional neural networks for classification of breast carcinomas in whole-slide histopathology images. Journal of Medical Imaging 2017;4(4). 044504-1-8.

[36] Steiner DF, et al. Impact of deep learning assistance on the histopathologic review of lymph nodes for metastatic breast cancer. The American Journal of Surgical Pathology 2018;42:1636−46.

[37] Bejnordi BE, et al. Diagnostic assessment of deep learning algorithms for detection of lymph node metastases in women with breast cancer. Journal of the American Medical Association 2017;318(22):2199−210.

[38] Bychkov D, et al. Deep learning based tissue analysis predicts outcome in colorectal cancer. Scientific Reports 2018;8:3395.

[39] Nirschl JJ, et al. A deep-learning classifier identifies patients with clinical heart failure using whole-slide images of H&E tissue. PLoS One 2018;13(4):e0192726.

[40] Fedorov A, et al. 3D slicer as an image computing platform for the quantitative imaging network. Magnetic Resonance Imaging 2012;30(9):1323−41.

[41] Lee G, et al. Supervised multi-view canonical correlation analysis (sMVCCA): integrating histologic and proteomic features for predicting recurrent prostate cancer. IEEE Transactions on Medical Imaging 2015;34:284−97.

[42] Savage RS, Yuan Y. Predicting chemosensitivity in breast cancer with 'omics/digital pathology data fusion. Royal Society Open Science 2016;3:14051.

[43] Gallas BD, Gravrielides MA. Assessment of digital pathology. 2018. Available from: https://www.fda.gov/medical-devices/cdrh-research-programs/assessment-digital-pathology. [Accessed 14 September 2019].

Index

Printed and bound by CPI Group (UK) Ltd, Croydon, CR0 4YY

03/10/2024

01040300-0004